*Eighth Edition*

APPLETON & LANGE
REVIEW OF

# PHARMACY

**Gary D. Hall, MS**
Professor of Pharmaceutics
Albany College of Pharmacy
Union University
Albany, New York

**Barry S. Reiss, PhD**
Professor Emeritus
Albany College of Pharmacy
Union University
Albany, New York

**Appleton & Lange Reviews/McGraw-Hill**
Medical Publishing Division

New York  Chicago  San Francisco  Lisbon  London  Madrid  Mexico City  Milan
New Delhi  San Juan  Seoul  Singapore  Sydney  Toronto

**Appleton & Lange Review of Pharmacy, Eighth Edition**

Previous editions copyright © 2001 by The McGraw-Hill Companies, Inc.; ©1997, 1993, 1990, 1985 by Appleton & Lange; ©1980, 1976 by Arco Publishing, Inc.

1 2 3 4 5 6 7 8 9 0   QPD/QPD   0 9 8 7 6 5 4

SET ISBN: 0-07-142543-8
BOOK ISBN: 0-07-144104-2
CD-ROM ISBN: 0-07-144105-0

This book was set in Palatino by International Typesetting and Composition.
The editors were Michael J. Brown and Christie Naglieri.
The production supervisor was Phil Galea.
Project management was provided by International Typesetting and Composition.
Quebecor World Dubuque was printer and binder.

This book is printed on acid-free paper.

---

**Notice**

Medicine is an ever-changing science. As new research and clinical experience broaden our knowledge, changes in treatment and drug therapy are required. The authors and the publisher of this work have checked with sources believed to be reliable in their efforts to provide information that is complete and generally in accord with the standards accepted at the time of publication. However, in view of the possibility of human error or changes in medical sciences, neither the authors nor the publisher nor any other party who has been involved in the preparation or publication of this work warrants that the information contained herein is in every respect accurate or complete, and they disclaim all responsibility for any errors or omissions or for the results obtained from use of the information contained in this work. Readers are encouraged to confirm the information contained herein with other sources. For example and in particular, readers are advised to check the product information sheet included in the package of each drug they plan to administer to be certain that the information contained in this work is accurate and that changes have not been made in the recommended dose or in the contraindications for administration. This recommendation is of particular importance in connection with new or infrequently used drugs.

---

**Library of Congress Cataloging-in-Publication Data**

Hall, Gary D.
    Appleton & Lange review of pharmacy / Gary D. Hall, Barry S. Reiss.–8th ed.
        p. ; cm.
    Rev. ed. of: Appleton & Lange's review of pharmacy. 7th ed. 2001.
    Includes bibliographical references and index.
    ISBN 0-07-142543-8
    1. Pharmacy—Examinations, questions, etc. I. Title: Appleton and Lange review of
pharmacy. II. Title: Review of pharmacy. III. Hall, Gary D. Appleton & Lange's
review of pharmacy. IV. Reiss, Barry S., 1944– V. Title.
    [DNLM: 1. Pharmacy—Examination Questions. QV 18.2 H1761a 2004]
RS97 .H35 2004
615′ .4′076—dc22
                                                            2003061426

# Contents

# Preface

Pharmacy licensing examinations are designed to determine whether a candidate has the minimum competencies required to enter and then carry out the responsibilities of the profession. A candidate preparing for the licensing examination must be prepared to demonstrate competence in many areas, any one of which may be the subject for in-depth questioning.

This book is designed as a self-testing tool for the pharmacy student to identify individual areas of strength and weakness, to suggest areas for further review, and to impart new concepts and other information useful to both the student and the practicing pharmacist. The book consists of three major sections: Chapters 1 through 6 concentrate on specific disciplines in order to improve the student's competence in each. Within each chapter, some questions dealing with related subject matter have been grouped together, whereas others have intentionally not been categorized, necessitating a return to certain areas of study in later questions to reinforce prior learning. In each chapter, questions are followed by an Answers and Explanations section, which we think is the keystone of our book. Some comments are quite extensive and represent miniature reviews, whereas others are limited to brief specifics. In every instance, the cited references offer a way for more extensive review.

Chapter 7 consists of patient profiles, each accompanied by a series of related questions. Information obtained from the questions and commentaries in Chapters 1 through 6 will probably aid in answering questions in Chapter 7.

A self-assessment disk is included in this eighth edition to help in preparing you for the computerized format of the NAPLEX. A description of the computer-based examination is provided on page xii.

There are also three appendices: the first lists more than 200 drugs by generic names that the authors consider most likely to be dispensed by pharmacists. Included in the table are trade or brand names, manufacturing companies, a brief description of therapeutic uses, and common dosage forms and strengths. It is *not* necessary to memorize the name of the company manufacturing a certain product, especially with the numerous company name changes; however, many individuals find it easier to relate a trade name to a company. The second appendix supplements the first by presenting some drugs that are mainly dispensed in hospital settings. To complete the cycle, the third appendix serves as a cross-reference of trade names with generic names.

We trust that this book will not be viewed as simply a means to review material for the licensing examination. Passing this examination does not guarantee continued competence throughout a long professional career. Practicing pharmacists must not only retain their previously acquired knowledge and skill, but must remain up to date on contemporary modes of practice. We hope that this book will serve both as a means for self-assessment of competence to practice as well as a valuable guided review. A statement listing professional competency in pharmacy originally prepared by the California State Board of Pharmacy appears on page xi. Many of the test items in this book relate to these competencies.

# Acknowledgments

We would like to thank Christie Naglieri, Editorial Coordinator, and Michael J. Brown, Executive Editor, for their editorial guidance throughout the development of this newly revised edition. We would also like to recognize and encourage all pharmacy students who aspire to enter and excel in their chosen profession.

*Gary D. Hall, MS*
*Barry S. Reiss, PhD*

# How to Use This Book

A competent pharmacist is one who is able to confer with a physician about the care and treatment of his or her patient. The pharmacist should appreciate the essentials of the clinical diagnosis and understand the medical management of the patient. He or she should also be informed about the drugs that may be used in the treatment of the patient—their mechanism of action; their combinations and dosage forms; the fate and disposition of the drugs (if known); the factors that may influence the physiological availability and biological activity of the drugs from their dosage forms; how age, sex, or secondary disease states might influence the course of treatment; and how other drugs, foods, and diagnostic procedures may interact to modify the activity of the drug.

A competent pharmacist is one whose overall function is to ensure optimum drug therapy. He or she should know the appropriate indications and dosage regimen for the drug therapy being undertaken as well as the contraindications and potential untoward reactions that may result during therapy. He or she should also be informed as to the proprietary products that might interact adversely with or be useful adjuncts to drug therapy, facilitating administration or improving overall patient care.

A competent pharmacist must be aware of the proposed therapeutic actions of proprietary medications, their composition, and any unique applications or potential limitations of their dosage forms. He or she should be able to objectively appraise advertising claims. At the patient's request, he or she should be able to ascertain the probable therapeutic usefulness of a certain drug in resolving the patient's complaints.

A competent pharmacist should be able to review a scientific publication and summarize the practical implications of the findings as they may relate to the clinical use of drugs. He or she should be able to analyze a published report of a clinical trial in terms of the appropriateness of the study design and the validity of the statistical analysis, and should be able to prepare an objective summary of the significance of the data and the authors' conclusions.

A competent pharmacist is a specialist as to the stability characteristics and storage requirements of drugs and drug products, the factors that influence the release of drugs from dosage forms, and the effect of the site of administration or its environment within the body on the absorption of a drug from the administered dosage form. Most importantly, the pharmacist understands the effect of the interaction of all these factors on the onset, intensity or duration of therapeutic action.

A competent pharmacist should be precisely informed as to the legal limitations on procurement, storage, distribution, and sale of drugs; the approved use of a drug as specified by federal authorities and acceptable medical practice; and his or her legal responsibilities to the patient when drugs are used in experimental therapeutic procedures.

A competent pharmacist should be able to recommend the drug and dosage form that are most likely to fulfill a particular therapeutic need, supporting his or her choice objectively with appropriate source material. In addition, he or she should be capable of identifying a drug, within a reasonable period of time, on the basis of its color, shape, and proposed use, as described in reference books or other sources.

On the basis of symptoms described in an interview with the patient, a competent pharmacist should know what additional information he or she must obtain from the patient. Based on this information, he or she should be able to refer the patient to the proper medical practitioner, specialist, or agency that would be of most help.

A competent pharmacist should be aware of drug toxicities, as well as the most effective means of treatment for them.

A competent pharmacist should be able to instruct patients on the proper administration of prescription and proprietary drugs. He or she should know which restrictions should be placed on food intake, other medication, and physical activity.

A competent pharmacist should be able to communicate with other healthcare professionals or laymen on appropriate subjects, ensuring that the recipient understands the contents of the message being communicated.

A competent pharmacist should be capable of compounding appropriate drugs or drug combinations in acceptable dosage forms.

Finally, a competent pharmacist is a person who takes appropriate measures to maintain his or her level of competency in each of the areas described above.

## Computer-Based Examinations

Following the lead of the nursing profession, many professions have reorganized their entry-level professional examinations to a computer-adaptive test (CAT) format. Qualified candidates have the opportunity to take their exam anytime during the year at a geographical location convenient for them. The actual exam format for pharmacy consists mainly of patient profiles followed by a series of questions that may or may not require reviewing the patient's profile. Using the computer keyboard or mouse, the candidate can scroll back to the profile for any needed information to answer a specific question. The questions will be presented one at a time and must be answered in sequence—that is, one may not skip or skim questions with the intention of returning to them later. Also, once the candidate has selected an answer and entered it into the computer, it is NOT possible to retrieve the answer and make changes. Be sure that you are satisfied with

your answer before entering it into the computer. Once entered, forget about that question even if later questions lead you to believe that you gave a wrong answer.

Remember that no one is expected to answer all questions correctly. Instead, the examining body has set reasonable goals based on both easy and more difficult questions or concepts. The examination is designated as a computer-adaptive test because the system evaluates each individual candidate by varying the question difficulty depending on the candidate's response to previous questions. Thus, different candidates at the same testing site may be answering different questions of varying difficulty. The scoring will be based at least partially on the number of questions answered correctly and the relative level of question difficulty.

When preparing for computer-based exams, the candidate should review material in the exact manner as for any other examination. It is suggested that the candidate participate in any tutorial session offered at the exam site just prior to the actual examination. These sessions will include instruction in the mechanics of operating the computer system being used. However, any anxiety about the use of the computer will soon be overcome once the exam has started. In addition, you are likely to benefit by receiving your grade and pharmacist license much earlier!

## Helpful Hints

There are several ways to maximize learning from this review book. For example, the reader could answer a short series of questions before looking for the answers at the end of each chapter. Keeping score will make these chapters function as miniature tests. Unfortunately, when challenged by multiple-choice questions, even in the nonthreatening environment of a self-learning program, our behavioral response is often predictable. When more than 75% of the questions are answered correctly, satisfaction and confidence dominate. As the percentage of missed questions increases, frustration and even panic develop. Such reactions lead to a self-limiting response: namely, the quick memorization of answers. Keep in mind, however, that although you may have increased your knowledge by one fact, you may not have maximized your learning experience. Do you really expect to see the same question on another examination? Do you realize why the other answer choices are not correct? Have you read the explanations of all the questions, even those you answered correctly? Hopefully, these explanations will contain additional tidbits of information that will increase your knowledge base. If the question mentions a drug with which you are not familiar, be sure to look up the drug in one of the reference sources at your disposal. The next time you see that drug may be when it is the subject of a question. Some questions may concern topics with which you are not familiar. This is a perfect opportunity for learning!

Rather than blindly guessing at the answers, seek information in the cited reference or other sources and then attempt to answer the question. If your answer does not agree with the one given in this book, check further in another source. Keep digging—learning cannot be passive. Recognize that a question stating "which of these does *not*" or "all of these *except*" gives you four positive facts or statements. These, in themselves, have expanded your knowledge base.

# References

The references listed represent a small number of sources available in most pharmacy libraries. The individual pharmacist or pharmacy could accumulate a collection to fit their needs but economically the cost would be high. Instead, many pharmacists now depend on the internet for information to supplant their private collections.

Because of the increasing costs and frequent issuing of new editions, the authors of *Appleton & Lange Review of Pharmacy* have attempted to limit the total number of books cited but realize that there are many other textbooks containing similar material. To maintain an up-to-date personal library, the reader should obtain at least a general pharmaceutical science book (e.g., Ref. 1 or 24), a pharmacology book (Ref. 6 being the classic), a book with a clinical pharmacy orientation, and a book devoted to discussions of drug therapy in managing certain disease states (Refs. 5 and 16). To keep current with new drugs, drug products, and recent developments in drug therapy, it is necessary to have publications that are updated periodically (monthly for Ref. 3 and yearly for Refs. 9 and 25). Monthly journals, such as *U.S. Pharmacist*, *Drug Topics*, and *American Druggist*, offer up-to-date information as well as continuing education programs.

The method of citing references in this edition of the *Review of Pharmacy* differs from previous editions. Each citation will be for the individual book but not individual pages. This will reduce confusion if the reader has an older edition and will find the material on pages differing from those that would be cited in a newer edition. The exception will be citations to journals such as the *U.S. Pharmacist*. These citations will include the month and year since many students and pharmacists collect previous issues of the journal.

1. Gennaro AR. *Remington: The Science and Practice of Pharmacy*, 20th ed. Philadelphia, PA: Lippincott Williams & Wilkins, 2000.
2. *Handbook of Nonprescription Drugs*, 13th ed. Washington, DC: American Pharmacists Association, 2000.
3. *Facts and Comparisons Loose-leaf with monthly updates or online*. Wolters Kluwer Health, Inc., 2003.
4. Thompson, JE: *A Practical Guide to Contemporary Pharmacy Practice*. Baltimore, MD: Lippincott Williams & Wilkins, 1998.
5. Dipiro JT, et al.: *Pharmacotherapy. A Pathophysiologic Approach*, 5th ed. New York, NY: McGraw-Hill, 2002.
6. Hardman JG, Limbird LE: *Goodman and Gilman's Pharmacological Basis of Therapeutics*, 10th ed. New York, NY: McGraw-Hill, 2001.
7. Katzung BG: *Basic & Clinical Pharmacology*, 8th ed. New York, NY: McGraw-Hill, 2001.
8. Tatro DS: *Drug Interactions Facts*. Lippincott Williams & Wilkins, 1998.
9. *AHFS Drug Information 03*. Bethesda, MD: American Society of Health-System Pharmacists, 2003.
10. Product literature drug package inserts current in 2003.
11. Pray WS: *Nonprescription Product Therapeutics*. Philadelphia, PA: Lippincott Williams & Wilkins, 1999.
12. Amiji, M and Sandmann, B, *Physical Pharmacy*, New York, NY: McGraw-Hill, 2003. Martin A: *Physical Pharmacy*, 4th ed. Philadelphia, PA: Lippincott Williams & Wilkins, 1993.
13. Turco SJ: *Sterile Dosage Forms*, 4th ed. Philadelphia, PA: Lippincott Williams & Wilkins, 1994.

14. Braunwald, E, et al.: *Harrison's Principles of Internal Medicine*. New York: McGraw-Hill, 2001.

15. Rowland M, Tozer TN: *Clinical Pharmacokinetics*, 3rd ed. Baltimore, MD: Lippincott Williams & Wilkins, 1995.

16. Beers MH, Berkow R: *The Merck Manual of Diagnosis and Therapy*. Whitehouse Station, NJ: Merck Research Labs, 1999.

17. Shargel L, Yu ABC: *Applied Biopharmaceutics and Pharmacokinetics*, 4th ed. New York, NY, McGraw-Hill, 1999.

18a. USP Convention Inc. *USP DI Volume I—Drug Information for the Health Care Professional*, 22nd ed. Rockville, MD: USPC Inc., 2002.

18b. USP Convention Inc. *USP DI Volume II—Advice for the Patient*, 22nd ed. Rockville, MD: USPC Inc., 2002.

18c. USP Convention Inc. *USP DI Volume III—Approved Drug Products and Legal Requirements*, 22nd ed. Rockville, MD: USPC Inc., 2002.

19. Allen, LV: *The Art, Science, and Technology of Pharmaceutical Compounding*, 2nd ed. Washington, DC: American Pharmacists Association, 2002.

20. Trissel LA: *Stability of Compounded Formulations*, 2nd ed. Washington, DC: American Pharmacists Association, 2000.

21. Trissel LA: *Handbook on Injectable Drugs*, 12th ed. Bethesda, MD: American Society of Health-System Pharmacists, 2003.

22. Catania PN, Rosner M: *Home Health Care Practice*, 2nd ed. Palo Alto, CA: Health Market Research, 1994.

23. Ansel HC, Stoklosa MJ : *Pharmaceutical Calculations*, 11th ed. Baltimore, MD: Lippincott Williams & Wilkins, 2001.

24. Ansel HC, Allen LV Popovich NG: *Pharmaceutical Dosage Forms and Drug Delivery Systems*, 7th ed. Baltimore, MD: Lippincott Williams & Wilkins, 1999.

25. *Physician's Desk Reference*, 57th ed. Montvale, NJ: Medical Economics Co., 2003.

26. Di Piro. *J.T. Pharmacist's Drug Handbook*. Springhouse, PA, 2001.

27. Thomas CL: *Taber's Cyclopedic Medical Dictionary*, 18th ed. Philadelphia, PA: F.A. Davis Co., 1997.

28. *U.S. Pharmacist*. New York: Jobson Publishing.

# CHAPTER 1

# Pharmacology

Since 1940, the first edition of the book cited in the references as reference 6 has been known to successive classes of pharmacy students as simply Goodman and Gilman. On page 1 of the current edition, the following statement can be found: "In its entirety, pharmacology embraces the knowledge of the history, source, physical and chemical properties, compounding, biochemical and physiological effects, mechanisms of action, absorption, distribution, biotransformation and excretion, and therapeutic and other uses of drugs. Since a drug is broadly defined as any chemical agent that affects processes of living, the subject of pharmacology is obviously quite extensive."

The test items in this chapter deal with some of these areas of pharmacology. Related questions may be found in chapters on biopharmaceutics and pharmacokinetics and on pharmaceutical care.

# Questions

**DIRECTIONS (Questions 1 through 185):** Each of the numbered items or incomplete statements in this section is followed by answers or by completions of the statement. Select the ONE lettered answer or completion that is BEST in each case.

1. Sulfones such as dapsone are employed commonly in the treatment of

    (A) Bright's disease
    (B) Hansen's disease
    (C) schizophrenia
    (D) atrial flutter
    (E) psoriasis

2. A patient with allergic rhinitis may be treated with a topical nasal corticosteroid such as

    (A) diphenhydramine
    (B) cetirizine
    (C) prednisone
    (D) zafirlukast
    (E) budesonide

3. Which of the following statements is (are) true of atorvastatin calcium?

    I. It may be administered orally or parenterally.
    II. It is utilized for the treatment of candidiasis.
    III. It is used for the same indication as nicotinic acid.

    (A) I only
    (B) III only
    (C) I and II only

    (D) II and III only
    (E) I, II, and III

4. A pharmacist is about to dispense torsemide 20 mg tablets? Which of the following concerns would be considered in using this product?

    I. Potassium supplementation may be required.
    II. Ototoxicity may occur.
    III. Patients with sulfahypersensitivity should not use this product.

    (A) I only
    (B) III only
    (C) I and II only
    (D) II and III only
    (E) I, II, and III

5. Quetiapine is used for the same indication as

    (A) pilocarpine
    (B) quinidine
    (C) nifedipine
    (D) celecoxib
    (E) risperidone

6. Which of the following statements is (are) true of ticlopidine HCl (Ticlid)?

    I. inhibits platelet aggregation
    II. dissolves blood clots
    III. only administered parenterally

    (A) I only
    (B) III only
    (C) I and II only

(D) II and III only

(E) I, II, and III

7. Gabapentin is indicated for the treatment of

I. Parkinsons disease

II. postherpetic neuralgia

III. epilepsy

(A) I only

(B) III only

(C) I and II only

(D) II and III only

(E) I, II, and III

8. The primary reason why clavulanate potassium is combined with amoxicillin is to

I. provide greater gram-negative coverage

II. act as a buffer to prevent GI decomposition of the amoxicillin

III. prevent destruction of amoxicillin activity by beta-lactamase

(A) I only

(B) III only

(C) I and II only

(D) II and III only

(E) I, II, and III

9. Mr. Harris has just begun treatment with metformin. He should be monitored for the development of which of the following?

I. lactic acidosis

II. respiratory distress

III. hypercalcemia

(A) I only

(B) III only

(C) I and II only

(D) II and III only

(E) I, II, and III

10. As an antiarrhythmic drug, tocainide is most similar in action to which one of the following agents?

(A) amiodarone

(B) mexiletine

(C) digoxin

(D) verapamil

(E) propranolol

11. A pharmacist dispenses *ortho*-tri-cyclen to Janice Brown, a 19-year-old new user of this product. The patient reads the patient package insert (PPI) and asks how the norgestimate component of this product works. Which of the following would be an appropriate response by the pharmacist?

I. It prevents ovulation.

II. It increases the viscosity of cervical fluids.

III. It prevents implantation of a fertilized egg onto the uterine wall.

(A) I only

(B) III only

(C) I and II only

(D) II and III only

(E) I, II, and III

12. Clonidine may best be described as a (an)

(A) alpha-adrenergic blocker

(B) beta-adrenergic blocker

(C) MAO inhibitor

(D) alpha-adrenergic agonist

(E) beta-adrenergic agonist

13. Minoxidil is an antihypertensive agent that works by

(A) directly dilating peripheral blood vessels

(B) potentiating GABA activity

(C) blocking alpha-adrenergic receptors

(D) inhibiting COMT

(E) blocking beta-adrenergic receptors

**14.** Agent(s) indicated for the treatment of depression include(s)

    I.   bupropion
   II.  venlafaxine
  III.  citalopram

(A) I only
(B) III only
(C) I and II only
(D) II and III only
(E) I, II, and III

**15.** A common adverse effect associated with the use of antacids containing calcium carbonate is

(A) nausea and vomiting
(B) gastrointestinal bleeding
(C) flatulence
(D) diarrhea
(E) hypoparathyroidism

**16.** Reduced clotting ability of the blood is associated with the administration of

    I.   filgrastim
   II.  abciximab
  III.  clopidogrel

(A) I only
(B) III only
(C) I and II only
(D) II and III only
(E) I, II, and III

**17.** Carbidopa can best be classified as a drug that

(A) reverses symptoms of Parkinson's disease
(B) exerts an anticholinergic action
(C) is a dopaminergic agent
(D) is a dopa-decarboxylase inhibitor
(E) is a COMT inhibitor

**18.** Selegeline can best be described as a (an)

(A) MAO-B inhibitor
(B) anticholinergic
(C) COMT inhibitor
(D) dopamine antagonist
(E) alpha$_1$ agonist

**19.** Which of the following is (are) true of fentanyl?

    I.   available as a transdermal system
   II.  available as a transmucosal dosage form
  III.  may be used as a cough suppressant

(A) I only
(B) III only
(C) I and II only
(D) II and III only
(E) I, II, and III

**20.** Lactase enzyme is commercially available for the treatment of

(A) lactose intolerance
(B) galactokinase deficiency
(C) cystic fibrosis
(D) phenylketonuria
(E) Crohn's disease

**21.** Isotretinoin (Accutane) is a drug employed in the treatment of severe recalcitrant cystic acne. Which one of the following is NOT an adverse effect associated with its use?

(A) hypertriglyceridemia
(B) fetal abnormalities
(C) pseudotumor cerebri
(D) conjunctivitis
(E) hyponatremia

**22.** Which of the following is (are) true of valsartan (Diovan)?

    I.   Should NOT be used in women during the third trimester of pregnancy.
   II.  Should NOT be administered with hydrochlorothiazide.
  III.  It is an ACE inhibitor.

(A) I only
(B) III only
(C) I and II only
(D) II and III only
(E) I, II, and III

23. Endorphins are

    (A) endogenous neurotransmitters
    (B) a new class of topical anti-inflammatory agents
    (C) endogenous opioid peptides
    (D) biogenic amines believed to cause schizophrenia
    (E) neuromuscular blocking agents

24. Which of the following statements is (are) true of "crack"?

    I.   It is generally injected intravenously.
    II.  Its use results in CNS depression.
    III. It is a free-base form of cocaine.

    (A) I only
    (B) III only
    (C) I and II only
    (D) II and III only
    (E) I, II, and III

25. A uricosuric drug is one that

    (A) promotes excretion of uric acid in the urine
    (B) decreases flow of urine
    (C) blocks excretion of uric acid in the urine
    (D) aids in the tubular reabsorption of uric acid
    (E) increases the flow of urine

26. Reteplase (Retavase) is employed clinically as a (an)

    (A) xanthine oxidase inhibitor
    (B) plasminogen activator
    (C) COMT inhibitor
    (D) antihypertensive agent
    (E) proteolytic enzyme

27. A disadvantage in the use of cimetidine (Tagamet) is its ability to cause

    (A) cheilosis
    (B) aplastic anemia
    (C) gastric hyperparesis
    (D) inhibition of hepatic enzyme activity
    (E) decreased prolactin secretion

28. A drug that decreases the formation of uric acid is

    (A) tolcapone
    (B) allopurinol
    (C) probenecid
    (D) ketamine
    (E) propylthiouracil

29. Hypoparathyroidism is a disorder that would most logically be treated with

    I.   dihydrotachysterol
    II.  calcium carbonate
    III. liotrix

    (A) I only
    (B) III only
    (C) I and II only
    (D) II and III only
    (E) I, II, and III

30. Drugs employed in reducing elevated serum lipid levels include(s)

    I.   colestipol
    II.  nicotinic acid
    III. psyllium

    (A) I only
    (B) III only
    (C) I and II only
    (D) II and III only
    (E) I, II, and III

31. The agent most similar in pharmacologic action to miglitol is

    (A) acarbose
    (B) lispro insulin
    (C) pioglitazone
    (D) repaglinide
    (E) glipizide

32. Xenical (Orlistat) is believed to work by acting as a (an)

    (A) CNS stimulant
    (B) proton pump inhibitor
    (C) acetylcholinesterase inhibitor
    (D) amylase inhibitor
    (E) lipase inhibitor

33. Patients receiving amiodarone (Cordarone) should be monitored for the development of

    (A) pseudomembranous enterocolitis
    (B) pulmonary toxicity
    (C) ptosis
    (D) stasis dermatitis
    (E) tinnitus

34. Methadone is a (an)

    I.   narcotic antagonist
    II.  controlled substance
    III. analgesic drug

    (A) I only
    (B) III only
    (C) I and II only
    (D) II and III only
    (E) I, II, and III

35. Which of the following is an example of a pure narcotic antagonist?

    I.   buprenorphine (Subutex)
    II.  nalbuphine (Nubain)
    III. naltrexone (ReVia)

    (A) I only
    (B) III only
    (C) I and II only
    (D) II and III only
    (E) I, II, and III

36. Tegaserod (Zelnorm) is used in the treatment of IBS. It can best be classified as a (an)

    (A) $5HT_3$-receptor antagonist
    (B) anti-inflammatory agent
    (C) $5HT_4$-receptor agonist
    (D) $H_2$-receptor antagonist
    (E) anticholinergic

37. Morphine can be expected to produce which of the following pharmacological effects?

    I.   pupillary dilation
    II.  respiratory depression
    III. constipation

    (A) I only
    (B) III only
    (C) I and II only
    (D) II and III only
    (E) I, II, and III

38. Which of the following are active metabolites of primidone (Mysoline)?

    I.   phenobarbital
    II.  phenylethylmalonamide
    III. gamma-aminobutyric acid

    (A) I only
    (B) III only
    (C) I and II only
    (D) II and III only
    (E) I, II, and III

39. Tiludronate disodium (Skelid) is indicated for the treatment of

    (A) Paget's disease
    (B) Meniere's syndrome
    (C) Crohn's disease
    (D) Hansen's disease
    (E) Parkinson's disease

40. Repaglinide (Prandin) is believed to work by

    (A) decreasing the absorption of carbohydrates
    (B) decreasing hepatic gluconeogenesis
    (C) reducing glucagon secretion from the pancreas
    (D) increasing hepatic gluconeogenesis
    (E) stimulating the release of insulin from the pancreas

41. Prednisone is an agent that is employed in the treatment of

    I.   fungal infections
    II.  Crohn's disease
    III. rheumatic disorders

    (A) I only
    (B) III only
    (C) I and II only
    (D) II and III only
    (E) I, II, and III

42. Jimmy K. is an 11-year-old boy who has been diagnosed with ADHD. He has been using Ritalin 5 mg tablets BID for the past six months but is embarrassed about taking one of his tablets at noon when his classmates and teachers are present. Which of the following might be a better choice for Jimmy?

    I.   Concerta
    II.  Paxil
    III. Xanax

    (A) I only
    (B) III only
    (C) I and II only
    (D) II and III only
    (E) I, II, and III

43. Helene T. is a 45-year-old female who is 5 ft 6 in tall and weighs 185 lb. She has failed to lose weight on several "crash" diets. Which of the following would be appropriate to prescribe for Helene?

    I.   sibutramine
    II.  mazindol
    III. benzphetamine

    (A) I only
    (B) III only
    (C) I and II only
    (D) II and III only
    (E) I, II, and III

44. Colesevelam can best be classified as a (an)

    (A) HMG-CoA reductase inhibitor
    (B) bile acid sequestrant
    (C) potassium-sparing diuretic
    (D) ACE inhibitor
    (E) vasopressor

45. Epoetin-alpha would be appropriate to use in order to raise levels of which of the following?

    I.   RBCs
    II.  hematocrit
    III. platelets

    (A) I only
    (B) III only
    (C) I and II only
    (D) II and III only
    (E) I, II, and III

46. The anxiolytic action of benzodiazepines is usually attributed to their ability to

    (A) alter the sodium ion influx into the CNS
    (B) potentiate the effects of GABA
    (C) alter the calcium ion influx into the CNS
    (D) interfere with the amine pump
    (E) inhibit the action of monoamine oxidase

47. Which of the following is a COMT inhibitor?

    (A) selegiline
    (B) carbidopa
    (C) pramipexole
    (D) ropinerole
    (E) entacapone

48. Henry M. visits his pharmacy and indicates to the pharmacist that he has a painful cold sore. Which of the following ingredients would be helpful for the treatment of Henry's cold sore?

    I.   docosanol
    II.  nystatin
    III. bacitracin

    (A) I only
    (B) III only
    (C) I and II only
    (D) II and III only
    (E) I, II, and III

49. Which of the following is (are) employed in the treatment of onychomycosis?

    I.   gentamicin
    II.  amikacin
    III. terbinafine

    (A)  I only
    (B)  III only
    (C)  I and II only
    (D)  II and III only
    (E)  I, II, and III

50. Timothy R. is a 14-year-old asthmatic. He has heard about several drugs that are used in treating asthma and wishes to know which one(s) could be used to treat an acute asthma attack. Which of the following drugs is (are) indicated for the treatment of an acute attack?

    I.   salmeterol
    II.  bitolterol
    III. pirbuterol

    (A)  I only
    (B)  III only
    (C)  I and II only
    (D)  II and III only
    (E)  I, II, and III

51. Which of the following agents is (are) indicated for use in the treatment of emesis?

    I.   granisetron (Kytril)
    II.  dronabinol (Marinol)
    III. zoledronic acid (Zometa)

    (A)  I only
    (B)  III only
    (C)  I and II only
    (D)  II and III only
    (E)  I, II, and III

52. Amrinone (Inocor) is most similar in action to

    (A)  digoxin (Lanoxin)
    (B)  lidocaine (Xylocaine)
    (C)  amiodarone (Cordarone)
    (D)  disopyramide (Norpace)
    (E)  benazepril (Lotensin)

53. Which of the following is true of butenafine?

    I.   It is only used topically.
    II.  It is used in treating impetigo.
    III. Containers of the drug must be refrigerated.

    (A)  I only
    (B)  III only
    (C)  I and II only
    (D)  II and III only
    (E)  I, II, and III

54. Lactulose (Cephulac, Chronulac)

    I.   decreases blood ammonia levels
    II.  is a laxative
    III. is an artificial sweetener

    (A)  I only
    (B)  III only
    (C)  I and II only
    (D)  II and III only
    (E)  I, II, and III

55. Which of the following can be classified as an osmotic laxative?

    (A)  castor oil
    (B)  senna
    (C)  bisacodyl
    (D)  docusate sodium
    (E)  milk of magnesia

56. The dose of liothyronine sodium that is approximately equivalent to 100 µg of levothyroxine sodium USP is

    (A)  25 µg
    (B)  0.4 µg
    (C)  250 µg
    (D)  120 µg
    (E)  100 µg

57. Phosphate binding is likely to occur when which of the following antacids are administered?

    I.   calcium carbonate
    II.  sodium bicarbonate
    III. aluminum hydroxide

(A) I only
(B) III only
(C) I and II only
(D) II and III only
(E) I, II, and III

58. Which of the following agents is indicated for the treatment of chronic inflammatory bowel disease?

(A) misoprostol (Cytotec)
(B) tegaserod (Zelnorm)
(C) rabeprazole (Aciphex)
(D) metoclopramide (Reglan)
(E) mesalamine (Asacol)

59. Patients who are hypersensitive to aspirin should avoid the use of

I. codeine
II. oxaprozin
III. ibuprofen

(A) I only
(B) III only
(C) I and II only
(D) II and III only
(E) I, II, and III

60. Aspirin is believed to inhibit clotting by its action on which of the following endogenous substances?

(A) cyclooxygenase
(B) xanthine oxidase
(C) fibrinogen
(D) endorphin A
(E) serotonin

61. The primary site of action of triamterene (Dyrenium) and spironolactone (Aldactone) is the

(A) glomerulus
(B) descending loop of Henle
(C) ascending loop of Henle
(D) proximal tubule
(E) distal tubule

62. Which of the following beta-adrenergic blocking agents also exhibit alpha$_1$-adrenergic blocking action?

I. timolol (Blocadren)
II. sotalol (Betapace)
III. labetalol (Normodyne, Trandate)

(A) I only
(B) III only
(C) I and II only
(D) II and III only
(E) I, II, and III

63. Which one of the following drugs is employed in treating acute attacks of gout?

(A) hyoscyamine sulfate (Nulev)
(B) ergonavine maleate (Ergotrate)
(C) buspirone (Buspar)
(D) naproxen (Anaprox)
(E) allopurinol (Zyloprim)

64. Prolonged activity (8 to 10 h) is an advantage in the use of which of the following topical decongestants?

I. xylometazoline
II. oxymetazoline
III. phenylephrine

(A) I only
(B) III only
(C) I and II only
(D) II and III only
(E) I, II, and III

65. Auranofin (Ridaura) is employed in the treatment of

(A) rheumatoid arthritis
(B) multiple sclerosis
(C) ulcerative colitis
(D) recalcitrant cystic acne
(E) ear infections

66. Which of the following agents is NOT likely to reduce blood sugar in a patient with type II diabetes mellitus?

    I.   glucagon
    II.  diazoxide
    III. repaglinide

    (A) I only
    (B) III only
    (C) I and II only
    (D) II and III only
    (E) I, II, and III

67. After oral administration, the greatest amount of iron absorption occurs in the

    (A) ascending colon
    (B) stomach
    (C) duodenum
    (D) transverse colon
    (E) sigmoid colon

68. Iron is required by the body to maintain normal

    (A) leukocyte development
    (B) ascorbic acid absorption
    (C) oxygen transport
    (D) immune function
    (E) bone growth

69. Prolonged use of organic nitrates (e.g., nitroglycerin) is likely to result in the development of

    (A) hepatotoxicity
    (B) nephrotoxicity
    (C) aplastic anemia
    (D) tolerance
    (E) megaloblastic anemia

70. Which of the following statements is (are) true of regular insulin?

    I.   It is a suspension.
    II.  It is shorter acting than lispro insulin.
    III. It may be administered either SC or IV.

    (A) I only
    (B) III only

    (C) I and II only
    (D) II and III only
    (E) I, II, and III

71. An agent that would be most likely to cause drug-induced bronchospasm is

    (A) sotalol
    (B) zileuton
    (C) isoproterenol
    (D) ephedrine
    (E) cromolyn

72. A physician calls a pharmacist and asks which of the following drugs are likely to cause dry mouth? Which of the following would you choose?

    I.   theophylline
    II.  montelukast sodium
    III. ipratropium bromide

    (A) I only
    (B) III only
    (C) I and II only
    (D) II and III only
    (E) I, II, and III

73. Which of the following is (are) true of dobutamine (Dobutrex)?

    I.   beta$_1$ agonist
    II.  only administered parenterally
    III. antidepressant

    (A) I only
    (B) III only
    (C) I and II only
    (D) II and III only
    (E) I, II, and III

74. Which of the following is (are) anticholinergic anti-Parkinson agents?

    I.   ropinirole (Requip)
    II.  pergolide (Permax)
    III. procyclidine (Kemadrin)

    (A) I only
    (B) III only

(C) I and II only

(D) II and III only

(E) I, II, and III

75. A pharmacist is about to dispense budesonide (Pulmicort) to an asthmatic patient. Which of the following is (are) true of this product?

 I. It is available as an inhalation powder.

 II. It is indicated for the treatment of acute asthma attacks.

 III. The patient should be advised not to eat, drink, or rinse his mouth for 30 min after the drug has been administered.

(A) I only

(B) III only

(C) I and II only

(D) II and III only

(E) I, II, and III

76. Which of the following drugs is (are) $H_1$-histamine receptor antagonists?

 I. loratadine

 II. fexofenadine

 III. nizatidine

(A) I only

(B) III only

(C) I and II only

(D) II and III only

(E) I, II, and III

77. Which of the following are considered to be prokinetic agents?

 I. lansoprazole

 II. diphenoxylate

 III. metoclopramide

(A) I only

(B) III only

(C) I and II only

(D) II and III only

(E) I, II, and III

78. Effects expected as a result of inhaling the smoke of cannabis (marijuana) include

 I. decreased pulse rate

 II. perceptual changes

 III. vascular congestion of the eye

(A) I only

(B) III only

(C) I and II only

(D) II and III only

(E) I, II, and III

79. Of the following glucocorticoids, which one has the greatest anti-inflammatory potency when administered systemically?

(A) hydrocortisone (Cortef)

(B) prednisone (Meticorten)

(C) triamcinolone (Aristocort)

(D) betamethasone (Celestone)

(E) cortisone (Cortone)

80. Tretinoin is commonly employed in the treatment of

(A) acne

(B) pinworms

(C) seborrheic dermatitis

(D) trichomoniasis

(E) psoriasis

81. Which of the following is (are) true of infliximab (Remicade)?

 I. used in treating Crohn's disease

 II. a monoclonal antibody

 III. administered intravenously

(A) I only

(B) III only

(C) I and II only

(D) II and III only

(E) I, II, and III

82. Simvastatin (Zocor) is contraindicated for use in patients who

    I. are type I diabetics
    II. have liver disease
    III. are pregnant

    (A) I only
    (B) III only
    (C) I and II only
    (D) II and III only
    (E) I, II, and III

83. Which of the following drugs are available in a transdermal dosage form?

    I. fentanyl
    II. clonidine
    III. latanoprost

    (A) I only
    (B) III only
    (C) I and II only
    (D) II and III only
    (E) I, II, and III

84. Which one of the following drugs is indicated for the treatment of primary nocturnal enuresis?

    (A) ritodrine (Yutopar)
    (B) amoxapine (Asendin)
    (C) desmopressin acetate (DDAVP)
    (D) metolazone (Zaroxolyn)
    (E) mannitol (Osmitrol)

85. Which of the following drugs is (are) classified as a selective serotonin reuptake inhibitor (SSRI)?

    I. citalopram
    II. nefazodone
    III. venlafaxine

    (A) I only
    (B) III only
    (C) I and II only
    (D) II and III only
    (E) I, II, and III

86. Which one of the following antimicrobial agents would be MOST useful in the treatment of an infection caused by beta-lactamase–producing staphylococci?

    (A) dicloxacillin
    (B) bacampicillin
    (C) cephalexin
    (D) amoxicillin
    (E) cephapirin

87. Gastric intrinsic factor is a glycoprotein that is required for the gastrointestinal absorption of

    (A) pyridoxine
    (B) folic acid
    (C) iron
    (D) cyanocobalamin
    (E) ascorbic acid

88. Hirsutism is an adverse effect associated with the use of

    (A) minoxidil (Loniten)
    (B) ethinyl estradiol
    (C) ginseng root
    (D) chlorpromazine (Thorazine)
    (E) ofloxacin (Floxin)

89. Latanoprost (Xalatan) is a drug used in the treatment of glaucoma. Which one of the following best describes its pharmacologic action?

    (A) miotic
    (B) peripheral vasodilator
    (C) inhibits action of carbonic anhydrase
    (D) mydriatic
    (E) prostaglandin agonist

90. Cardioselectivity is a property of which of the following beta-adrenergic blocking agents?

    I. timolol (Timoptic)
    II. metipranolol HCl (OptiPranolol)
    III. levobetaxolol (Betaxon)

    (A) I only
    (B) III only
    (C) I and II only
    (D) II and III only
    (E) I, II, and III

91. Which of the following is true of pilocarpine?

    I. ingredient in Ocusert ocular therapeutic system
    II. direct-acting mydriatic
    III. similar pharmacological action to dorzolamide (Trusopt)

    (A) I only
    (B) III only
    (C) I and II only
    (D) II and III only
    (E) I, II, and III

92. Which one of the following statements best describes the mechanism of action of nizatidine (Axid)?

    (A) Interferes with the synthesis of histamine in the body.
    (B) Forms an inactive complex with histamine.
    (C) Stimulates the metabolism of endogenous histamine.
    (D) Blocks the receptor sites on which histamine acts.
    (E) Directly inhibits the action of mucin in the stomach.

93. Haloperidol (Haldol) differs from chlorpromazine (Thorazine) in that haloperidol

    I. does not produce extrapyramidal effects
    II. cannot be administered parenterally
    III. is not a phenothiazine

    (A) I only
    (B) III only
    (C) I and II only
    (D) II and III only
    (E) I, II, and III

94. Tamoxifen (Nolvadex) can best be characterized as a(an)

    (A) gonadotropin-releasing hormone analog
    (B) estrogen
    (C) progestin
    (D) antiestrogen
    (E) androgen

95. Which of the following is true of permethrin?

    I. only used topically
    II. used to treat topical fungal infections
    III. is used to enhance permeation of drugs through the skin

    (A) I only
    (B) III only
    (C) I and II only
    (D) II and III only
    (E) I, II, and III

96. Advantages of acetaminophen over aspirin include all of the following EXCEPT

    (A) no alteration of bleeding time
    (B) less gastric irritation
    (C) no occult blood loss
    (D) no appreciable effect on uric acid excretion
    (E) greater anti-inflammatory action

97. The use of clozapine (Clozaril) has been associated with the development of

    (A) thrombocytopenia
    (B) hypocalcemia
    (C) meningitis
    (D) agranulocytosis
    (E) hematuria

98. Didanosine can best be described as a (an)

    (A) nonnucleoside reverse transcriptase inhibitor
    (B) nucleoside reverse transcriptase inhibitor
    (C) protease inhibitor
    (D) pyrimidine antagonist
    (E) purine antagonist

99. Respiratory damage is most likely to occur with the use of which of the following antineoplastic agents?

    (A) bleomycin
    (B) cytarabine
    (C) actinomycin
    (D) vincristine
    (E) flutamide

100. The anti-inflammatory effect of NSAIDS is due to their ability to

    I.   inhibit prostaglandin synthesis
    II.  inhibit the stimulation of the chemoreceptor trigger zone (CTZ)
    III. reset the hypothalamic "setpoint"

    (A) I only
    (B) III only
    (C) I and II only
    (D) II and III only
    (E) I, II, and III

101. The "first-dose" effect is characterized by marked hypotension and syncope on taking the first few doses of medication. This effect is seen with the use of

    I.   sotalol (Betapace)
    II.  enalapril (Vasotec)
    III. doxazosin (Cardura)

    (A) I only
    (B) III only
    (C) I and II only
    (D) II and III only
    (E) I, II, and III only

102. Carbon monoxide exerts its toxic effects primarily by

    (A) inhibiting the gag reflex
    (B) paralyzing the muscles of the diaphragm
    (C) reacting with amino acids in the body to form ammonia
    (D) reacting with body enzymes to produce respiratory acidosis
    (E) decreasing the oxygen-carrying capacity of the blood

103. The most serious potential consequence of ingestion of a liquid hydrocarbon such as kerosene or gasoline is

    (A) inactivation of hepatic enzymes
    (B) the corrosive action of the poison on the stomach lining
    (C) the aspiration of the poison into the respiratory tract
    (D) dissolution of the mucus coat of the esophagus
    (E) the paralysis of peristaltic motion of the GI tract

104. Deferoxamine mesylate is considered to be a specific antidote for the treatment of poisoning caused by

    (A) anticholinergic agents
    (B) heavy metals
    (C) benzodiazepines
    (D) iron-containing products
    (E) carbon monoxide

105. Which of the following agents is (are) classified pharmacologically as carbonic anhydrase inhibitors?

    I.   nilutamide
    II.  dacarbazine
    III. dorzolamide

    (A) I only
    (B) III only
    (C) I and II only
    (D) II and III only
    (E) I, II, and III only

106. Thiazide diuretics decrease the excretion of

    I.   sodium
    II.  chloride
    III. uric acid

    (A) I only
    (B) III only
    (C) I and II only
    (D) II and III only
    (E) I, II, and III only

107. The renal excretion of amphetamines can be diminished by alkalinizing the urine. Which of the following would tend to diminish the excretion rate of amphetamine sulfate?

   I.  methenamine mandelate
   II. ammonium chloride
   III. potassium citrate

   (A) I only
   (B) III only
   (C) I and II only
   (D) II and III only
   (E) I, II, and III only

108. Cyclophosphamide (Cytoxan) is an example of a (an)

   (A) antibiotic
   (B) estrogen antagonist
   (C) antimetabolite
   (D) alkylating agent
   (E) prostaglandin inhibitor

109. Which of the following drugs may interfere with ethanol metabolism?

   I.  metronidazole (Flagyl)
   II. chlorpropamide (Diabinese)
   III. disulfiram (Antabuse)

   (A) I only
   (B) III only
   (C) I and II only
   (D) II and III only
   (E) I, II, and III only

110. Which of the following is (are) classified as a monoamine oxidase inhibitor?

   I.  phenylzine
   II. selegeline
   III. gemcitabine

   (A) I only
   (B) III only
   (C) I and II only
   (D) II and III only
   (E) I, II, and III only

111. A drug indicated for the treatment of both diarrhea and constipation is

   (A) polycarbophil
   (B) lactulose
   (C) bisacodyl
   (D) senna
   (E) magnesium hydroxide

112. Which of the following agents is (are) classified as a leukotriene receptor antagonist?

   I.  ipratropium bromide
   II. salmeterol
   III. montelukast sodium

   (A) I only
   (B) III only
   (C) I and II only
   (D) II and III only
   (E) I, II, and III only

113. The thiazide derivative diazoxide (Hyperstat)

   (A) is not a diuretic
   (B) is a stronger diuretic than hydrochlorothiazide
   (C) produces about the same diuretic response as an equal dose of hydrochlorothiazide
   (D) is used in the treatment of shock
   (E) must be used with a potassium supplement

114. Which of the following is (are) classified as a broad-spectrum antifungal agent?

   I.  caspofungin
   II. ciclopirox
   III. miconazole

   (A) I only
   (B) III only
   (C) I and II only
   (D) II and III only
   (E) I, II, and III

115. Which of the following drugs are sulfonamides?

    (A) mafenide
    (B) tacrolimus
    (C) tramadol
    (D) busulfan
    (E) milrinone

116. Which of the following drugs may be used in the treatment of diabetes insipidus?

    (A) hydrochlorothiazide
    (B) lypressin
    (C) miglitol
    (D) glyburide
    (E) glucagon

117. In the treatment of cardiac arrhythmias, sotalol (Betapace) is most similar in action to

    (A) tocainide
    (B) verapamil
    (C) amiodarone
    (D) digoxin
    (E) flecainide

118. Pioglitazone (Actos) is believed to exert its hypoglycemic effect by

    (A) stimulating the release of insulin from the pancreas
    (B) inhibiting the breakdown of endoge-nous insulin
    (C) decreasing the absorption of dietary glucose
    (D) increasing the sensitivity of insulin receptors
    (E) decreasing the desire for sugar con-sumption

119. Which of the following is true of finasteride?

    I.  It is useful in treating BPH.
    II. It is used to treat some types of alopecia.
    III. It is a prostaglandin.

    (A) I only
    (B) III only
    (C) I and II only

    (D) II and III only
    (E) I, II, and III only

120. Vidarabine (Vira-A) is an antiviral agent indi-cated for the treatment of

    (A) rubella
    (B) AIDS
    (C) influenza
    (D) herpes simplex encephalitis
    (E) *pneumocystis carinii* pneumonia (PCP)

121. Zosyn is a product that contains piperacillin sodium and tazobactam sodium. Tazobactam sodium

    (A) is a renal dipeptidase inhibitor
    (B) prevents the urinary excretion of piperacillin sodium
    (C) prevents first-pass metabolism of piperacillin sodium
    (D) is a COMT inhibitor
    (E) is a beta-lactamase inhibitor

122. Which one of the following hormones is (are) released from the posterior pituitary gland?

    I.   human growth hormone
    II.  follicle-stimulating hormone (FSH)
    III. oxytocin

    (A) I only
    (B) III only
    (C) I and II only
    (D) II and III only
    (E) I, II, and III

123. During ovulation, peak plasma concentra-tion(s) of which of the following hormone(s) will be reached?

    I.   luteinizing hormone (LH)
    II.  follicle-stimulating hormone (FSH)
    III. progesterone

    (A) I only
    (B) III only
    (C) I and II only
    (D) II and III only
    (E) I, II, and III

124. Liotrix is a thyroid preparation that contains

    I.   desiccated thyroid
    II.  levothyroxine sodium
    III. liothyronine sodium

    (A) I only
    (B) III only
    (C) I and II only
    (D) II and III only
    (E) I, II, and III

125. Propylthiouracil is used for the same therapeutic indication as

    (A) methoxsalen
    (B) danazol
    (C) methimazole
    (D) omeprazole
    (E) azathioprine

126. Most antipsychotic drugs can be said to have which of the following actions?

    (A) cholinergic
    (B) dopamine agonist
    (C) COMT antagonist
    (D) dopamine antagonist
    (E) alpha$_1$-adrenergic agonist

127. Which of the following agents are indicated for the treatment of convulsive disorders?

    I.   topiramate
    II.  tiagabine
    III. clonidine

    (A) I only
    (B) III only
    (C) I and II only
    (D) II and III only
    (E) I, II, and III

128. Which of the following antianxiety agents causes the least sedation?

    (A) diazepam (Valium)
    (B) lorazepam (Ativan)
    (C) chlordiazepoxide (Librium)
    (D) oxazepam (Serax)
    (E) buspirone (Buspar)

129. Which of the following drugs are classified as protease inhibitors?

    I.   nelfinavir
    II.  acyclovir
    III. cidofovir

    (A) I only
    (B) III only
    (C) I and II only
    (D) II and III only
    (E) I, II, and III

130. Which of the following are classified as aminopenicillins?

    I.   bacampicillin
    II.  amoxicillin
    III. ampicillin

    (A) I only
    (B) III only
    (C) I and II only
    (D) II and III only
    (E) I, II, and III

131. Dalteparin sodium acts in the body to

    (A) regulate menstrual activity
    (B) prevent blood clot formation
    (C) inhibit thyroid function
    (D) inhibit viral replication
    (E) manage preterm labor

132. Oseltamivir is indicated for the treatment of patients with

    I.   influenza
    II.  herpes simplex type 1
    III. human immunodeficiency virus (HIV)

    (A) I only
    (B) III only
    (C) I and II only
    (D) II and III only
    (E) I, II, and III

133. Which one of the following statements is true of alteplase (Activase)?

    (A) It is an anticoagulant.
    (B) It is administered intramuscularly.
    (C) It is derived from porcine tissue.
    (D) It is a thrombolytic agent.
    (E) It is derived from bovine tissue.

134. Which of the following bronchodilators act by inhibiting phosphodiesterase?

    I.   dyphylline (Lufyllin)
    II.  salmeterol (Serevent)
    III. nedocromil sodium (Tilade)

    (A) I only
    (B) III only
    (C) I and II only
    (D) II and III only
    (E) I, II, and III

135. Valdecoxib (Bextra) is most similar in action to

    (A) buspirone (Buspar)
    (B) oxaprozin (Daypro)
    (C) chlorzoxazone (Paraflex)
    (D) dicyclomine (Bentyl)
    (E) mecamylamine (Inversine)

136. Which of the following is likely to have the shortest duration of hypnotic action?

    (A) flurazepam
    (B) zaleplon
    (C) estazolam
    (D) phenobarbital
    (E) temazepam

137. Which of the following calcium channel blockers may be employed parenterally in the treatment of cardiac arrhythmias?

    I.   amlodipine (Norvasc)
    II.  isradipine (DynaCirc)
    III. verapamil (Isoptin, Calan)

    (A) I only
    (B) III only
    (C) I and II only

    (D) II and III only
    (E) I, II, and III

138. Which one of the following antibiotics is a third-generation cephalosporin?

    (A) cefoxitin (Mefoxin)
    (B) cefonicid (Monocid)
    (C) cefixime (Suprax)
    (D) cephalexin (Keflex)
    (E) cefaclor (Ceclor)

139. Reflex tachycardia is an adverse effect most likely to be associated with the use of which of the following drugs?

    (A) minoxidil (Loniten)
    (B) losartan (Cozaar)
    (C) moexipril (Univasc)
    (D) nadolol (Corgard)
    (E) clonidine (Catapres)

140. Which of the following statements is TRUE of buprenorphine (Buprenex)?

    I.   It is used in the treatment of narcotic dependence.
    II.  It is only administered parenterally.
    III. It is a meperidine derivative.

    (A) I only
    (B) III only
    (C) I and II only
    (D) II and III only
    (E) I, II, and III

141. Which one of the following is NOT a progestin?

    (A) norethynodrel
    (B) norethindrone
    (C) ethynodiol diacetate
    (D) levonorgestrel
    (E) mestranol

142. Which one of the following beta-adrenergic blocking agents has the greatest lipid solubility?

    (A) esmolol (Brevibloc)
    (B) atenolol (Tenormin)
    (C) pindolol (Visken)

(D)  acebutolol (Sectral)

(E)  propranolol HCl (Inderal)

143.  Danazol (Danocrine) can best be classified as a (an)

(A)  anabolic steroid

(B)  estrogen

(C)  progestin

(D)  endometriosis treatment

(E)  ovulatory stimulant

144.  Torsemide (Demadex) is most similar in action to

(A)  bumetanide (Bumex)

(B)  risperidone (Risperdal)

(C)  spironolactone (Aldactone)

(D)  chlorthalidone (Hygroton)

(E)  acetazolamide (Diamox)

145.  Potassium depletion is LEAST likely to occur in a patient using

(A)  ethacrynic acid (Edecrin)

(B)  amiloride (Midamor)

(C)  torsemide (Demadex)

(D)  acetazolamide (Diamox)

(E)  chlorthalidone (Hygroton)

146.  Valacyclovir (Valtrex) is indicated for the treatment of

(A)  multiple sclerosis

(B)  psoriasis

(C)  HIV infection

(D)  shingles

(E)  mononucleosis

147.  Which of the following barbiturates is likely to be the shortest acting?

(A)  amobarbital sodium

(B)  methohexital sodium

(C)  pentobarbital sodium

(D)  mephobarbital

(E)  phenobarbital

148.  Which of the following agents decreases the production of hydrochloric acid in the stomach?

I.  olsalazine

II.  magnesium hydroxide

III.  pantoprazole

(A)  I only

(B)  III only

(C)  I and II only

(D)  II and III only

(E)  I, II, and III

149.  Which of the following is (are) an indication for the use of metoclopramide?

I.  diabetic gastroparesis

II.  symptomatic gastroesophageal reflux

III.  prevention of postoperative nausea and vomiting

(A)  I only

(B)  III only

(C)  I and II only

(D)  II and III only

(E)  I, II, and III

150.  Olsalazine sodium (Dipentum) is employed in the treatment of

(A)  diabetes mellitus

(B)  duodenal ulcers

(C)  urinary tract infections

(D)  ulcerative colitis

(E)  diabetes insipidus

151.  Which of the following agents would be most appropriate to use in the treatment of narcolepsy?

(A)  bupropion (Wellbutrin)

(B)  buspirone (BuSpar)

(C)  ziprasidone (Geodon)

(D)  modafinil (Provigil)

(E)  rivastigmine (Exelon)

**152.** Mifepristone is indicated for the

(A) treatment of rheumatoid arthritis

(B) treatment of alopecia

(C) termination of early pregnancy

(D) protection of the GI lining

(E) treatment of carcinoma of the breast

**153.** Ramipril HCl can best be classified as a (an)

(A) angiotensin II antagonist

(B) $H_2$-receptor antagonist

(C) calcium channel blocker

(D) angiotensin-converting enzyme inhibitor

(E) alpha-adrenergic blocking agent

**154.** Which of the following statements is TRUE of beclomethasone dipropionate (Beclovent, Vanceril) aerosol?

(A) It should only be used in the treatment of an acute asthmatic attack.

(B) It should not be used in a patient who is currently using a theophylline product.

(C) Beclomethasone is not systemically absorbed by this route.

(D) The aerosol form is indicated in the treatment of status asthmaticus.

(E) If used in conjunction with a bronchodilator administered by inhalation, the bronchodilator should be used first.

**155.** Which of the following is true of naratriptan (Amerge)?

I. It is a 5-$HT_1$-receptor antagonist.

II. It must be used regularly to prevent migraines.

III. It may be administered orally or by inhalation.

(A) I only

(B) III only

(C) I and II only

(D) II and III only

(E) I, II, and III

**156.** Which of the following cancer chemotherapeutic agents is (are) classified as an antimetabolite?

I. cladribine (Leustatin)

II. fluorouracil (Adrucil)

III. fludarabine (Fludara)

(A) I only

(B) III only

(C) I and II only

(D) II and III only

(E) I, II, and III

**157.** Which one of the following antihistamines would be LEAST likely to cause sedation?

(A) azatadine (Optimine)

(B) dimenhydrinate (Dramamine)

(C) clemastine (Tavist)

(D) loratidine (Alavert)

(E) tripelennamine (PBZ)

**158.** The pharmacologic properties of which one of the following agents is similar to amphetamine?

(A) zonisamide

(B) lithium carbonate

(C) methylphenidate

(D) haloperidol

(E) methoxsalen

**159.** Which of the following agents is (are) classified as macrolides?

I. netilmicin

II. clarithromycin

III. azithromycin

(A) I only

(B) III only

(C) I and II only

(D) II and III only

(E) I, II, and III

**160.** Stavudine (Zerit) is an antiviral agent employed in the treatment of

(A) lupus erythematosus

(B) influenza A virus

(C) HIV infection

(D) herpes zoster

(E) herpes simplex

161.  Beta carotene is considered to be a precursor for

(A)  betaseron
(B)  beta interferon
(C)  tocopherol
(D)  vitamin A
(E)  carteolol

162.  Simvastatin (Zocor) acts by

(A)  inhibiting xanthine oxidase
(B)  inhibiting HMG-CoA reductase
(C)  inhibiting acetylcholinesterase
(D)  acting as a bile sequestrant
(E)  acting as a lipase inhibitor

163.  Which of the following is a commercially available dosage form of fentanyl?

I.   transmucosal
II.  transdermal patch
III. suppository

(A)  I only
(B)  III only
(C)  I and II only
(D)  II and III only
(E)  I, II, and III

164.  Which of the following agents is an anabolic steroid?

I.   oxandrolone
II.  stanozolol
III. fluorometholone

(A)  I only
(B)  III only
(C)  I and II only
(D)  II and III only
(E)  I, II, and III

165.  Amrinone is a drug that produces

(A)  bronchodilation
(B)  antidepressant action
(C)  control of focal seizures
(D)  narcotic antagonism
(E)  positive inotropism

166.  Which of the following statements is (are) true of potassium?

I.   It is a monovalent anion.
II.  It facilitates the utilization of glucose by cells.
III. It is the principal intracellular ion.

(A)  I only
(B)  III only
(C)  I and II only
(D)  II and III only
(E)  I, II, and III

167.  Oxybutynin can best be described as a (an)

(A)  androgen inhibitor
(B)  antispasmodic
(C)  bleaching agent
(D)  sedative
(E)  urinary antiseptic

168.  Which of the following agents have cortical stimulant action?

I.   cocaine
II.  pemoline
III. methamphetamine

(A)  I only
(B)  III only
(C)  I and II only
(D)  II and III only
(E)  I, II, and III

169.  Lactulose is used to treat

I.   constipation
II.  portal-systemic encephalopathy
III. renal tubular necrosis

(A)  I only
(B)  III only
(C)  I and II only
(D)  II and III only
(E)  I, II, and III

170. The primary function of simethicone in antacid products is to act as a (an)

    (A) suspending agent
    (B) adsorbent
    (C) buffer
    (D) antiflatulent
    (E) flavoring agent

171. Which of the following is (are) true of penta-midine isethionate?

    I. It may be administered by inhalation.
    II. It may be administered parenterally.
    III. It may be used to treat PCP.

    (A) I only
    (B) III only
    (C) I and II only
    (D) II and III only
    (E) I, II, and III

172. Which of the following statements is (are) true of metronidazole?

    I. It is a pediculocide.
    II. It has disulfiram-like activity.
    III. It has antiprotozoal activity.

    (A) I only
    (B) III only
    (C) I and II only
    (D) II and III only
    (E) I, II, and III

173. Which of the following is indicated for the prevention of thrombotic stroke?

    (A) oprelvekin
    (B) filgrastim
    (C) sargramostim
    (D) ticlopidine
    (E) cilostazol

174. Cinchonism is an adverse effect associated with

    (A) quinidine
    (B) procainamide
    (C) clozapine
    (D) vinblastine
    (E) clindamycin

175. Which of the following is (are) true of the use of Strattera?

    I. an amphetamine deriviative
    II. should not be used with an MAOI
    III. norepinephrine reuptake inhibitor

    (A) I only
    (B) III only
    (C) I and II only
    (D) II and III only
    (E) I, II, and III

176. Which of the following antimicrobial products are prodrugs?

    I. dirithromycin
    II. cefpodoxime proxetil
    III. clindamycin

    (A) I only
    (B) III only
    (C) I and II only
    (D) II and III only
    (E) I, II, and III

177. Levofloxacin is an example of a drug in which of the following categories?

    (A) monobactam
    (B) anthelmintic
    (C) aminoglycoside
    (D) macrolide
    (E) fluoroquinolone

178. Two hundred milligrams of penicillin G is equivalent to approximately how many units of penicillin G activity?

    (A) 480,000
    (B) 320,000
    (C) 1600
    (D) 270,000
    (E) 960,000

**179.** Which one of the following agents is most similar in action to cloxacillin?

(A) amoxicillin (Amoxil)
(B) bacampicillin (Spectrobid)
(C) penicillin V potassium (Pen Vee K)
(D) nafcillin (Unipen, Nallpen)
(E) ticarcillin (Ticar)

**180.** Which of the following agents is (are) classified as antiseptics or germicides?

I. benzalkonium chloride
II. chlorhexidine gluconate
III. glutaraldehyde

(A) I only
(B) III only
(C) I and II only
(D) II and III only
(E) I, II, and III

**181.** Which of the following is (are) true of valdecoxib (Bextra)?

I. COX-2 agonist
II. stimulates prostaglandin synthesis
III. indicated for treatment of osteoarthritis and rheumatoid arthritis

(A) I only
(B) III only
(C) I and II only
(D) II and III only
(E) I, II, and III

**182.** Which of the products listed below are vaccines?

I. fluzone
II. enerix-B
III. tripedia

(A) I only
(B) III only
(C) I and II only
(D) II and III only
(E) I, II, and III

**183.** Which of the following drugs are NOT used in treating migraine headaches?

I. naratriptan
II. methysergide
III. propofol

(A) I only
(B) III only
(C) I and II only
(D) II and III only
(E) I, II, and III

**184.** Which of the following morphine derivatives is most likely to cause dependence?

(A) diacetylmorphine
(B) ethylmorphine
(C) methylmorphine
(D) hydrocodone
(E) oxycodone

**185.** Sulfonamides exert their antimicrobial effect by competitively inhibiting the action of

(A) monoamine oxidase
(B) DNA polymerase
(C) pyrimidine
(D) serotonin
(E) *p*-aminobenzoic acid

# Answers and Explanations

1. **(B)** Dapsone is a sulfone that is bactericidal and bacteriostatic against *Mycobacterium leprae*, the organism believed to be the cause of leprosy (Hansen's disease). *(6)*

2. **(E)** Budesonide (Rhinocort) is a corticosteroid that is used intranasally either as a nasal inhaler or spray. Either may be used for the treatment of allergic rhinitis. Side effects may include epistaxis (nosebleed), cough, or nasal and throat irritation. *(10)*

3. **(B)** Atorvastatin (Lipitor) is an HMG-CoA reductase inhibitor used orally for the treatment of hyperlipidemia. By inhibiting this enzyme the drug interferes with an early step in cholesterol synthesis, thereby resulting in lowered LDL and triglyceride levels and an increase in HDL levels. Nicotinic acid (niacin) is also used to treat hyperlipidemia but appears to work by a different mechanism of action. *(10)*

4. **(E)** Torsemide (Demadex) is a loop diuretic that is similar in action to furosemide (Lasix), ethacrynic acid (Edecrin), and bumetanide (Bumex). Loop diuretics inhibit the reabsorption of sodium, chloride, and potassium ions in the ascending loop of Henle and may, therefore, cause hypokalemia and other electrolyte disturbances. They may also cause ototoxicity. All of these drugs are chemically related to the sulfonamides and may cause adverse reactions in patients who have a history of sulfonamide hypersensitivity. *(6)*

5. **(E)** Quetiapine (Seroquel) is an atypical antipsychotic drug that is chemically classified as a dibenzothiazepine. The only choice provided

that is also an antipsychotic drug is risperidone (Risperdal), another atypical antipsychotic agent. *(6)*

6. **(A)** Ticlopidine HCl (Ticlid) is an orally administered platelet aggregation inhibitor, which prolongs bleeding time. It acts by inhibiting ADP-induced platelet-fibrinogen binding and subsequent platelet-platelet adhesion. The effect on platelet function is irreversible for the life of the platelet. Ticlopidine is indicated for reducing risk of thrombotic stroke (fatal or nonfatal) in patients who have experienced stroke precursor symptoms and in patients who have had a completed thrombotic stroke. *(10)*

7. **(D)** Gabapentin (Neurontin) is an anticonvulsant that is structurally related to the neurotransmitter gamma-aminobutyric acid (GABA). It is indicated as an adjunct in the treatment of partial seizures in adults and for the management of postherpetic neuralgia. *(6)*

8. **(B)** The purpose of combining amoxicillin with clavulanate sodium (e.g., Augmentin) is to reduce the potential destruction of the amoxicillin by beta-lactamase enzymes. Clavulanate and similar agents such as sulbactam are, therefore, classified as beta-lactamase inhibitors. *(10)*

9. **(A)** Metformin is part of the chemical group known as the biguanides. These compounds are associated with the development of lactic acidosis. *(6)*

10. **(B)** Tocainide (Tonocard) is most similar to mexiletine (Mexitil). Both are classified as Group IB antiarrhythmic drugs. These are

agents that slightly depress phase 0 and may shorten the duration of the action potential. *(6)*

11. **(D)** Norgestimate is a progestin compound. While estrogens tend to work by preventing ovulation, progestins work primarily by increasing the viscosity of cervical mucous and by altering the endometrial lining (the inner lining of the uterus) to prevent implantation of a fertilized egg. *(6)*

12. **(D)** Clonidine is a central alpha-adrenergic stimulant. Its primary action is to stimulate alpha$_2$-adrenergic receptors to reduce sympathetic outflow from the CNS, thereby reducing peripheral vascular resistance and reducing heart rate and blood pressure. *(6)*

13. **(A)** Minoxidil is a direct-acting peripheral vasodilator. Because of its potential for producing a number of serious adverse effects, minoxidil is not a first-choice antihypertensive agent. Its ability to produce excess hair growth (hypertrichosis) has led to its topical use as the product Rogaine for the treatment of alopecia. *(10)*

14. **(E)** Bupropion (Wellbutrin), venlafaxine (Effexor), and citalopram (Celexa) are each antidepressants. *(6)*

15. **(C)** Calcium carbonate—containing antacids may cause flatulence because when carbonate comes in contact with the acid pH of the stomach, carbon dioxide gas is formed. *(6)*

16. **(D)** Clopidogrel (Plavix) and abciximab (ReoPro) are platelet aggregation inhibitors. Filgrastim (Neupogen) is a human granulocyte colony stimulating factor. *(6)*

17. **(D)** Carbidopa is a dopa-decarboxylase inhibitor that prevents peripheral decarboxylation of levodopa in the body. This reduces the adverse effects associated with peripheral dopa decarboxylation and reduces the dose of levodopa required to control a patient with Parkinson's disease. Carbidopa is available alone (Lodosyn) or in combination with levodopa (Sinemet). *(6)*

18. **(A)** Selegeline (Eldepryl) is an MAO-B inhibitor that is used in the adjunctive treatment of Parkinson's disease. *(10)*

19. **(C)** Fentanyl is a potent narcotic agonist analgesic used IM or IV to promote analgesia during anesthesia. It is also available in a transmucosal (Fentanyl Oralet, Actiq) and transdermal (Duragesic) dosage form. *(6)*

20. **(A)** Lactase enzyme is effective in treating symptoms of lactose intolerance. These symptoms are most evident shortly after consuming a lactose-containing food and may include bloating and diarrhea. Lactase enzyme is available as a liquid (LactAid), caplets (LactAid), capsules (Lactrase), or as chewable tablets (Dairy Ease). It is also added to some commercial dairy products. *(6)*

21. **(E)** Hyponatremia is not a problem commonly associated with the use of isotretinoin (Accutane). Cheilitis (cracked margins of the lips), conjunctivitis, and dry mouth occur in a large proportion of patients receiving this drug. Hypertriglyceridemia and pseudotumor cerebri have also been reported. Isotretinoin is classified in pregnancy category X and will, therefore, potentially cause fetal abnormalities. *(6)*

22. **(A)** Valsartan (Diovan) is an angiotensin II-receptor blocker. It should not be administered to women during the second and third trimester of pregnancy because of the potential for fetal harm during that period. This drug may be combined with a diuretic such as hydrochlorothiazide in order to potentiate its antihypertensive effect. *(10)*

23. **(C)** Endorphins are endogenous (naturally found in the body) opioid peptides that are released in response to stress. *(6)*

24. **(B)** Crack is a free-base form of cocaine. It is generally smoked and rapidly absorbed through the respiratory membranes. Within seconds, it reaches the brain and produces central nervous system stimulation and euphoria. Dependence may occur with only a single dose of the drug. *(6)*

25. **(A)** A uricosuric drug is one that promotes the excretion of uric acid in the urine. Uricosuric agents such as probenecid (Benemid) and sulfinpyrazone (Anturane) inhibit tubular reabsorption of urate and promote urate excretion. They are used to treat hyperuricemia associated with gout or gouty arthritis. *(6)*

26. **(B)** Reteplase (Retavase) is a plasminogen activator produced by recombinant DNA technology. It is used in the management of acute myocardial infarction. Once injected into the circulation, reteplase catalyzes the conversion of plasminogen to plasmin. Plasmin then produces local fibrinolysis and assists in reopening a blocked blood vessel. *(10)*

27. **(D)** Cimetidine (Tagamet) is an $H_2$-histamine receptor antagonist used to decrease gastric acid secretion in patients with peptic ulcer disease. It has been shown to inhibit the hepatic metabolism of drugs metabolized via the cytochrome P450 pathway, thereby delaying metabolism and increasing serum levels. Cimetidine may affect the metabolism of drugs such as theophylline, some benzodiazepines, phenytoin, and warfarin. *(6)*

28. **(B)** Allopurinol (Zyloprim) is a xanthine oxidase inhibitor that does not exert a uricosuric effect but does prevent the conversion of hypoxanthine to uric acid. It is employed in the treatment of gout as well as in the management of patients receiving therapy for leukemia and other malignancies that increase uric acid formation. *(6)*

29. **(C)** Dihydrotachysterol is a synthetic product of tachysterol, a substance similar to vitamin D. It is used in combination with calcium supplements in the treatment of hypoparathyroidism. *(6)*

30. **(E)** Colestipol (Colestid) binds bile acids in the intestine, thereby reducing fat absorption. Nicotinic acid (niacin, Niaspan) also reduces cholesterol, LDL and triglyceride levels and raises HDL levels. Psyllium (Metamucil) is a soluble fiber product that prevents the absorption of fats and also reduces lipid levels. *(6)*

31. **(A)** Acarbose (Precose) and miglitol (Glyset) are both alpha-glucosidase inhibitors. Since they act to reduce the GI absorption of carbohydrates, they are best taken three times a day with the first bite of each main meal. *(6)*

32. **(E)** Xenical (Orlistat) is a lipase inhibitor that reduces the amount of dietary fat that is absorbed from the GI tract by binding some of the gut lipase. If the use of this drug is accompanied by a reduction in fat intake, the combination can result in weight loss. Consumption of high amounts of dietary fat while taking this drug may cause diarrhea and other adverse GI effects. *(10)*

33. **(B)** Amiodarone (Cordarone) is an antiarrhythmic agent used in treating ventricular arrhythmias. It may cause a number of serious adverse effects, the most serious being pulmonary toxicity. Baseline chest x rays and pulmonary function studies should be performed before therapy begins. Studies should be repeated at three- to six-month intervals. *(10)*

34. **(D)** Methadone (Dolophine) is a narcotic agonist analgesic with actions similar to those of morphine. It is twice as potent when used parenterally as when used orally. It is employed in the treatment of severe pain and in maintenance treatment of narcotic addiction. *(10)*

35. **(B)** A pure narcotic antagonist is one that reverses the effects of opioids without producing agonist action of its own. Naltrexone (ReVia) is an example of a pure narcotic antagonist. Other drugs listed have agonist and some antagonist activity. *(6)*

36. **(C)** Tegaserod (Zelnorm) is the first of a new class of agents that work as $5HT_4$-receptor agonists. These agents tend to increase the motility of the GI tract, increase intestinal secretions, and inhibit sensitivity of the GI lining. This drug is specifically indicated for the treatment of irritable bowel syndrome (IBS) in women whose primary IBS bowel symptom is constipation. *(10)*

37. **(D)** Constipation is a common effect because morphine decreases peristaltic activity in the GI tract. Constriction of the pupils, CNS and respiratory depression, and nausea and vomiting are also effects associated with morphine use. *(6)*

38. **(C)** Primidone (Mysoline) is an anticonvulsant drug used in grand mal, psychomotor, and focal epileptic seizures. Primidone as well as its two active metabolites, phenobarbital and phenylethylmalonamide (PEMA), have anticonvulsant activity. *(10)*

39. **(A)** Tiludronate (Skelid) is an agent used in treating Paget's disease of the bone, a condition characterized by abnormal bone resorption and the development of fractures. The use of the drug seems to decrease the dissolution of hydroxyapatite crystals, the building blocks of bone tissue. *(6)*

40. **(E)** Repaglinide (Prandin) acts by stimulating the release of insulin from the pancreas. *(6)*

41. **(D)** The naturally occurring adrenal cortical steroids exert both salt-retaining (mineralocorticoid) and anti-inflammatory (glucocorticoid) activity. The synthetic steroids prednisone and prednisolone exert similar actions on the body. The use of these agents is often associated with fluid and sodium retention. Crohn's disease and rheumatic disorders are generally characterized by an inflammatory component and will, therefore, often respond to anti-inflammatory drug therapy. *(6)*

42. **(A)** Concerta would be a better choice because it is a sustained-release form of methylphenidate, the active ingredient in Ritalin. The use of a single dose of Concerta in the morning, before leaving for school, would provide action throughout the school day and diminish the need for an additional dose during school hours. *(10)*

43. **(E)** Sibutramine (Meridia), mazindol (Sanorex, Mazanor) and benzphetamine (Didrex) are central nervous system stimulants used as anorexiants, i.e., they are used to reduce appetite. *(6)*

44. **(B)** Colesevelam (Welchol) is an anion exchange resin that binds bile acids, particularly glycocholic acid, the major bile acid in humans. The drug binds bile acids in the intestine, causing them to be removed in the feces. This causes further breakdown of cholesterol to bile acids, as well as a decrease in low-density lipoproteins (LDL) and serum cholesterol levels. *(10)*

45. **(C)** Epoetin-alpha is a glycoprotein that is manufactured using recombinant DNA technology. It is similar to the glycoprotein erythropoietin produced by the kidney. Both of these compounds act to stimulate red blood cell production, thereby raising the level of RBCs as well as hematocrit (proportional to the volume of red blood cells in whole blood). Red blood cell production tends to diminish in patients with chronic renal failure (because of the reduction in erythropoietin production) and in patients who are HIV positive and those who are undergoing cancer chemotherapy. After administration of epoetin-alpha by SC or IV routes, it normally takes two to six weeks to see a significant clinical change in red blood cell production. *(6)*

46. **(B)** Benzodiazepines are believed to act by potentiating the effects of gamma-aminobutyric acid (GABA), an inhibitory amino acid in the CNS. Some benzodiazepines are also used for the treatment of muscle spasms and convulsive disorders. *(6)*

47. **(E)** Entacapone (Comtan) is a reversible inhibitor of catechol-O-methyltransferase (COMT) used as an adjunct to levodopa/carbidopa in the treatment of Parkinson's disease. When used with a combination of levodopa and carbidopa (e.g., Sinemet) entacapone increases the AUC of levodopa by about 35% and the elimination half-life of levodopa is almost doubled. Entacapone has no significant anti-Parkinson effects when used alone. Entacapone should not be used with nonspecific MAO inhibitors, such as tranylcypromine or phenelzine, but may be used with selective MAO-B inhibitors such as selegiline. *(6)*

48. **(A)** Docosanol (Abreva) is a topically applied antiviral medication used to treat cold sore

infections caused by the herpes simplex virus. Docosanol acts by shortening the healing time, and the length-of-time symptoms are present. *(10)*

49. **(B)** Onychomycosis is a fungal infection that causes fingers or toenails to become thickened, discolored, disfigured, and/or split. Terbinafine (Lamisil) is an antifungal compound that is administered orally. Its antifungal action is believed to be the result of its ability to inhibit a key enzyme needed in the sterol synthesis of fungi. Gentamicin and amikacin are aminoglycoside antimicrobial agents that only have antibacterial action. *(10)*

50. **(D)** Bitolterol (Tornalate) and pirbuterol (Maxair) are rapidly-acting selective beta$_2$-agonist bronchodilators. Because of their rapid action, their use is suitable for the treatment of acute asthma attacks as well as for the prevention of attacks. Salmeterol (Serevent) is also a selective beta$_2$-agonist; however, it has a relatively slower onset and longer duration of action. Salmeterol would, therefore, not be appropriate to use in treating an acute asthma attack but would be useful in the prevention of asthma attacks. *(6)*

51. **(C)** Dronabinol (Marinol) is a marijuana derivative and granisetron (Zofran) is a selective serotonin receptor antagonist used for the prevention of nausea and vomiting associated with cancer chemotherapy. Zoledronic acid (Zometa) is indicated for the treatment of hypercalcemia in malignancy. *(10)*

52. **(A)** Amrinone (Inocor), like digoxin, is a drug that produces a positive inotropic effect. In addition, amrinone also produces vasodilation. The drug is used for the short-term management of congestive heart failure in patients who have not responded adequately to digoxin, diuretics, or vasodilators. Use of the drug has been associated with the development of thrombocytopenia, arrhythmias, and GI upset. It is administered by IV bolus or infusion. *(10)*

53. **(A)** Butenafine (Mentax, Lotrimin Ultra) is an antifungal drug useful in the topical treatment of superficial dermatophyte infections, including tinea pedis (athlete's foot), tinea corporis (ringworm), and tinea cruris (jock itch). It should be stored at controlled room temperature. *(10)*

54. **(C)** Lactulose (Cephulac, Chronulac), a synthetic disaccharide, is an analog of lactose. Unlike lactose, which is hydrolyzed enzymatically to its monosaccharide components, oral doses of lactulose pass to the colon virtually unchanged. In the colon, bacteria chemically convert the lactulose to low-molecular-weight acids and carbon dioxide. The acids produce an osmotic effect that draws water into the colon and makes the stools more watery. They also permit ammonia in the body to be converted to ammonium ion in the acidic colon and allow it to be eliminated in the stool. *(6)*

55. **(E)** Milk of magnesia contains magnesium hydroxide as its active ingredient. This acts osmotically to produce a laxative effect. Castor oil, senna, and bisacodyl contain stimulant laxatives while docusate sodium is a surfactant stool softener. *(6)*

56. **(A)** Liothyronine sodium (Cytomel) is a synthetic form of the natural thyroid hormone T3. Approximately 25 µg of liothyronine sodium is equivalent to 100 µg of levothyroxine sodium (T4). *(6)*

57. **(B)** Aluminum hydroxide reacts with phosphate ion in the intestine to form insoluble aluminum phosphate, which is eliminated in the feces. This may be of value in treating hyperphosphatemia in chronic renal failure. *(6)*

58. **(E)** Mesalamine (Asacol) or 5-aminosalicylic acid (5-ASA) is a break down product of sulfasalazine that is believed to be useful in treating chronic ulcerative colitis. *(6)*

59. **(D)** Ibuprofen (Motrin) and oxaprozin (Daypro) are nonsteroidal anti-inflammatory agents (NSAID) and should be avoided in patients who are sensitive to aspirin because of possible cross-sensitivity reactions. *(6)*

60. **(A)** Single aspirin doses are known to inhibit platelet aggregation. This is believed to occur by the acetylation of platelet cyclooxygenase by aspirin. This, in turn, prevents the synthesis of thromboxane A2, a prostaglandin that is a potent vasoconstrictor and an inducer of platelet aggregation. *(6)*

61. **(E)** Both triamterene (Dyrenium) and spironolactone (Aldactone) inhibit sodium reabsorption in the distal tubule. Spironolactone is an aldosterone antagonist that prevents the formation of a protein important for sodium transport in the distal tubule. Triamterene inhibits sodium reabsorption induced by aldosterone and inhibits basal sodium reabsorption. Triamterene is not an aldosterone antagonist. *(6)*

62. **(B)** Labetalol (Normodyne, Trandate) is a nonselective beta-adrenergic blocking agent primarily used for the management of hypertension. In addition to its beta-blocking action, labetalol is also able to block alpha$_1$-adrenergic receptors. This lowers standing blood pressure and may result in hypotension and syncope. *(10)*

63. **(D)** NSAIDs reduce the inflammation caused by deposits of uric acid crystals seen in gout but have no effect on the amount of uric acid in the body. The NSAIDs most commonly prescribed for gout are Indomethacin (Indocin) and naproxen (Anaprox, Naprosyn), which are taken orally every day. *(6)*

64. **(C)** Oxymetazoline (Afrin, Duration) and xylometazoline (Otrivin), when used as topical nasal decongestants, produce an effect that may persist for 8 to 12 h. This is in sharp contrast to other topical nasal decongestant drugs such as phenylephrine, naphazoline, and tetrahydrozoline, which require dosing at 3- to 4-h intervals. *(6)*

65. **(A)** The use of gold compounds such as auranofin (Ridaura), gold sodium thiomalate (Myochrysine), and aurothioglucose (Solganal), while effective in many patients with rheumatoid arthritis, have been associated with a wide variety of adverse effects, including blood dyscrasias, dermatitis, and renal disorders. Patients using such compounds must be monitored constantly for adverse effects. *(6)*

66. **(C)** Glucagon is a polypeptide secreted by the pancreas. It acts to enhance gluconeogenesis and glycogenolysis, thereby causing higher levels of glucose in the blood. Glucagon is used to treat severe hypoglycemia. It is generally administered intramuscularly or intravenously. Diazoxide for parenteral use (Hyperstat) is used to reduce blood pressure in cases of hypertensive emergency. When given orally, diazoxide (Proglycem) tends to increase blood glucose levels by decreasing insulin release in the pancreas. Repaglinide (Prandin) is an oral antidiabetic agent that reduces blood sugar levels. *(6)*

67. **(C)** Iron is primarily absorbed in the duodenum and the jejunum by an active transport mechanism. The ferrous salt form is absorbed approximately three times more readily than the ferric form. The presence of food, particularly dairy products, eggs, coffee, and tea, in the GI tract may decrease the absorption of iron significantly, although the concurrent administration of vitamin C maintains iron in the ferrous state, thereby enhancing its absorption from the GI tract. *(6)*

68. **(C)** Iron is an essential component of hemoglobin, myoglobin, and several enzymes. Approximately two-thirds of total body iron is in the circulating red blood cells as part of hemoglobin, the most important carrier of oxygen in the body. *(6)*

69. **(D)** The development of tolerance to the action of nitroglycerin and other organic nitrates may occur with repeated use or with the use of sustained-release products. Sensitivity to the action of nitroglycerin is generally restored after several hours of withdrawal from the drug. *(6)*

70. **(B)** Regular insulin is secreted by the beta cells of the pancreas. In its unmodified form, regular insulin is clear, has a short (0.5 to 1 h) onset of action, and a relatively short (6 to 8 h) duration of action. Lispro insulin solution has a

more rapid onset and shorter duration of action than regular insulin. Because regular insulin is a clear product, it can be administered either SC or IV. *(6)*

71. **(A)** Sotalol (Betapace) is a selective beta-adrenergic blocking agent used for the treatment of life-threatening ventricular arrhythmias. As is the case with all other beta-adrenergic blockers, sotalol should not be used in patients with a history of bronchospastic disease. *(10)*

72. **(B)** Ipratropium bromide (Atrovent) is an anticholinergic compound that produces a bronchodilator effect when administered by inhalation. It is used either alone or with beta-adrenergic compounds to treat bronchospasm associated with COPD. Because of its anticholinergic effect, it can be expected to produce dry mouth in some patients. *(10)*

73. **(C)** Dobutamine (Dobutrex) is a parenterally administered agent that is chemically related to dopamine. It acts by stimulating primarily beta$_1$-adrenergic receptors to produce an inotropic effect. It is commonly employed in the treatment of shock syndrome. Unlike dopamine, dobutamine does not cause the endogenous release of norepinephrine. *(10)*

74. **(B)** Procyclidine (Kemadrin) is an anticholinergic drug used to treat Parkinson's disease. Ropinirole (Requip) and pergolide (Permax) are dopaminergic agents that enhance dopamine activity and provide palliative treatment of Parkinson's disease. *(10)*

75. **(A)** Budesonide (Pulmicort) is an anti-inflammatory corticosteroid that is useful in the prevention of asthma attacks. It probably works by inhibiting mast cells and mediators such as histamine, leukotrienes, and cytokines involved in allergic and nonallergic causes of asthma attacks. *(10)*

76. **(C)** Loratadine (Claritin) and fexofenadine (Allegra) are histamine H$_1$-receptor antagonists used for the treatment of seasonal allergic rhinitis. Unlike older H$_1$-receptor antagonists such as chlorpheniramine or diphenhydramine, these drugs tend to be less sedating and are better tolerated. Nizatidine (Axid) is an H$_2$-receptor antagonist, particularly at the parietal cells, which is used in the maintenance treatment of duodenal ulcer. *(10)*

77. **(B)** Metoclopramide (Reglan) is a prokinetic agent, i.e. it stimulates the motility of the upper GI tract, thereby increasing duodenal and jejunal peristalsis as well as the rate of stomach emptying. It is used for the short-term treatment of gastroesophageal reflux and for the treatment of diabetic gastroparesis. It may also be useful in controlling nausea and vomiting in postoperative patients and in those receiving emetogenic cancer chemotherapy. *(10)*

78. **(D)** Upon inhaling the smoke of cannabis (marijuana) perceptual changes, vascular congestion of the eye, and increased heart rate generally occur. These effects generally continue for about 1 to 2 h after smoke inhalation; however, one of cannabis' active components, tetra-hydrocannabinol (THC), may remain in the body for as long as 10 days. *(10)*

79. **(D)** Betamethasone is about 25 times as potent as hydrocortisone, five to six times as potent as prednisone, four to six times as potent as triamcinolone, and about 30 times as potent as cortisone. *(6)*

80. **(A)** Tretinoin (Retin-A) is a derivative of vitamin A. It is used in the treatment of mild to moderate acne. It is believed that tretinoin acts by irritating the skin and causing the skin cells in the area to which it is applied to turn over more rapidly. This causes removal of comedones and prevents their reoccurrence. Tretinoin has also been used to treat sun-damaged skin and to reduce the signs of aging on the skin. *(10)*

81. **(E)** Infliximab (Remicade) is a monoclonal antibody produced by recombinant technology. It acts by inhibiting the binding of Tumor Necrosis Factor (specifically TNF$_\alpha$) to its receptor sites, thereby reducing inflammation within the colon. It is administered intravenously as a

single dose in the treatment of moderate to severe Crohn's disease. *(10)*

82. **(D)** Simvastatin (Zocor) is a cholesterol-lowering agent in the "statin" group of drugs. It is contraindicated for use during pregnancy because of its great potential for causing fetal harm. The drug is in FDA pregnancy category X. Its use is also contraindicated in active liver disease because of its potential for elevating liver enzyme concentrations. *(6)*

83. **(C)** Transdermal dosage forms are generally formulated from potent, low-dose drugs that will easily pass through the skin. Fentanyl (Duragesic), a potent opioid analgesic, is available in a transdermal form that has a duration of action of about 72 h. Clonidine (Catapres TTS) is a transdermal product which exerts a centrally-acting alpha$_2$-adrenergic agonist action that will provide an antihypertensive effect that will have about a one-week duration. *(10)*

84. **(C)** Desmopressin acetate is the synthetic analog of naturally occurring human antidiuretic hormone (ADH) produced by the posterior pituitary gland. It is administered intranasally (Stimate) or orally (DDA VP) for the treatment of primary nocturnal enuresis. A single dose of the drug will produce an antidiuretic effect lasting from 8 to 20 h. *(6)*

85. **(A)** Citalopram (Celexa) is classified as an SSRI. Venlafaxine (Effexor) and Nefazodone (Serzone) are not SSRIs or tricyclic antidepressants. They act to inhibit neuronal uptake of serotonin and norepinephrine. *(6)*

86. **(A)** Dicloxacillin (Dynapen, Pathocil) is a beta-lactamase–resistant penicillin and would be suitable for treating an infection caused by beta-lactamase–producing staphylococci. Other penicillins that would also be suitable include oxacillin (Prostaphlin, Bactocill), cloxacillin (Cloxapen, Tegopen) and nafcillin (Nafcil, Unipen). All of these products are available for oral use. *(6)*

87. **(D)** Cyanocobalamin, or vitamin B$_{12}$, is essential for proper growth, cell reproduction, formation of blood components, and many other functions. In order for cyanocobalamin to be absorbed properly from the GI tract, it must combine with a glycoprotein called intrinsic factor. In the absence of proper levels of intrinsic factor, cyanocobalamin is administered parenterally or intranasally. *(6)*

88. **(A)** Minoxidil (Loniten) is an antihypertensive drug that can produce excessive hair growth or hirsutism. Recognition of this fact resulted in the marketing of a topical form of minoxidil (Rogaine). *(10)*

89. **(E)** Latanoprost (Xalatan) is a prostaglandin F$_{2a}$ analog that reduces intraocular pressure by increasing the outflow of aqueous humor. *(6)*

90. **(B)** Levobetaxolol (Betaxon) is a beta-adrenergic blocking agent used ophthalmically to reduce intraocular pressure, particularly, in patients with chronic open-angle glaucoma. Levobetaxolol and betaxolol are ophthalmic beta-blockers that are more specific for beta$_1$-adrenergic receptors than for beta$_2$-receptors, making them less likely to affect respiratory function. *(6)*

91. **(A)** Pilocarpine (Isopto Carpine, Pilostat) is a direct-acting miotic agent used to decrease elevated intraocular pressure. By causing miosis (constriction of the pupil), greater outflow of aqueous humor is promoted and intraocular pressure falls. Dorzolamide (Trusopt) acts by inhibiting the action of carbonic anhydrase. *(10)*

92. **(D)** Nizatidine (Axid) and other histamine H$_2$-receptor antagonists competitively block H$_2$-receptor sites, particularly those found in gastric parietal cells. These agents do not block histamine release, antibody production, or antigen–antibody reactions and they do not bind histamine. *(6)*

93. **(B)** Haloperidol (Haldol) is an antipsychotic agent available in oral and parenteral forms. It has pharmacological actions similar to the phenothiazines (sedation, extrapyramidal effects,

etc.). Chemically, haloperidol is a butyrophenone. *(10)*

94. **(D)** Tamoxifen (Nolvadex) is an agent that has potent antiestrogenic effects because of its ability to compete with estrogen for binding sites in target tissues such as the breast. It is used in the treatment of metastatic breast cancer in women, particularly in patients with tumors that are estrogen-receptor–positive. It is also used to reduce the incidence of breast cancer in high-risk women. *(6)*

95. **(A)** Permethrin (Nix, Elimite) is a topical scabicide and pediculocide. It acts by disrupting the nerve cell membranes of parasites, resulting in their paralysis. *(6)*

96. **(E)** Acetaminophen (Tylenol, APAP) is an agent with analgesic and antipyretic actions similar to aspirin. Unlike aspirin, acetaminophen does not significantly inhibit peripheral prostaglandin synthesis, which may account for its relative lack of anti-inflammatory activity. Acetaminophen does not inhibit platelet function, affect prothrombin time, or produce GI distress. *(6)*

97. **(D)** Clozapine (Clozaril) is an antipsychotic agent indicated for use in patients who do not respond to standard antipsychotic therapy (phenothiazines, etc.). Use of clozapine has been associated with the development of agranulocytosis, a potentially life-threatening blood disorder. Patients being treated with clozapine must have a baseline white blood cell (WBC) and differential count performed before initiation of treatment as well as a WBC count every week during treatment and for four weeks after discontinuing therapy. *(10)*

98. **(B)** Didanosine (Videx) is a nucleoside reverse transcriptase inhibitor that is active against the human immunodeficiency virus (HIV). Its use has been associated with the development of peripheral neuropathy and pancreatitis. *(6)*

99. **(A)** Bleomycin (Blenoxane) is an antineoplastic drug in the antibiotic group. The most serious adverse effect associated with this drug is

pulmonary fibrosis and about 10% of patients on this drug experience some form of pulmonary toxicity. *(10)*

100. **(A)** The anti-inflammatory and analgesic action of NSAIDS is believed to result from inhibition of prostaglandin synthesis. *(6)*

101. **(B)** Doxazosin (Cardura) is an alpha1-adrenergic blocking agent used in the treatment of hypertension. By causing dilation of arterioles and veins, the drug causes the lowering of both supine and standing blood pressures. The "first-dose" effect is the development of marked hypotension and syncope (fainting) on administration of the first few doses of the drug. Administering low initial doses of the drug at bedtime can minimize this effect. Dosage may be increased gradually until the drug is better tolerated. *(6)*

102. **(E)** Carbon monoxide is a colorless and odorless product of the incomplete combustion of hydrocarbons. When it is inhaled and carried to the blood, it reacts with hemoglobin to form carboxyhemoglobin. This reaction dramatically reduces the oxygen-carrying capacity of the blood and, unless corrected quickly, results in the death of the individual. *(6)*

103. **(C)** Aspiration of a liquid hydrocarbon, such as gasoline or kerosene, may result in severe inflammation of pulmonary tissues, interference with gas exchange, pneumonitis, and possible death. Emesis or gastric lavage is avoided in such patients to avoid aspiration. Catharsis using magnesium or sodium sulfate may be attempted. Supportive therapy is generally recommended for such patients. *(6)*

104. **(D)** Deferoxamine mesylate (Desferal) is a chelating agent that has a high affinity for ferric iron and a relatively low affinity for calcium. It is usually administered parenterally in the treatment of acute iron poisoning. *(10)*

105. **(B)** Dorzolamide (Trusopt) is a carbonic anhydrase inhibitor used clinically in the treatment of chronic open-angle glaucoma. Systemically used carbonic anhydrase inhibitors increase

the excretion of sodium, potassium, bicarbonate, and water, and may cause the alkalinization of the urine. *(6)*

106. **(B)** Thiazide diuretics such as hydrochlorothiazide (Esidrix, HydroDIURIL) increase the renal excretion of sodium, chloride, and potassium while decreasing the excretion of calcium and uric acid. These drugs compete with uric acid for secretion in the kidney. *(6)*

107. **(B)** Potassium citrate (Urocit-K) and sodium bicarbonate are urinary alkalinizers. Ammonium chloride and ascorbic acid are urinary acidifiers. *(6)*

108. **(D)** Cyclophosphamide (Cytoxan) is an alkylating agent related to the nitrogen mustards. Patients using this agent should be advised to take the drug on an empty stomach. Since hemorrhagic cystitis may occur with the use of this drug, patients should be advised to drink lots of fluids. *(6)*

109. **(E)** All of these drugs are aldehyde dehydrogenase inhibitors. They cause intolerance to alcohol so that consumption of even a small amount may produce a broad array of unpleasant effects. These include flushing, throbbing headaches, nausea, sweating, and palpitations. Disulfiram is used in the management of selected chronic alcoholics. The drug should only be used with the full knowledge and understanding of the patient. *(6)*

110. **(C)** Phenylzine (Nardil) and selegeline (Eldepryl) are MAO inhibitors. Patients using them should avoid tyramine-containing foods as well as most cold and allergy products. *(6)*

111. **(A)** Polycarbophil (Mitrolan, Equalactin) is a synthetic hydrophilic compound that is capable of absorbing large amounts of water. It is indicated for use as a bulk laxative in the treatment of constipation. It is also employed in the treatment of diarrhea, in which it absorbs excess free fecal water and helps create formed stools. *(10)*

112. **(B)** Montelukast sodium (Singulair) is a leukotriene receptor antagonist. Since leukotrienes are associated with causing asthmatic symptoms, the use of such drugs reduces the likelihood of asthma attacks. They are, therefore, used to prevent attacks, not to treat an acute attack. *(6)*

113. **(A)** Diazoxide (Hyperstat) is a nondiuretic antihypertensive agent structurally related to the thiazides. It is used in the emergency reduction of elevated blood pressure. Because diazoxide is rapidly and extensively bound to serum protein, it must be administered by rapid IV injection (bolus). Repeated administration of the drug may cause sodium and water retention and the need for adjuvant diuretic therapy. An oral form of diazoxide (Proglycem) is used in the management of hypoglycemia. *(6)*

114. **(B)** Miconazole (Micatin, Monistat) is a broad-spectrum antifungal agent effective against yeast infections (*Candida albicans*) as well as dermatophyte infections (*tinea cruris, tinea corporis*). Ciclopirox (Penlac) is primarily used for the topical treatment of onychomycosis and caspofungin (Cancidas) is indicated only for the treatment of invasive aspergillosis. *(10)*

115. **(A)** Mafenide (Sulfamylon) is a bacteriostatic agent that is active against many gram-positive and gram-negative organisms. Topical products containing mafenide are applied to second and third degree burns in order to reduce the chance of infection and increase the speed of healing. *(6)*

116. **(B)** Lypressin (Diapid) is a synthetic vasopressin analog, possessing antidiuretic activity without producing a pressor or oxytocic effect. It is used clinically in the management of symptoms of diabetes insipidus. Lypressin is administered as a nasal spray. *(6)*

117. **(C)** Sotalol (Betapace) and amiodarone (Cordarone) are both Group III antiarrhythmic agents. This means that they both act to prolong the repolarization phase (phase 3). *(6)*

118. **(D)** Pioglitazone (Actos) appears to reduce blood glucose levels by increasing the target cell response to insulin. Because its mechanism is different from the sulfonylureas or metformin, pioglitazone may be used in combination with these other drugs to control blood glucose levels. *(10)*

119. **(C)** Finasteride (Propecia, Proscar) is an androgen hormone inhibitor used to treat benign prostatic hyperplasia (BPH) as well as male pattern hair loss (alopecia). *(6)*

120. **(D)** Vidarabine (Vira-A) is an antiviral agent that possesses activity against herpes simplex virus. It is administered by slow IV infusion for the treatment of herpes simplex encephalitis and is used ophthalmically for the treatment of herpes simplex infections of the eye. *(6)*

121. **(E)** Tazobactam sodium is a broad spectrum beta-lactamase inhibitor. It is used in combination with penicillins such as piperacillin sodium in order to enhance the activity of the penicillin to include the treatment of infection caused by beta-lactamase–producing organisms. *(6)*

122. **(B)** Oxytocin is an endogenous hormone produced by the posterior pituitary gland. It is a uterine stimulant that promotes uterine contractions, particularly during labor. The other hormones listed are released by the anterior pituitary gland. *(6)*

123. **(C)** During the menstrual cycle, levels of follicle-stimulating hormone (FSH) and luteinizing hormone (LH) vary widely. At the time of ovulation, the plasma concentration of each of these hormones reaches a peak, coinciding with the release of the ovum and the complete development of a mature endometrial wall. The plasma level of progesterone generally reaches a peak much later in the menstrual cycle. *(6)*

124. **(D)** Liotrix consists of a uniform mixture of synthetic levothyroxine sodium (T4) and liothyronine sodium (T3) in a ratio of 4:1 by weight. It is used in products such as Euthroid and Thyrolar as a thyroid hormone supplement. *(10)*

125. **(C)** Propylthiouracil and methimazole (Tapazole) are antithyroid agents that inhibit the synthesis of thyroid hormone and are, therefore, useful in the treatment of hyperthyroidism. *(6)*

126. **(D)** Most antipsychotic agents are believed to act by antagonizing dopamine receptors. They may also cause some blockade of cholinergic, alpha$_1$-adrenergic, and histamine receptors. *(6)*

127. **(C)** Tiagabine (Gabitril) and topiramate (Topamax) are anticonvulsants primarily utilized for the treatment of partial seizures. *(6)*

128. **(E)** Buspirone (Buspar) is an antianxiety agent that, unlike the benzodiazepines, barbiturates, and carbamates, does not produce significant sedative, muscle relaxant, or anticonvulsant effects. *(6)*

129. **(A)** Nelfinavir (Viracept) is the only protease inhibitor. Cidofovir is an inhibitor of DNA polymerase that is used for the treatment of CMV retinitis. Acyclovir (Zovirax) also acts by interfering with DNA polymerase and is used for the treatment of herpes simplex and herpes zoster infections. *(6)*

130. **(E)** All of these are aminopenicillins. They are easily recognized by the "...am..." in their name. *(6)*

131. **(B)** Dalteparin sodium (Fragmin) is a low molecular weight heparin derivative most commonly used in preventing deep vein thrombosis. *(6)*

132. **(A)** Oseltamivir (Tamiflu) is an antiviral compound that is used to treat illness caused by influenza in patients one year or older. It is only effective if used within two days of the outbreak of symptoms. *(10)*

133. **(D)** Alteplase (Activase) is a tissue plasminogen activator produced by recombinant DNA technology. It is used intravenously in the

management of acute myocardial infarction (AMI) patients in order to lyse thrombi-obstructing coronary arteries. It is administered as soon as possible after the onset of AMI. *(6)*

134. **(A)** Dyphylline is a theophylline derivative. These agents act by inhibiting the enzyme phosphodiesterase, thereby increasing cyclic-AMP levels and producing bronchodilation. Salmeterol is a beta$_2$-adrenergic agonist, and nedocromil sodium is an agent that inhibits mediator release from a variety of inflammatory cell types including mast cells. *(10)*

135. **(B)** Valdecoxib (Bextra) and oxaprozin (Daypro) are both nonsteroidal anti-inflammatory drugs (NSAIDs). Valdecoxib is a COX-2 inhibitor while oxaprozin is a COX-1 inhibitor. It is believed that COX-2 inhibitors may produce less GI upset than COX-1 inhibitors. *(6)*

136. **(B)** Zaleplon (Sonata) is a short-acting hypnotic agent that has a terminal half-life of approximately one hour. It is particularly useful for decreasing the time to sleep onset. It is not useful for prolonging total sleep time or for decreasing the number of awakenings. *(10)*

137. **(B)** Verapamil (Calan, Isoptin) is a calcium channel–blocking agent used orally and parenterally in the treatment of cardiac arrhythmias. The other calcium channel–blocking agents listed are used in the treatment of angina pectoris and/or essential hypertension. Oral verapamil is also used for these indications. *(10)*

138. **(C)** Cefixime (Suprax) is a third-generation cephalosporin. Third-generation cephalosporins generally have greater gram-negative activity, less gram-positive activity, greater efficacy against resistant organisms, and higher cost than cephalosporins in first- or second-generation groups. *(6)*

139. **(A)** Reflex tachycardia is commonly seen with the use of peripheral vasodilators such as minoxidil (Loniten) and hydralazine (Apresoline). The drop in blood pressure produced by the use of these agents causes

increased renin secretion, heart rate, and output as well as sodium and water retention. This may worsen both angina and congestive heart failure. These adverse effects observed with the use of peripheral vasodilators may be managed by the concurrent administration of a beta-adrenergic blocking agent and/or a diuretic. *(6)*

140. **(C)** Buprenorphine (Buprenex) is an opioid narcotic agonist-antagonist. As an analgesic, it is about 30 times as potent as morphine. It is administered intramuscularly or intravenously for the relief of moderate to severe pain and in the treatment of narcotic dependence. *(6)*

141. **(E)** Mestranol is an estrogen commonly employed in several oral contraceptive products (e.g., Norinyl, Ortho-Novum). *(6)*

142. **(E)** Propranolol (Inderal) is a nonspecific beta-adrenergic blocking agent that exhibits a high degree of lipid solubility. As a result, it is more likely than other beta-blockers to enter the CNS and produce CNS-adverse effects. *(6)*

143. **(D)** Danazol (Danocrine) is a synthetic compound that suppresses the pituitary-ovarian axis by inhibiting the production of pituitary gonadotropins. It is used clinically in the treatment of endometriosis, in which it causes the normal and ectopic endometrial tissue to become inactive and atrophic. Danazol is also employed in the prevention of attacks related to hereditary angioedema. *(10)*

144. **(A)** Torsemide (Demadex) and bumetanide (Bumex) are both loop diuretics. *(6)*

145. **(B)** Amiloride (Midamor) is one of the three potassium-sparing diuretics currently on the market. The others include spironolactone (Aldactone) and triamterene (Dyrenium). These drugs are primarily used to enhance the action and counteract the potassium-depleting effect of thiazides and loop diuretics. *(6)*

146. **(D)** Valacyclovir (Valtrex) is an antiviral agent used in the treatment of shingles, a painful disorder caused by the herpes zoster virus. *(10)*

147. **(B)** Methohexital sodium (Brevital Sodium) is a highly lipid soluble barbiturate. It can, therefore, rapidly cross the blood-brain barrier and produce a rapid onset of action and a short duration. Methohexital is employed for the induction and maintenance of anesthesia. *(6)*

148. **(B)** Pantoprazole (Protonix) is a proton pump inhibitor that dramatically reduces the secretion of hydrochloric acid in the stomach. Magnesium hydroxide is an antacid that neutralizes existing hydrochloric acid. *(6)*

149. **(E)** Metoclopramide (Reglan) is a prokinetic agent that increases the motility of the upper GI tract without stimulating gastric, biliary, or pancreatic secretions. It is employed in the treatment of diabetic gastroparesis, symptomatic gastroesophageal reflux, prevention of postoperative nausea and vomiting, radiological examination, and other clinical situations where greater GI motility is desirable. *(6)*

150. **(D)** Olsalazine sodium (Dipentum) is a salicylate compound that is converted to 5-aminosalicylic acid (5-ASA) in the colon. This exerts an anti-inflammatory effect useful in treating ulcerative colitis. Because it does not contain a sulfa component, it is particularly useful in treating patients who cannot tolerate sulfasalazine. *(10)*

151. **(D)** Modafinil (Provigil) is a drug that is useful in promoting wakefulness in patients with excessive daytime sleepiness associated with narcolepsy. Its mechanism of action is not clear. *(10)*

152. **(C)** Mifepristone (Mifeprex) is an anti-progesterone drug that competes with progesterone at receptor sites. It is indicated for the medical termination of pregnancy during the first 49 days of pregnancy. If a complete abortion has not occurred within two days of taking three 200 mg tablets of Mifeprex, the patient must take 200 µg of misoprostol (Cytotec) to facilitate abortion. *(10)*

153. **(D)** Ramipril (Altace) is an angiotensin-converting enzyme inhibitor indicated for the treatment of hypertension. When administered orally, antihypertensive action generally occurs within 1 to 2 h. The drug's action persists for 24 h. This permits single daily dosing. *(6)*

154. **(E)** Beclomethasone dipropionate (Beclovent, Vanceril) is a synthetic corticosteroid used by inhalation to control bronchial asthma. It is generally reserved for patients in whom bronchodilators and other nonsteroidal medications have not been totally successful in controlling asthmatic attacks. When used with a bronchodilator administered by inhalation, the beclomethasone dipropionate should be administered several minutes after the bronchodilator in order to enhance the penetration of the beclomethasone into the bronchial tree. *(6)*

155. **(A)** Naratriptan (Amerge) is a 5-$HT_1$-receptor antagonist used orally to treat acute migraine headaches. It is not used prophylactically. *(6)*

156. **(E)** Antimetabolites are a diverse group of compounds that interfere with normal metabolic processes and thereby disrupt nucleic acid synthesis and normal cell function. *(6)*

157. **(D)** Loratidine (Alavert, Claritin), cetirizine (Zyrtec) and fexofenadine (Allegra) are peripherally selective antihistamines that produce a low degree of sedation. The other agents are much more likely to produce sedation as an adverse effect. *(6)*

158. **(C)** Methylphenidate (Ritalin) is an amphetamine-like cortical stimulant employed in treating attention deficit disorders as well as narcolepsy. Nervousness and insomnia are common adverse effects associated with methylphenidate use. *(10)*

159. **(D)** Azithromycin (Zithromax) is a macrolide antimicrobial agent related to erythromycin, clarithromycin (Biaxin), and dirithromycin (Dynabac). Netilmicin (Netromycin) is an aminoglycoside antimicrobial agent. *(6)*

160. **(C)** Stavudine (Zerit) is an antiviral agent used in treating patients with HIV. Its use has been associated with the development of peripheral neuropathy. *(6)*

161. **(D)** Beta carotene is also known as provitamin A. It is a precursor that is converted to vitamin A in the body. *(6)*

162. **(B)** Simvastatin (Zocor) is an HMG-CoA reductase inhibitor. It and similar agents such as fluvastatin, lovastatin, atorvastatin, and pravastatin inhibit HMG-CoA reductase, an enzyme that catalyzes an early step in the synthesis of cholesterol in the body. *(6)*

163. **(C)** Fentanyl is a narcotic agonist analgesic that is significantly more potent than morphine. It may be administered parenterally (IM or IV) for induction or as an adjunct to general anesthesia. It may also be used transdermally (Duragesic) to manage chronic pain for up to 72 h. It is also available as a transmucosal system (Actiq). Because of its potency, Actiq should only be used in patients who are opioid tolerant. *(6)*

164. **(C)** Anabolic steroids are related to androgens. Their use results in enhanced tissue building. They are used in the treatment of certain types of anemia and in treating metastatic breast cancer in women. Fluorometholone is an anti-inflammatory corticosteroid. *(6)*

165. **(E)** Amrinone (Inocor) is an agent that produces a positive inotropic effect as well as vasodilation. It is used to treat congestive heart failure (CHF) in patients who have not responded adequately to digitalis glycosides, diuretics, or vasodilators. *(10)*

166. **(D)** Potassium is the principal intracellular cation of a number of body tissues. It is essential for proper transmission of nerve impulses; contraction of cardiac, skeletal, and smooth muscles; and in the transport of glucose across cell membranes. *(6)*

167. **(B).** Oxybutynin is an antispasmodic most commonly used to decrease muscle spasms of the bladder and the frequent urge to urinate caused by such spasms. The drug exerts a direct antispasmodic effect on smooth muscle and inhibits the muscarinic action of acetylcholine on smooth muscle. It is available as the

product Ditropan and Ditropan XL. The XL form utilizes osmotic pressure to deliver oxybutynin hydrochloride over a 24-h period. *(6)*

168. **(E)** Pemoline (Cylert), methamphetamine (Desoxyn) and cocaine stimulate the central nervous system and increase alertness and a heightened awareness of surroundings. High doses may produce hyperactivity, autonomic effects on the heart, and muscle tremor. *(6)*

169. **(C)** Lactulose is a synthetic disaccharide that is broken down by gut bacteria to low molecular weight acids and carbon dioxide. These cause an osmotic laxative effect. The acidity produced also causes ammonia to be converted to ammonium ion. Ammonium ion cannot be reabsorbed, so it is eliminated from the body. This effect may be useful in patients with portal-systemic encephalopathy to prevent ammonia accumulation in the body. *(10)*

170. **(D)** Simethicone is a mixture of inert silicon polymers. It is employed as an ingredient in antacid products because of its defoaming action in the GI tract. It acts to reduce the surface tension of gas bubbles, thereby causing them to break and release their entrapped gases. *(6)*

171. **(E)** Pentamidine isethionate (Pentam, NebuPent) is an agent that has activity against *Pneumocystis carinii*, the cause of *Pneumocystis carinii* pneumonia (PCP). It is administered by inhalation to prevent PCP in high-risk HIV patients. It is administered parenterally to treat PCP. *(6)*

172. **(D)** Metronidazole (Flagyl) is an agent that is primarily used because of its antiprotozoal activity, particularly, in the treatment of trichomoniasis. It is also employed as an antibacterial in treating certain anaerobic bacterial infections. Patients using metronidazole should avoid alcoholic beverages to avoid disulfiram-like effects when the combination is used. *(6)*

173. **(D)** Ticlopidine (Ticlid) is an inhibitor of platelet aggregation that is administered orally, with food, in doses of 250 mg twice daily.

Patients using this drug should have a complete blood count (CBC) with differential performed every two weeks for three months to detect neutropenia (decreased number of white blood cells). The drug's antiplatelet effects are not maximal until at least 8 to 11 days of therapy have been completed. *(10)*

174. **(A)** Quinidine is an antiarrhythmic agent derived from the bark of the cinchona tree. As does quinine, quinidine may cause an array of adverse effects collectively referred to as cinchonism. *(6)*

175. **(D)** Atomoxetine (Strattera) is a selective norepinephrine reuptake inhibitor that is indicated for the treatment of attention deficit hyperactivity disorder (ADHD) in children, adolescents, and adults. Because this drug affects drug monoamine concentrations, it should not be used within two weeks of using any MAOI drug. Unlike most ADHD drugs, atomoxetine is not a controlled substance and does not have amphetamine-like effects such as CNS stimulation. *(10)*

176. **(C)** Cefpodoxime proxetil (Vantin) and dirithromycin (Dynabac) are prodrugs, i.e., they are pharmacologically inactive until they are enzymatically converted to their active forms in the body. *(6)*

177. **(E)** Levofloxacin and other "floxacin" drugs such as ciprofloxacin, ofloxacin, and levofloxacin are considered to be fluoroquinolones. These agents are particularly useful in the treatment of UTIs, gonorrhea, and respiratory infections. *(6)*

178. **(B)** The strength of penicillin G is usually measured in milligrams or units. Each milligram of the pure drug is equivalent to 1600 units of activity. Thus, 200 mg of penicillin G is approximately equivalent to 320,000 units of activity. *(6)*

179. **(D)** Nafcillin and cloxacillin are both beta-lactamase–resistant penicillins. They are employed primarily in treating infections caused by beta-lactamase–producing staphylococci. Other beta-lactamase–resistant penicillins include oxacillin and dicloxacillin. *(6)*

180. **(E)** Chlorhexidine gluconate (Hibiclens, Betasept), glutaraldehyde (Cidex), and benzakonium chloride (Zephiran) are antiseptic agents used either as surgical scrubs or for the disinfection of surgical and dental equipment. *(6)*

181. **(B)** Valedecoxib (Bextra) is a drug that is indicated for the treatment of symptoms related to osteoarthritis, rheumatoid arthritis, and dysmenorrhea. Its action is believed to be due to inhibition of prostaglandin synthesis primarily through inhibition of cyclooxygenase-2 (COX-2). *(10)*

182. **(E)** Fluzone (Aventis Pasteur) is an influenza vaccine. Enerix-B (Glaxo Smith Kline) is a hepatitis-B vaccine. Tripedia (Aventis Pasteur) is a diphtheria, tetanus, and acellular pertussis vaccine. *(10)*

183. **(B)** Propofol (Diprivan) is a sedative-hypnotic agent used to induce and maintain general anesthesia. Naratriptan (Amerge) is a 5-hydroxytryptamine-1 subtype agonist used for treating acute migraine attacks. It is typical of the "triptan" group of drugs. Methysergide (Sansert) is an ergot alkaloid used to prevent migraine attacks. *(10)*

184. **(A)** Diacetylmorphine is another name for heroin. Because of its great ability to cause dependence, diacetylmorphine may not be legally prescribed in the United States. *(6)*

185. **(E)** Sulfonamides exert their antimicrobial action by competitively antagonizing $p$-aminobenzoic acid (PABA). Sulfonamide resistance may occur if an organism produces excessive amounts of PABA, or if PABA-containing products are used concurrently with a sulfonamide drug. *(6)*

# CHAPTER 2

# Pharmaceutical Calculations

While the number of prescriptions being compounded in community and institutional settings has diminished during the past decade, the importance of pharmaceutical calculations has not declined. There is a continued necessity for accurate compounding of some prescriptions and medical orders, especially for pharmacists preparing parenteral admixtures in both institutional and community settings. The concern over medication errors has made it imperative that the pharmacist be competent in handling pharmaceutical calculations. In addition, the pharmacist must be able to comprehend and evaluate the mathematics included in the scientific literature.

There are several textbooks dealing with pharmaceutical calculations that present the reader with many problems to solve. We have attempted to present this topic with a sampling of pharmaceutical calculations that are relevant to current pharmacy practice. Following the lead of the USP/NF, the metric system is the basis for this chapter. Any problems from previous editions that involved the apothecary system have been dropped. Obviously, units that are commonly referred to as "household measures" have been retained.

# Questions

DIRECTIONS (Questions 1 through 70): Each of the numbered items or incomplete statements in this section is followed by answers or by completions of the statement. Select the ONE lettered answer or completion that is BEST in each case.

1. Micro, nano, atto, and mega are prefixes associated with which of the following measuring systems?

   I. avoirdupois
   II. metric
   III. Systeme International

   (A) I only
   (B) III only
   (C) I and II only
   (D) II and III only
   (E) I, II, and III

2. One hundred (100) micrograms equals

   I. 100,000 ng
   II. 0.1 mg
   III. 0.001 g

   (A) I only
   (B) III only
   (C) I and II only
   (D) II and III only
   (E) I, II, and III

3. A patient's serum cholesterol value is reported as 4 mM/L. What is this concentration expressed in terms of mg/dL? (mol wt cholesterol = 386):

   (A) 0.154 mg/dL
   (B) 1.54 mg/dL
   (C) 154 mg/dL
   (D) 596 mg/dL
   (E) 1540 mg/dL

4. What is the minimum amount of a potent drug that may be weighed on a prescription balance with a sensitivity requirement of 6 mg if at least 95% accuracy is required?

   (A) 6 mg
   (B) 120 mg
   (C) 180 mg
   (D) 200 mg
   (E) 300 mg

5. Which of the following occur(s) when the sensitivity requirement of a balance increases?

   I. The accuracy of the balance increases.
   II. The minimum mass weighed with a certain degree of accuracy increases.
   III. The potential error in any given weighing increases.

   (A) I only
   (B) III only
   (C) I and II only
   (D) II and III only
   (E) I, II, and III

6. The upper therapeutic drug concentration for vancomycin is considered to be 40 μg/mL. Express this value in terms of mg/dL.

   (A) 0.04 mg/dL
   (B) 0.4 mg/dL
   (C) 4 mg/dL

(D)  40 mg/dL

(E)  400 mg/dL

7.  Calculate the dose of a drug to be administered to a patient if the dosing regimen is listed as 2 mg/kg/day. The patient weighs 140 lb.

(A)  65 mg

(B)  130 mg

(C)  300 mg

(D)  350 mg

(E)  600 mg

8.  A package insert lists a drug dose for a neonate as being 10 μg/kg/day. The age range for a neonate is considered to be

(A)  birth to 1 month

(B)  1 month to 6 months

(C)  1 month to 1 year

(D)  birth to 1 week

(E)  1 year through 5 years

9.  A child's dose of a drug is reported as 1.2 mg/kg body weight. What is the appropriate dose for a child weighing 60 lb?

(A)  6 mg

(B)  9 mg

(C)  32 mg

(D)  72 mg

(E)  126 mg

10.  The infusion rate of theophylline established for an infant is 0.08 mg/kg/h. How many mg of drug are needed for a 12-h infusion bottle if the body weight is 16 lb?

(A)  0.58 mg

(B)  14 mg

(C)  30 mg

(D)  150 mg

(E)  7 mg

11.  How many mg of codeine phosphate are being consumed daily by a patient taking the following prescription as directed?

| Rx | |
|---|---|
| Codeine Phosphate | 200 mg |
| Dimetapp Elix | qs 120 mL |

Sig: z i t.i.d. p.c. & h.s.

(A)  6.25 mg

(B)  8.25 mg

(C)  19 mg

(D)  25 mg

(E)  33 mg

12.  How many mg of codeine base is in each dose of the cough product used in Question 11? (Mol. wts: codeine = 299, codeine phosphate = 406.)

(A)  6 mg

(B)  8 mg

(C)  11 mg

(D)  16 mg

(E)  24 mg

13.  The adult dose of a drug is 250 mg. What would be the approximate dose for a 6-year-old child weighing 60 lb? (Use Young's rule.)

(A)  60 mg

(B)  85 mg

(C)  100 mg

(D)  125 mg

(E)  180 mg

14.  The USP contains nomograms for estimating body surface area (BSA) for both children and adults. Which of the following measurements must be known in order to use these nomograms?

(A)  age and height

(B)  age and weight

(C)  height and creatinine clearance

(D)  height and weight

(E)  weight and sex

15. The adult dose of a drug is 200 mg. What is an appropriate dose for an 8-year-old child whose BSA is calculated to be 0.6 m²?

   (A) 25 mg
   (B) 40 mg
   (C) 50 mg
   (D) 70 mg
   (E) 80 mg

16. The usual dose for paclitaxel intravenous is 135 mg/m². How many mg should be administered to a 40-year-old female weighing 120 lb if her body surface area was calculated to be 1.5 m²?

   (A) 110
   (B) 120
   (C) 135
   (D) 180
   (E) 200

17. Blood pressure measurements were made for one week on five patients with the following averages:

| Patient | 1 | 2 | 3 | 4 | 5 |
|---------|-------|--------|--------|--------|--------|
| BP | 140/70 | 160/84 | 180/88 | 190/90 | 150/70 |

What is the median systolic pressure?

   (A) 80
   (B) 83
   (C) 84
   (D) 160
   (E) 164

18. Using the above data, determine the approximate mean diastolic blood pressure value.

   (A) 80
   (B) 84
   (C) 100
   (D) 115
   (E) 160

19. After one month of therapy, all of the patients listed in Question 16 had a systolic blood pressure reduction of 10 mm with a standard deviation (SD) of ±5 mm. What percentage of patients had a reduction between 5 and 15 mm?

   (A) 20%
   (B) 40%
   (C) 50%
   (D) 70%
   (E) 90%

20. A pharmacist adds 1 pt of alcohol USP to 1 L of a mouthwash formula. What is the new percentage of alcohol present if the original mouthwash was labeled as 12% v/v ethanol?

   (A) 30%
   (B) 38%
   (C) 45%
   (D) 57%
   (E) 59%

21. A prescription calls for the dispensing of a 4% Pilocar solution with the directions of "gtt i OU TID." How many mg of pilocarpine hydrochloride is being used per day? Assume that the dropper is calibrated to deliver 20 drops to the mL.

   (A) 4 mg
   (B) 6 mg
   (C) 12 mg
   (D) 24 mg
   (E) 60 mg

22. The adult intravenous (IV) dose of zidovudine is 2 mg/kg q4h six times daily. How many mg will a 180-lb patient receive daily?

   (A) 12 mg
   (B) 164 mg
   (C) 650 mg
   (D) 980 mg
   (E) 2160 mg

23. A pharmacist dilutes 100 mL of Clorox with sufficient water to make one quart of solution. Express the concentration of sodium hypochlorite in the final dilution as a w/v ratio. Commercial Clorox contains 5.25% w/v sodium hypochlorite.

    (A) 1/10
    (B) 1/90
    (C) 1/100
    (D) 1/180
    (E) 1/200

**Questions 24 and 25 relate to the following hospital formula for T-A-C solution.**

| Cocaine HCl | 4% |
|---|---|
| Tetracaine HCl 2% | 0.5 mL |
| Epinephrine HCl | 1/2000 |
| Sodium chloride injection | qs 4 mL |

24. How many mg of cocaine HCl are in the final solution?

    (A) 4 mg
    (B) 8 mg
    (C) 20 mg
    (D) 40 mg
    (E) 160 mg

25. How many mL of Epinephrine HCl solution (0.1%) may be used to prepare the solution?

    (A) 0.002 mL
    (B) 0.04 mL
    (C) 1 mL
    (D) 2 mL
    (E) 5 mL

**Questions 26 and 27 relate to the following hospital order.**

| Parenteral Admixture Order | |
|---|---|
| For: Alex Sanders | Room: M 704 |
| Cefazolin sodium | 400 mg in 100 mL N/S |
| Infuse over 20 min q6h ATC for 3 days | |

Available in the pharmacy are cefazolin sodium 1-g vials with reconstitution directions of "addition of 2.5 mL SWFI will give 3.0 mL of solution."

26. How many mL of the reconstituted solution are required for each day of therapy?

    (A) 1.2 mL
    (B) 4.8 mL
    (C) 3 mL
    (D) 6 mL
    (E) 12 mL

27. What infusion rate in mL/min should the nurse establish for each bottle?

    (A) 0.15 mL/min
    (B) 0.28 mL/min
    (C) 1.1 mL/min
    (D) 2 mL/min
    (E) 5 mL/min

28. An ICU medical order reads "KCl 40 mEq in 1 L N/S. Infuse at 0.5 mEq/min." How many minutes will this bottle last on the patient?

    (A) 20
    (B) 80
    (C) 500
    (D) 1000
    (E) 2000

29. The attending physician changes the flow rate of the above solution (KCl 40 mEq/1 L N/S) to 2 mEq/h. What will be the approximate flow rate in mL/min?

    (A) 0.8
    (B) 1.5
    (C) 8
    (D) 10
    (E) 50

30. How many mL of N/S should be mixed in a syringe with 1 mL of a 1:1000 strength solution in order to obtain a 1:2500 dilution?

    (A)  1.0
    (B)  1.5
    (C)  2.0
    (D)  2.5
    (E)  4.5

31. Dopamine (intropin) 200 mg in 500 mL of normal saline at 5 µg/kg/min is ordered for a 155-lb patient. What is the final concentration of solution in µg/mL?

    (A)  0.4 µg/mL
    (B)  2.5 µg/mL
    (C)  40 µg /mL
    (D)  400 µg/mL
    (E)  25 µg/mL

32. Referring to Question 31, at what rate (mL/min) should the solution be infused to deliver the desired dose of 5 µg/kg/min?

    (A)  0.35 mL/min
    (B)  0.40 mL/min
    (C)  0.88 mL/min
    (D)  2.0 mL/min
    (E)  5.0 mL/min

33. A 250-mL infusion container contains 5.86 g of potassium chloride (KCl). How many milliequivalents (mEq) of KCl are present? (Mol weight KCl = 74.6.)

    (A)  12.7 mEq
    (B)  20 mEq
    (C)  78.5 mEq
    (D)  150 mEq
    (E)  157 mEq

34. A medication order reads "Aclovate Oint 0.05% 15 g—dilute to 0.02% with white pet and apply to hands t.i.d." How many grams of white petrolatum should the pharmacist use?

    (A)  15
    (B)  20
    (C)  22.5

    (D)  37.5
    (E)  360

35. Calcium chloride ($CaCl_2 \cdot 2H_2O$) has a formula weight of 147. What weight of the chemical is needed to obtain 40 mEq of calcium? (Ca = 40.1, Cl = 35.5, $H_2O$ = 18)

    (A)  0.80 g
    (B)  2.22 g
    (C)  1.47 g
    (D)  2.94 g
    (E)  5.88 g

36. A floor nurse requests a 50-mL minibottle to contain heparin injection 100 units/mL. The number of mL of heparin injection 10,000 units/mL needed for this order will be

    (A)  0.1 mL
    (B)  0.5 mL
    (C)  1 mL
    (D)  2.5 mL
    (E)  5 mL

**Questions 37 through 39 relate to the following order received by a home infusion pharmacy.**

---

Morphine sulfate 500 mg in a 100 mL PCA unit to deliver 0.05 mg/min

Dosing to start at 08:00 a.m. tomorrow.

---

37. How many mL of a commercial morphine sulfate vial (25 mg/mL) is needed to fill this order?

    (A)  10
    (B)  20
    (C)  25
    (D)  30
    (E)  50

38. What flow rate must be programmed into the PCA unit to obtain the desired amount of morphine per minute?

    (A)  0.01 mL/min
    (B)  0.05 mL/min
    (C)  0.1 mL/min

(D)  0.1 mL/h

(E)  1.0 mL/min

39.  Upon consultation, the prescriber decides to allow bolus PRN dosing of 2 mg with a lockout of 1 h intervals. Assuming that the patient uses all bolus dosing intervals, approximately how long will the PCA last?

(A)  <2.5 days

(B)  4 days

(C)  7 days

(D)  10 days

(E)  >14 days

**Questions 40 through 43 relate to the following formula for a psoriasis lotion.**

| | |
|---|---|
| Coal tar solution | 5 mL |
| Salicylic acid | |
| Urea | aa 5% |
| Triamcinolone acetonide | 0.25 g |
| Alcohol USP | 20 mL |
| Propylene glycol | qs 120 mL |

40.  What weight of salicylic acid is needed to prepare 1 pt of the formula listed?

(A)  11.8 g

(B)  12 g

(C)  23.7 g

(D)  24 g

(E)  25 g

41.  What percent v/v concentration of alcohol would be listed on the label?

(A)  8%

(B)  15.8%

(C)  16.7%

(D)  19%

(E)  20%

42.  How many mL of triamcinolone acetonide aqueous injection (40 mg/mL) could be used to prepare 240 mL of the formula?

(A)  6.3 mL

(B)  12.5 mL

(C)  1.2 mL

(D)  10 mL

(E)  15 mL

43.  Propylene glycol was purchased at a cost of $24.00 per pound. What is the cost of 100 mL of the liquid? (Specific gravity = 1.04.)

(A)  $2.60

(B)  $2.64

(C)  $2.75

(D)  $5.50

(E)  $13.00

44.  A pharmacist adds 2 mL of tobramycin injection (40 mg/mL) to 4 mL of tobramycin ophthalmic solution 0.3%. The concentration of tobramycin in the final mixture will be _____ g/mL.

(A)  0.012

(B)  0.015

(C)  0.03

(D)  0.052

(E)  0.092

45.  The hospital protocol calls for additional dosing when the trough level of tobramycin (mol wt = 470) approaches 2 μg/mL. The concentration may also be expressed as how many micromoles per liter?

(A)  2.1

(B)  4.2

(C)  6.4

(D)  8.5

(E)  0.04

46.  A physician requests 1 lb of bacitracin ointment containing 200 U of bacitracin per gram. How many grams of bacitracin ointment (500 U/g) must be used to make this ointment?

(A)  182 g

(B)  200 g

(C)  227 g

(D)  362 g

(E)  400 g

47. A total parenteral nutrition (TPN) order requires 500 mL of $D_{30}W$. How many mL of $D_{50}W$ should be used if the $D_{30}W$ is not available?

    (A) 125 mL
    (B) 300 mL
    (C) 375 mL
    (D) 400 mL
    (E) 200 mL

48. How many grams of 1% hydrocortisone cream must be mixed with 0.5% hydrocortisone cream if one wishes to prepare 60 g of a 0.8% w/w preparation?

    (A) 6 g
    (B) 12 g
    (C) 24 g
    (D) 36 g
    (E) 48 g

49. How many grams of pure hydrocortisone powder must be mixed with 60 g of 0.5% hydrocortisone cream if one wishes to prepare a 2.0% w/w preparation?

    (A) 0.90 g
    (B) 0.92 g
    (C) 0.30 g
    (D) 1.2 g
    (E) 1.53 g

50. How much sodium chloride is needed to adjust the following prescription to isotonicity? (E value for sodium thiosulfate is 0.31.)

    | Rx | |
    | --- | --- |
    | Sodium thiosulfate | 1.2% |
    | Sodium chloride | qs |
    | Purified water | qs 100 mL |

    (A) 0.37 g
    (B) 0.45 g
    (C) 0.53 g
    (D) 0.31 g
    (E) 0.90 g

51. How many mg of sodium chloride should be added to the following medication order to maintain isotonicity? "Atrovent Inhalation Solution 0.02% 5 mL + SWF Injection 25 mL – Place in nebulizer ut dict" [Note: Atrovent Inhalation Solution is isotonic.]

    (A) 45 mg
    (B) 225 mg
    (C) 270 mg
    (D) 900 mg
    (E) 0 (Since sterile water for injection is already isotonic.)

52. How many mg of sodium chloride are needed to adjust 30 mL of a 4% cocaine HCl solution to isotonicity. The freezing point depression of a 1% solution of cocaine HCl is 0.09°C.

    (A) 62
    (B) 83
    (C) 108
    (D) 120
    (E) 270

53. Estimate the milliosmolarity (mOsm/L) for normal saline (Na = 23, Cl = 35.5).

    (A) 150 mOsm/L
    (B) 300 mOsm/L
    (C) 350 mOsm/L
    (D) 400 mOsm/L
    (E) 600 mOsm/L

54. How many milliosmoles are present in a solution prepared by dissolving 1000 mg of sodium chloride in 100 mL $D_5W$? (Na = 23, Cl = 35.5, hydrous dextrose = 198.)

    (A) 30
    (B) 60
    (C) 150
    (D) 300
    (E) 600

55. A nurse in a nursing home setting mixes 240 mL of a dietary supplement formula (400 mOsm/L) with 250 mL of $D_{10}W$ and 200 mL of water containing 5 g calcium chloride (mol wt = 111).

(Mol wt of dextrose = 180) What is the osmolarity of this solution expressed as mOsm/L?

(A)  280

(B)  370

(C)  410

(D)  470

(E)  540

56. How much elemental iron is present in every 300 mg of ferrous sulfate ($FeSO_4 \cdot 7H_2O$)? (Atomic weights: iron = 55.9, S = 32, O = 16, H = 1. Iron has valences of 2 and 3.)

(A)  30 mg

(B)  60 mg

(C)  110 mg

(D)  120 mg

(E)  164 mg

57. Approximately how many milliequivalents of iron is present in every 300 mg of ferrous sulfate ($FeSO_4 \cdot 7H_2O$)? (Atomic weights: iron = 55.9, S = 32, O = 16, H = 1. Iron has valences of 2 and 3.)

(A)  1

(B)  2

(C)  3

(D)  4

(E)  6

58. What is the decay constant ($k$) of the radioisotope $^{32}P$ if its half-life is 14.3 days? Assume that radiopharmaceutical decay follows first-order kinetics.

(A)  0.048/day

(B)  0.07/day

(C)  0.097/day

(D)  0.1/day

(E)  0.15/day

59. A radiopharmacist prepares a solution of $^{99m}Tc$ (40 mCi/mL) at 06:00 a.m. If the solution is intended for administration at 12:00 p.m. at a dose of 20 mCi, how many mL of the original solution are needed? The half-life of the radioisotope is 6 h.

(A)  0.5 mL

(B)  1.0 mL

(C)  1.5 mL

(D)  2.0 mL

(E)  5.0 mL

60. What concentration of the original $^{99m}Tc$ solution described in Question 59 will remain 24 h after its original preparation?

(A)  15 mCi

(B)  10 mCi

(C)  7.5 mCi

(D)  5.0 mCi

(E)  2.5 mCi

**Questions 61 and 62 relate to the following formula for Citrate of Magnesia.**

| Rx | |
| --- | --- |
| Magnesium carbonate | 15 g |
| Citric acid (anhydrous) | 27.4 g |
| Syrup | 60 mL |
| Purified water | qs 350 mL |

61. How many grams of magnesium are present in every 350 mL dose? (Mg = 24.3, carbonate = 60)

(A)  2.5

(B)  4.32

(C)  6.08

(D)  6.7

(E)  8.6

62. What % w/v of hydrated citric acid could be listed in a formula if the anhydrous citric acid is not available? The hydrated form of citric acid contains 10% water. (Mol wt citric acid, anhydrous = 192 g/mol; water = 18 g/mol)

(A)  7.0

(B)  7.8

(C)  8.7

(D)  24.7

(E)  30.4

63. A nursing home patient is experiencing diarrhea from his enteral nutritional solution, which has an osmolarity of 520 mOsm/L. How many mL of purified water are needed to reduce 500 mL of this solution to an osmolarity of 300 mOsm/L?

    (A)  290 mL
    (B)  310 mL
    (C)  360 mL
    (D)  500 mL
    (E)  870 mL

64. The level of iron impurities in a water sample is 2 mg/L. Express this concentration in terms of ppm.

    (A)  0.2 ppm
    (B)  2 ppm
    (C)  20 ppm
    (D)  200 ppm
    (E)  2000 ppm

65. The concentration of mercury in a water sample is reported as 5 ppm. Express this concentration as a percentage.

    (A)  0.00005%
    (B)  0.0005%
    (C)  0.005%
    (D)  0.05%
    (E)  0.5%

66. A medication order in CCU reads "Heparin 20,000 units in NS 250 mL—infuse at 20 units/min." What flow rate in drops per minute should be established if a Buretrol delivering 60 drops to the mL is used?

    (A)  15
    (B)  20
    (C)  25
    (D)  30
    (E)  60

67. How many mL of isopropyl rubbing alcohol (70% v/v) will be needed to prepare one pint of 50% isopropyl alcohol?

    (A)  70
    (B)  170
    (C)  342
    (D)  400
    (E)  480

68. How many grams of glacial acetic acid (99.9% w/w) must be added to 1 gal purified water to prepare an irrigation solution containing 0.25% w/v acetic acid?

    (A)  1.2 g
    (B)  9.5 g
    (C)  12 g
    (D)  20 g
    (E)  95 g

69. A hospital clinic requests 2 lb of 2% hydrocortisone ointment. How many grams of 5% hydrocortisone ointment should be diluted with white petrolatum to prepare this order?

    (A)  18.2 g
    (B)  27.5 g
    (C)  45.4 g
    (D)  363 g
    (E)  545 g

70. For how many days will a 20 mL vial of Dilaudid (4 mg/mL) last if the home patient is ordered on 3 mg q6h ATC?

    (A)  4
    (B)  6
    (C)  8
    (D)  9
    (E)  12

# Answers and Explanations

1. **(D)** The metric system is used exclusively in most nations in the world except the United States. The prefixes in the metric system are based on increasing or decreasing magnitudes of 10, 100, or 1000. Converting from one set of quantities to another simply requires the movement of decimal points. For example, converting 1 kg to g requires moving the decimal point three places to the right. The metric system has been expanded into the Systeme International (SI) measuring system that encompasses all types of measures. The major prefixes in the order of magnitude include:

| Prefix | Magnitude | Example |
|---|---|---|
| mega | $1,000,000 \times$ | megagram |
| kilo | $1000 \times$ | kilogram |
| — | $1 \times$ | gram |
| centi | $0.01 \times$ | centigram |
| milli | $0.001 \times$ | milligram |
| micro | $1 \times 10^{-6} \times$ | microgram |
| nano | $1 \times 10^{-9} \times$ | nanogram |
| pico | $1 \times 10^{-12} \times$ | picogram |
| femto | $1 \times 10^{-15} \times$ | femtogram |
| atto | $1 \times 10^{-18} \times$ | attogram |

*(23)*

2. **(C)** In this example, consider 1 µg as equaling 1000 ng thus 100 µg = 100,000 ng. Since 1 mg equals 1000 µg, 100 µg equals 0.1 mg. If 1 mg equals .001 g, 0.1 mg or 100 µg equals 0.0001 g. It may be clearer if one solves this conversion using dimensional analysis.

$$100\,\mu g \times \frac{1\,mg}{1000\,\mu g} \times \frac{1\,g}{1000\,mg} = 0.00001\,g \;\; (1; 23)$$

3. **(C)** An increasing number of laboratory test values and drug doses are being reported in terms of millimoles (mM). Weight quantities expressed in molar amounts allow a more realistic evaluation of the actual number of drug molecules present, for example, when comparing salts of a drug. In this problem, the mM/L concentration is converted by recognizing that 1 mole of cholesterol weighs 386 g and 4 mmol equals 0.004 mol.

$$386 \times 0.004\,mol = 1.544\,g \text{ or } 1540\,mg/L$$

$$1540\,mg/L = 154\,mg/dL \qquad (1; 23)$$

4. **(B)** The minimum weight that can be measured on any balance can be determined if the balance's sensitivity requirement (SR) and the acceptable percentage of error has been established. The equation is

$$SR = (\text{minimum weighable amount}) \times (\text{acceptable error})$$

In this problem, the SR was given as 6 mg and an accuracy of at least 95% or an error of not more than 5% is permissible.

$$6\,mg = (x\,mg)\,(5\%)$$

$$6\,mg = (x\,mg)\,(0.05)$$

$$x = 120\,mg \qquad (1; 23)$$

5. **(B)** The larger the sensitivity requirement (SR) value for a balance, the less accurate the balance. This occurs since the SR is the smallest amount that causes a discernable visual movement of the balance indicator. If in the previous question, the SR of the balance was 10 mg, then the error in weighing 120 mg would be

$$SR = (\text{minimum weighable amount}) \times (\text{acceptable error})$$

$$10\,mg = 120\,mg \times (\text{acceptable error})$$

$$\text{error} = 0.08 \text{ or } 8\% \qquad (23)$$

6. **(C)** Since $1000\ \mu g = 1\ mg$ and $100\ mL = 1\ dL$, $40\ \mu g/mL = 0.04\ mg/mL$ or $4\ mg/dL$. This problem may be solved by dimensional analysis,

$$\frac{40\ \mu g}{1\ mL} \times \frac{1\ mg}{1000\ \mu g} \times \frac{100\ mL}{1\ dL} = 4\ mg/dL$$

Note that when dimensional analysis is used, all of the units cancel except those appropriate for the final answer. *(23; 13)*

7. **(B)** One kilogram = 2.2 lb.

$$140\ lb \times \frac{1\ kg}{2.2\ lb} = 64\ kg$$

$$64\ kg \times 2\ mg\ dose = 128\ mg \qquad (23)$$

8. **(A)** Neonates have an age span from birth to 1 month of age. Infants are 1 month to 1 year, early childhood is 1 to 5 years, and late childhood is 6 to 12 years. *(23)*

9. **(C)**

$$60\ lb \times \frac{1\ kg}{2.2\ lb} \times \frac{1.2\ mg}{kg} = 32\ mg \qquad (23)$$

10. **(E)** The body weight will be

$$16\ lb \times \frac{1\ kg}{2.2\ lb} = 7.27\ kg$$

$$\frac{0.08\ mg}{kg} \times 7.27\ kg = 0.58\ mg/h \times 12\ h$$

$$= 7\ mg\ in\ 12\ h$$

The low dosing of theophylline is correct because the metabolic pathway of theophylline in young babies has yet to develop sufficiently. *(19; 23)*

11. **(E)** In today's health practice, the symbol "z" is used to represent a 1 teaspoon dose. The symbol's original meaning as a drachm (weight) or fluidrachm (volume) quantities is archaic and should not be used. Because the volume of a standard teaspoon is considered to be 5 mL, the patient in this prescription is receiving four daily doses for a total of 20 mL.

$$\frac{200\ mg\ codeine}{120\ mL\ of\ Rx} = \frac{x\ mg\ codeine}{20\ mL\ of\ Rx} \qquad (23)$$

12. **(A)** The weight of codeine phosphate present in each dose is

$$\frac{200\ mg}{120\ mL} = \frac{x\ mg}{5\ mL}$$

$$x = 8.3\ mg\ per\ teaspoon$$

The relationship between codeine and codeine phosphate is easily seen when viewed as a chemical reaction.

$$(x\ mg) \qquad\qquad\qquad (8.3\ mg)$$
codeine + phosphoric acid → codeine phosphate
(mol wt = 299)        (mol wt = 406)

$$x = 6\ mg\ codeine\ base \qquad (1; 23)$$

13. **(B)** Young's rule relates a child's dose to the child's age.

$$Child's\ dose = \frac{Age\ (yr)}{(Age\ [yr] + 12)} \times Adult\ dose$$

$$Child's\ dose = \frac{6}{(6 + 12)} \times 250\ mg$$

$$Dose = 83.3\ or\ 85\ mg$$

Although well intended, rules like Young's (child's age), Cowling's (age at next birthday divided by 24), Clark's (weight divided by average weight of an adult [150 lb]) are only rough estimates. Pharmacists should check the literature for individual drug dosing for children. In some instances, the child's dose will be similar to that for the adult. *(1; 23)*

14. **(D)** The nomogram in the USP consists of three parallel vertical lines. The left line is calibrated with height measurements in both centimeters and inches, whereas the right line lists weights in kilograms and pounds. Using data based on the patient's measurements, a line is drawn between the two outside parallel lines. The intercept on the middle line, which is calibrated in square meters of body surface area, allows the estimation of the patient's BSA. *(23)*

15. **(D)** In this problem one of two methods could be used, Young's rule or a body surface area (BSA) calculation. Since the BSA is usually more accurate, it is the preferred method. The average adult BSA is estimated to be 1.73 m². A child's dose can be estimated by

$$\frac{\text{BSA (child)}}{\text{BSA (adult)}} \times \text{Adult dose} = \text{Child's dose}$$

In this question,

$$\frac{0.6\ \text{m}^2}{1.73\ \text{m}^2} \times 200\ \text{mg} = 69\ \text{or}\ 70\ \text{mg} \qquad (1;\ 23)$$

16. **(E)** Many drugs, especially chemotherapeutic agents, have their dosage expressed as mg/m² of body surface area. One simply has to multiply the dose by the specific patient's body surface area to obtain the dose.

$$135\ \text{mg/m}^2 \times 1.5\ \text{m}^2 = 202\ \text{mg} \qquad (23)$$

Answer (B) of 120 or 117 is incorrect since it involved the use of the surface area equation which was not needed.

Answer (A) of 110 or 108 is incorrect since it attempted to correct the dose based upon the patient's body weight.

17. **(D)** The median value in a series of numbers is that value in the middle (i.e., the number of values lower than the median value is equal to the number of values higher than the median value). The median may not be the same as the average or mean value, which is obtained by adding all of the values together and dividing by the number of values. *(23)*

18. **(B)** The mean value of a series of numbers is obtained by adding all of the values then dividing by the actual number of values. In this example, the diastolic readings were 70 + 84 + 88 + 90 + 70 = 402 divided by 5 = 80.4. *(23)*

19. **(D)** A standard deviation is calculated mathematically for experimental data. It shows the dispersion of numbers around the mean (average value). One SD will include approximately 67 to 70% of all values, whereas two SDs will include approximately 97 to 98%. *(1; 23)*

20. **(B)** Alcohol USP contains 95% v/v ethanol. Therefore,

$$473\ \text{mL} \times 95\% = 449\ \text{mL of ethanol}$$
$$1000\ \text{mL} \times 12\% = \underline{120\ \text{mL}}$$
$$\text{total} = 569\ \text{mL of ethanol}$$

$$\frac{569\ \text{mL}}{1473\ \text{mL}} = 38\%\ \text{v/v} \qquad (4;\ 23)$$

21. **(C)** The patient is placing one drop in each eye three times a day, thus a total of six drops. This equates to 0.3 mL, since the dropper calibration was 20 drops to an mL.

$$\frac{20\ \text{drops}}{1\ \text{mL}} = \frac{6\ \text{drops}}{x\ \text{mL}} \quad x = 0.3\ \text{mL}$$

Since a 4% Pilocar solution contains 4000 mg of drug per 100 mL.

$$\frac{4000\ \text{mg}}{100\ \text{mL}} = \frac{x\ \text{mg}}{0.3\ \text{mL}} \quad x = 12\ \text{mg} \qquad (23)$$

22. **(D)** First, convert the weight in pounds to kilograms.

$$180\ \text{lb} \times \frac{1\ \text{kg}}{2.2\ \text{lb}} = 82\ \text{kg}$$

Second, determine the total daily dose.

$$82\ \text{kg} \times 2\ \text{mg} \times 6\ \text{doses} = 980\ \text{mg} \qquad (23)$$

23. **(D)** One hundred mL of Clorox will contain 5.25 g of sodium hypochlorite. The final dilution will be 1 qt, which is 946 mL. The ratio strength will be

$$\frac{5.25\ \text{g}}{946\ \text{mL}} = \frac{1}{x} \quad x = 180,\ \text{or}\ 1{:}180\ \text{w/v}$$

of sodium hypochlorite.

In actual practice, Clorox is recommended as a disinfectant for HIV-contaminated equipment when used in a 1:10 dilution. However, this designation refers to 1 mL of *Clorox* in every 10 mL of final dilution. *(23)*

24. **(E)** Four milliliters of a 4% cocaine HCl solution will contain 0.16 g, or 160 mg, of cocaine HCl (4 mL × 4%), or, by proportions:

$$\frac{4000\ \text{mg}}{100\ \text{mL}} = \frac{x\ \text{mg}}{4\ \text{mL}} \quad x = 160\ \text{mg} \qquad (23)$$

**25. (D)** Use the equation of

$$Q_1 \times C_1 = Q_2 \times C_2$$

$$4 \text{ mL} \times \frac{1}{2000} = x \text{ mL} \times \frac{1}{1000}$$

$$\frac{4}{2000} = \frac{x}{1000}$$

$$x = 2 \text{ mL} \qquad (20; 23)$$

**26. (B)** The dosing regimen for this patient consists of 400 mg of cefazolin every 6 h. When the pharmacist reconstitutes the 1000-mg vials, the strength will be 1000 mg/3 mL of solution.

$$\frac{1000 \text{ mg}}{3 \text{ mL}} = \frac{1600 \text{ mg}}{x \text{ mL}} \qquad x = 4.8 \text{ mL} \qquad (23)$$

**27. (E)** The original order requested that the solution be infused over a 20-min time span. Therefore, 100 mL divided by 20 min equals 5 mL/min. *(23)*

**28. (B)** Determine the total time for the infusion by using the relationship of

$$\frac{40 \text{ mEq}}{x} = \frac{0.5 \text{ mEq}}{1 \text{ min}}$$

$$0.5x = 40 \text{ min}$$

$$x = 80 \text{ min} \qquad (4; 23)$$

**29. (A)** First determine the mL/h flow rate to obtain 2 mEq/h.

$$\frac{2 \text{ mEq}}{x \text{ mL}} = \frac{40 \text{ mEq}}{1000 \text{ mL}} \qquad x = 50 \text{ mL/h}$$

Now determine the equivalent flow per minute

$$\frac{50 \text{ mL}}{60 \text{ min}} = \frac{x \text{ mL}}{1 \text{ min}} \qquad x = 0.83 \text{ mL/min} \quad (23)$$

**30. (B)** This calculation may be done by several methods.

$$Q_1 \times C_1 = Q_2 \times C_2$$

$$1 \text{ mL} \times \frac{1}{1000} = x \text{ mL} \times \frac{1}{2500}$$

$$\frac{1}{1000} = \frac{x}{2500} \qquad x = 2.5 \text{ mL}$$

2.5 mL – 1 mL (original volume) = 1.5 mL *(23)*

**31. (D)** 200 mg dopamine in 500 mL = 0.4 mg/mL. Because 1 mg = 1000 µg, 0.4 mg = 400 µg; therefore, the final concentration of dopamine will be 400 µg/mL. *(23)*

**32. (C)**

$$155 \text{ lb} \times \frac{1 \text{ kg}}{2.2 \text{ lb}} \times \frac{5 \text{ µg}}{\text{kg/1 min}} = 352 \text{ µg/min}$$

Because the solution concentration is 400 µg/mL, divide the dosage rate by the concentration:

$$\frac{352 \text{ µg/min}}{400 \text{ µg/mL}} = 0.88 \text{ mL/min} \qquad (23)$$

**33. (C)** 1 equivalent weight of KCl = 74.6 g, therefore,

$$1 \text{ mEq} = 74.6 \text{ mg}$$

$$\frac{1 \text{ mEq}}{74.6 \text{ mg}} = \frac{x \text{ mEq}}{5860 \text{ mg}} \qquad x = 78.5 \text{ mEq}$$

Or the problem may be solved by using the equation:

$$\text{mg of chemical} = \frac{(\text{mEq}) (\text{mol wt})}{\text{valence}}$$

$$5860 \text{ mg} = \frac{(x) (74.6)}{1}$$

$$x = 78.5 \text{ mg} \qquad (23)$$

**34. (C)** $$Q_1 \times C_1 = Q_2 \times C_2$$

$$(15 \text{ g}) (0.05\%) = (x \text{ g}) (0.02\%)$$

$$0.02x = 0.75$$

$$x = 37.5 \text{ g (final weight)}$$

Therefore, 37.5 g – 15 g = 22.5 g $\qquad (23)$

**35. (D)** 1 equivalent of calcium chloride = 147 (mol wt) divided by 2 (valence of calcium) = 73.5 g and 1 mEq = 73.5 mg. Therefore, 40 mEq is 40 × 73.5 mg = 2940 mg, which is 2.94 g.

Or, the problem can be solved by the equation:

$$mg \text{ of chemical} = \frac{(mEq)(mol \ wt)}{valence}$$

$$x \ mg = \frac{(40 \ mEq)(147)}{2}$$

$$x = 2940 \ mg, \text{ or } 2.94 \ g$$

It must be remembered that 40 mEq of calcium combines with 40 mEq of chloride to form 40 mEq of calcium chloride. *(1; 23)*

(A—incorrect) This answer is obtained if one multiplies the 40 mEq desired by the atomic weight of calcium and then divides by the valence of 2. The use of the atomic weight of calcium is incorrect because the official hydrated calcium chloride is being weighed to obtain the correct amount of calcium. The right answer can be obtained by adding this step:

$$\frac{0.80 \ g \ (Ca)}{40 \ (atomic \ wt \ Ca)}$$

$$= \frac{x \ g \ (hydrated \ calcium \ chloride)}{147 \ (formula \ wt \ hydrated \ salt)}$$

$$x = 2.94 \ g \text{ hydrated calcium chloride}$$

(B—incorrect) The answer of 2.22 g is incorrect because it assumes that anhydrous calcium chloride (molecular weight of 111) was used. However, the problem specified that the official form, which contains two waters of hydration, was available.

(E—incorrect) The answer of 5.88 g is obtained if one ignores the +2 valence of calcium.

**36. (B)**    50 mL × 100 U/mL = 5000 U total

$$\frac{10,000 \ U}{1 \ mL} = \frac{5000 \ U}{x \ mL}$$

$$x = 0.5 \ mL \qquad (23)$$

**37. (B)**

$$\frac{500 \ mg}{x \ mL} = \frac{25 \ mg}{1 \ mL} \quad x = 20 \ mL \qquad (23)$$

**38. (A)**

$$\frac{0.05 \ mg}{x \ mL} = \frac{500 \ mg}{100 \ mL} \quad x = 0.01 \ mL/min \ (23)$$

**39. (B)** The maximum volume used per hour will be

$$0.01 \ mL/min \times 60 \ min = 0.6 \ mL$$

plus bolus dosing of

$$\frac{2 \ mg}{x \ mL} = \frac{500 \ mg}{100 \ mL} \quad x = 0.4 \ mL \text{ for a total of 1 mL}$$

Since the total volume in the PCA is 100 mL, it should last at least 100 h or 4.2 days. *(23)*

**40. (C)**

$$\frac{5 \ g \ salicylic \ acid}{100 \ mL \ of \ lotion} = \frac{x \ g}{473 \ mL \ of \ lotion}$$

$$x = 23.7 \ g \qquad (23)$$

**41. (B)** When concentrations of alcohol are listed on labels, the percent v/v is based on absolute alcohol (100% ethanol), although this form of alcohol is seldom used during manufacturing or compounding. Alcohol USP was specified for the formula. Its strength is 95% v/v.

$$20 \ mL \times 95\% = 19 \ mL$$

$$\frac{19 \ mL}{120 \ mL} = 15.8\% \ v/v \qquad (23)$$

**42. (B)**

$$\frac{0.25 \ g}{120 \ mL} = \frac{x \ g}{240 \ mL}$$

$$x = 500 \ mg \text{ pure triamcinolone}$$

$$\frac{40 \ mg}{1 \ mL} = \frac{500 \ mg}{x \ mL}$$

$$x = 12.5 \ mL \text{ of the injection solution} \ (23)$$

**43. (D)** The mL in 1 lb of propylene glycol can be calculated as

$$SG = \frac{W}{V}$$

$$1.04 = \frac{454 \text{ g}}{x \text{ mL}}$$

$$x = 436 \text{ mL of propylene glycol in 1 lb}$$

$$\frac{\$24.00}{436 \text{ mL}} = \frac{\$x}{100 \text{ mL}}$$

$$x = \$5.50 \qquad (1; 23)$$

**44. (B)** Total amount of pure tobramycin will be as follows:

In ophthalmic solution 4 mL × 0.3% = 0.012 g
In injection 2 mL × 40 mg/mL = 0.08 g
Total in solution of 6 mL = 0.092 g

$$\frac{0.092 \text{ g}}{6 \text{ mL}} = 0.0153 \text{ g/mL} \qquad (4)$$

**45. (B)** 1 mol of tobramycin = 470 g/L

1 mmol/L = 0.470 g or 470 mg or 470,000 µg
1 µmol/L = 470 µg
2 µg/mL = 2,000 µg/L

$$\frac{1 \text{ mmol}}{470 \text{ µg/L}} = \frac{x \text{ mmol}}{2000 \text{ µg/L}}$$

$$x = 4.25 \text{ µmol/L} \qquad (1; 23)$$

**46. (A)** One avoirdupois pound contains 454 g. The total number of bacitracin units required is

$$454 \text{ g} = 200 \text{ U/g} = 90,800 \text{ U}$$

$$\frac{500 \text{ U}}{1 \text{ g}} = \frac{90,800 \text{ U}}{x \text{ g}} \quad x = 182 \text{ g} \qquad (23)$$

**47. (B)** 500 mL of $D_{30}W$ will contain 150 g of dextrose while $D_{50}W$ contains 50 g of dextrose per 100 mL.

$$\frac{50 \text{ g dextrose}}{100 \text{ mL of solution}} = \frac{150 \text{ g dextrose}}{x \text{ mL of solution}}$$

$$x = 300 \text{ mL}$$

Or, this problem may be solved by using the equation:

$$Q_1 \times C_1 = Q_2 \times C_2$$

$$(x \text{ mL}) (50\%) = (500 \text{ mL}) (30\%)$$

$$x = 300 \text{ mL} \qquad (23)$$

**48. (D)** This problem can be solved by the alligation alternate or simple parts method

Thus, the final solution will contain 0.2 parts of the 0.5% hydrocortisone (HC) cream for every 0.3 parts of 1% HC cream for a total of 0.5 parts.

(One may refer to the above parts as 2 parts to every 3 parts for a total of 5 parts.)

$$1\% \text{ HC cream} = \frac{0.3 \text{ parts}}{0.5 \text{ parts}} \times 60 \text{ g} = 36 \text{ g}$$

$$0.5\% \text{ HC cream} = \frac{0.2 \text{ parts}}{0.5 \text{ parts}} \times 60 \text{ g} = 24 \text{ g} \quad (23)$$

**49. (B)** Because the amount of 0.5% hydrocortisone cream is exactly 60 g, the final weight of the cream will be greater when hydrocortisone powder is added. Therefore, the problem may be solved by the alligation alternate method or by simple algebra.

$$\frac{60 \text{ g of } 0.5\%}{98 \text{ parts}} = \frac{x \text{ g of } 100\%}{1.5 \text{ parts}}$$

$$x = 0.92 \text{ g}$$

Or, by algebra, let $x$ = weight of 100% HC powder, then

$$(x \text{ g}) (100\%) + (60 \text{ g}) (0.5\%) = (60 \text{ g} + x \text{ g}) (2\%)$$

$$x + 0.3 = 1.2 + 0.02 x$$

$$x = 0.92 \text{ g} \qquad (23)$$

50. **(C)** Step 1. Determine amount of sodium thiosulfate in the Rx.

$$100 \text{ mL} \times 1.2\% = 1.2 \text{ g, or } 1200 \text{ mg}$$

Step 2. Multiply the amount of chemical by its "E" value

$$1200 \text{ mg} \times 0.31 = 372 \text{ mg}$$

(equivalent amount of NaCl)

Step 3. Determine amount of NaCl needed as if no other chemical was present.

$$100 \text{ mL} \times 0.9\% = 900 \text{ mg}$$

Step 4. Subtract contribution by chemical (Step 2) from the amount of NaCl (Step 3)

$$900 \text{ mg} - 372 \text{ mg} = 528 \text{ mg}$$

(the amount of NaCl needed to render the solution isotonic) *(1)*

51. **(B)** Since the 5 mL of Atrovent Inhalation Solution is already isotonic, the pharmacist has to render the remaining volume of solution (diluent) isotonic.

$$30 \text{ mL} - 5 \text{ mL} = 25 \text{ mL}$$

$$25 \text{ mL} \times 0.9\% \text{ sodium chloride} = 225 \text{ mg}$$

*(1; 23)*

52. **(B)** The freezing point depression method for determining isotonicity calculations is more accurate than the sodium chloride equivalent method. It is based upon the premise that isotonic solutions have a reduction in freezing points of 0.52°C. This problem now becomes:

Step 1. What is the change in the freezing point of a 4% cocaine HCl solution if a 1% solution has a depression of 0.09°?

$$\frac{1\%}{0.09} = \frac{4\%}{x} \quad x = 0.36°$$

Step 2. Determine the amount of sodium chloride needed for a total freezing point depression of 0.52°.

Remember that a 0.9% concentration of sodium chloride is isotonic and must have a freezing point depression of 0.52° and that 4% cocaine HCl gave a depression of 0.36°; thus

the further reduction needed will be 0.52 − 0.36 = 0.16.

$$\frac{0.9\% \text{ NaCl}}{0.52 \text{ deg}} = \frac{x\% \text{ NaCl}}{0.16} \quad x = 0.277\% \text{ NaCl}$$

Step 3. Since 30 mL of solution is required, 30 mL × 0.277% = 0.083 g or 83 mg of sodium chloride. *(4)*

53. **(B)** One liter of normal saline contains 0.9% NaCl, or 9 g. To calculate the milliosmolarity of the solution, we have the following steps.

Step 1. Determine the moles present.

$$\frac{\text{Wt of chemical}}{\text{Mol wt}} = \frac{0.9}{58.5}$$

$$= 0.154 \text{ mol or } 154 \text{ mmol}$$

Step 2. Multiply the millimoles by the "i" value. The "i" value is the theoretical number of ions or particles formed by one molecule of chemical assuming complete ionization.

$$154 \text{ mmol} \times 2 = 308 \text{ mOsm/L} \quad (1; 23)$$

54. **(B)** Unlike the previous problem, this question asks for mOsm/100 mL and there are two chemicals present. It is best to calculate the mOsm of each separately, then add the amounts.

$$\text{NaCl} \quad \frac{1000 \text{ mg}}{58.5} = 17.1 \text{ mM} \times i \text{ value of 2}$$

$$= 34.2 \text{ mOsm}$$

$$\text{Dextrose} \quad \frac{5000 \text{ mg}}{198} = 25.3 \text{ mM} \times i \text{ value of 1}$$

$$= 25.3 \text{ mOsm}$$

Total will be 34.2 mOsm + 25.3 mOsm = 59.5 mOsm *(1; 23)*

55. **(E)** The final mixture consists of three solutions each contributing to its osmolarity.

(1) 240 mL of supplement formula with osmolarity of 400 mOsm/L.

$$\frac{400 \text{ mOsm}}{1000 \text{ mL}} = \frac{x \text{ mOsm}}{240 \text{ mL}} \quad x = 96 \text{ mOsm}$$

(2) 250 mL $D_{10}W$ = 25 g dextrose

$$\frac{25 \text{ g}}{180 \text{ g/mol}} = 0.14 \text{ mol or } 140 \text{ mmol}$$

140 mmol × i value of 1 = 140 mOsm

(3) $\dfrac{5 \text{ g } CaCl_2}{111 \text{ g/mol}} = 0.045$ mol or 45 mmol

45 mmol × i value of 3 = 135 mOsm

Total mOsm of 96 + 140 + 135 = 371 mOsm in a volume of 690 mL; therefore,

$$\frac{371}{690 \text{ mL}} = \frac{x}{1000 \text{ mL}} \quad x = 538 \text{ mOsm/L.}$$
$(1; 23)$

**56. (B)** The formula weight of ferrous sulfate is 278. The amount of iron present in 300 mg of the chemical will be

$$\frac{\text{Atomic wt Fe}}{\text{Form wt salt}} = \frac{55.9}{278} = \frac{x \text{ mg}}{300 \text{ mg}} \quad x = 60.4 \text{ mg}$$
$(23)$

Choices A or D would be obtained if the correct answer was either doubled or halved to reflect the +2 valence of iron. The valence of iron has no significance in this type of problem because only one atom of iron is present in each molecule of ferrous sulfate.

Choice C assumes that the ferrous sulfate is anhydrous with a molecular weight of 152. This is incorrect, because the 300-mg weight is based on a chemical formula containing seven waters of hydration.

Choice E is the amount of anhydrous ferrous sulfate present in each 300 mg. The question asks for iron (Fe) only.

**57. (B)**

$$mg = \frac{[\text{mEq}][\text{formula weight}]}{\text{valence}}$$

$$300 \text{ mg} = \frac{[x \text{ mEq}][278]}{2}$$

$$x = 2.2 \text{ mEq} \qquad (4; 23)$$

**58. (A)** First-order half-lives relate to kinetic constant rate values by the equation

$$t_{0.5} = \frac{0.693}{k}$$

$$14.3 \text{ days} = \frac{0.693}{k}$$

$$k = 0.048 \text{ per day, or } 4.8\% \text{ per day}$$
$(23)$

**59. (B)** Because the time interval between preparation and administration is 6 h, and the half-life of the radiopharmaceutical is 6 h, approximately one half of the original strength has decayed. Therefore, 1 mL of the solution which now assays at 20 mCi/mL is needed. $(23)$

**60. (E)** The loss in first-order kinetics is a constant fraction of the immediate past concentration. In this example, the half-life of 6 h allows a quick comparison of the amount of radioactivity remaining.

| | |
|---|---|
| Original activity | 40 mCi/mL |
| After 6 h | 20 mCi/mL |
| After 12 h | 10 mCi/mL |
| After 18 h | 5 mCi/mL |
| After 24 h | 2.5 mCi/mL    $(13; 23)$ |

**61. (B)** Magnesium carbonate has the structure of $MgCO_3$ therefore,

$$\frac{\text{Magnesium}}{MgCO_3} = \frac{24.3}{84.3} \times 15 \text{ g} = 4.32 \text{ g} \qquad (4)$$

**62. (C)** Since the written formula is based upon a total volume of 350 mL, reduce the amounts for a percentage formula based upon 100%.

$$\frac{27.4 \text{ g (anhydrous citric acid)}}{350 \text{ mL}}$$
$$= \frac{x \text{ g anhydrous citric acid}}{100 \text{ mL}}$$

$$x = 7.83 \text{ g anhydrous citric acid}$$

Since the hydrated form of citric acid contains 10% impurities (water!), an adjustment may be made by

$$Q_1 \times C_1 = Q_2 \times C_2$$

[7.83 g anhydrous citric acid] [100%]

$$= [x \text{ g hydrous}] [90\%]$$

$$x = 8.7 \text{ g of hydrated citric acid} \quad (1; 4; 23)$$

63. **(C)** One of the most convenient methods of solving this problem is using the equation:

$$Q_1 \times C_1 = Q_2 \times C_2$$

$$(500 \text{ mL})(520 \text{ mOsm/L}) = (x \text{ mL}) (300 \text{ mOsm/L})$$

$$300x = 260,000$$

$$x = 867 \text{ mL of final product}$$

Therefore, the amount of water diluent needed = 867 mL – 500 mL = 367 mL. *(1; 23)*

64. **(B)** Since the concentration expression parts per million is usually based upon 1 g of chemical in 1,000,000 mL of solution, conversion of 2 mg/L will involve

$$\frac{2 \text{ mg}}{L} = \frac{0.002 \text{ g}}{1000 \text{ mL}} = \frac{x \text{ g}}{1,000,000 \text{ mL}}$$

$$1000x = 2000 \quad x = 2 \text{ ppm} \quad (23)$$

65. **(B)** Mercury is a solid chemical. Thus, the 5 ppm concentration indicates 5 g of mercury per 1,000,000 mL of solution. Therefore, the grams present in 100 mL will be

$$\frac{5 \text{ g mercury}}{1,000,000 \text{ mL}} = \frac{x \text{ g}}{100 \text{ mL}}$$

$$1,000,000x = 500$$

$$x = 0.0005\% \quad (23)$$

66. **(A)** Step 1. Determine the drug concentration present in every milliliter.

$$\frac{20,000 \text{ U}}{250 \text{ mL}} = \frac{x \text{ U}}{1 \text{ mL}} \quad x = 80 \text{ U/mL}$$

Step 2. Determine the mL needed to obtain the concentration requested.

$$\frac{80 \text{ U}}{1 \text{ mL}} = \frac{20 \text{ U}}{x \text{ mL}} \quad x = 0.25 \text{ mL}$$

Step 3. Calculate the number of drops needed, based on the administration set being used, to obtain the required volume.

$$\frac{60 \text{ drops}}{1 \text{ mL}} = \frac{x \text{ drops}}{0.25 \text{ mL}} \quad x = 15 \text{ drops} \quad (23)$$

67. **(C)** This problem may be solved by alligation or by simply using the relationship:

$$Q_1 \times C_1 = Q_2 \times C_2$$

$$[480 \text{ mL}][50\%] = [x \text{ mL}][70\%]$$

$$x = 342 \text{ mL} \quad (4)$$

68. **(B)** One gallon contains 3785 mL; thus 3785 mL × 0.25% = 9.46 or 9.5 g.

Because the volume contributed by the acetic acid is insignificant when compared to 3785 mL, it does not enter into the calculation of the final volume. *(1; 23)*

69. **(D)** Two pounds would contain 454 × 2 = 908 g of ointment. The final preparation would contain 908 g × 2% = 18.18 g of pure hydrocortisone. Because the available hydrocortisone ointment is 5% strength, one would need:

$$\frac{5 \text{ g}}{100 \text{ g}} = \frac{18.6 \text{ g}}{x \text{ g}}$$

$$x = 363.2 \text{ g of the 5\% ointment}$$

Or, using the equation

$$Q_1 \times C_1 = Q_2 \times C_2$$

$$(908 \text{ g}) (2\% \text{ w/w}) = (x \text{ g}) (5\% \text{ w/w})$$

$$x = 363.2 \text{ g} \quad (23)$$

70. **(B)** The total content of the vial will be 20 mL × 4 mg/mL = 80 mg.

The total amount of Dilaudid prescribed per day = 3 mg × 4 (every 6 h around the clock) = 12 mg. 80 mg ÷ 12 mg = 6.67 days. The nearest answer is 6 whole days.

# CHAPTER 3

# Pharmacy

When one peruses the definitions of pharmacy as presented by various state boards of pharmacy, one notices an expansion from the traditional definition of "the art of preparing and dispensing drugs" to "the art or practice of preparing, preserving, compounding, and dispensing drugs plus administering drugs and discovering new drugs through research." With the expanding role of the pharmacist in health care, many states include wording allowing the pharmacist to diagnose and prescribe, usually under set protocols.

Today, pharmacy encompasses all aspects of drug preparation and dispensing, as well as evaluation of therapeutic effects in patients. The term "pharmaceutical care" is being used to stress the duty of the pharmacist to ensure that drug therapy produces maximum beneficial outcomes. This chapter includes basic material with which the practicing pharmacist should be familiar in order to dispense drug products successfully and to serve as the resource person to other health professionals and the general public. This includes knowledge of the manufacture and characteristics of the dosage form, trade names and generic names, drug strengths and commercial dosage forms, packaging, dispensing advice, recognition of significant drug interactions, and the selection of over-the-counter products. Actually, this chapter is intended to include topics and information not specifically designated in the other book chapters. Subsequent chapters stress the pharmacokinetics and therapeutic actions of drugs in the body, the selection of specific drugs to treat various diseases, and the evaluation of therapeutic outcomes.

# Questions

DIRECTIONS (Questions 1 through 203): Each of the numbered items or incomplete statements in this section is followed by answers or by completions of the statement. Select the ONE lettered answer or completion that is BEST in each case.

1. Official standards for individual drugs and chemicals formulated into dosage forms are published in the

    (A) *USP/NF*
    (B) *USP DI* Volume I
    (C) *USP DI* Volume II
    (D) *USP DI* Volume III
    (E) *PDR*

2. The agency in the United States responsible for selecting appropriate nonproprietary names for drugs is the

    (A) AMA
    (B) APhA
    (C) FDA
    (D) USAN
    (E) USP

3. Descriptions of the Federal Controlled Substances Act, Approved Drug Products with Therapeutic Equivalence Evaluations, and USP/NF dispensing requirements may be found in the

    (A) *USP DI* Volume I
    (B) *USP DI* Volume II
    (C) *USP DI* Volume III
    (D) *Facts and Comparisons*
    (E) *PDR*

4. Prescription drug descriptions expressed in layperson's terms and useful as handouts for patients may be photocopied from the

    (A) *USP DI* Volume I
    (B) *USP DI* Volume II
    (C) *USP DI* Volume III
    (D) *Facts and Comparisons*
    (E) *Remington's Pharmaceutical Sciences*

5. The most frequently dispensed dosage form in the United States is the

    (A) oral capsule
    (B) oral solution
    (C) parenteral solution
    (D) oral tablet
    (E) topical ointment or cream

6. Into which one of the following oral dosage forms should a pharmaceutical manufacturer formulate an experimental drug to assure the most rapid absorption from the GI tract?

    (A) capsule
    (B) solution
    (C) suspension
    (D) enteric coated tablet
    (E) compressed tablet

7. Which one of the following series correctly reflects the rates of disintegration for most commercial tablets?

    (A) coated tablets > sublingual tablets > uncoated tablets
    (B) coated tablets > uncoated tablets > sublingual tablets

(C) sublingual tablets > coated tablets > uncoated tablets

(D) sublingual tablets > uncoated tablets > coated tablets

(E) uncoated tablets > coated tablets > sublingual tablets

8. Which of the following types of tablet coatings is (are) used to mask the bitter taste of drugs?

   I. enteric

   II. film

   III. sugar

(A) I only

(B) III only

(C) I and II only

(D) II and III only

(E) I, II, and III

9. Advantages to the manufacturer for tablet film coating when compared to sugar coating include

   I. shorter production times

   II. less gross weight

   III. lower incidence in coat chipping

(A) I only

(B) III only

(C) I and II only

(D) II and III only

(E) I, II, and III

10. Which of the following is NOT used primarily as a diluent in tablet formulations?

(A) magnesium stearate

(B) dicalcium phosphate

(C) lactose

(D) mannitol

(E) starch

11. Which of the following is NOT a function of the lubricant in a tablet formulation?

(A) improving flow properties of granules

(B) reducing powder adhesion onto the dies and punches

(C) improving tablet wetting in the stomach

(D) reducing punch and die wear

(E) facilitating tablet ejection from the die

12. Which of the following trademarked dosage forms is enteric coated?

(A) Enduret

(B) Enseal

(C) Extentab

(D) Filmtab

(E) Spansule

13. A sweetener that is widely employed in chewable tablet formulations is

(A) aspartame

(B) glucose

(C) lactose

(D) mannitol

(E) sucrose

14. Starch may be included in tablet formulations as a

   I. binder

   II. disintegrant

   III. lubricant

(A) I only

(B) III only

(C) I and II only

(D) II and III only

(E) I, II, and III

15. Disintegration tests are required for which of the following types of tablets?

   I. sugar coated

   II. enteric coated

   III. buccal

(A) I only

(B) III only

(C) I and II only

(D) II and III only

(E) I, II, and III

16. Colloidal silicon dioxide is most likely to be included in what type of pharmaceutical dosage form?

    (A) capsules
    (B) parenteral solutions
    (C) pressurized aerosols
    (D) tablets
    (E) troches

17. Which one of the following general characteristics is NOT true for alkaloids?

    (A) contain nitrogen in the molecule
    (B) have good alcohol solubility
    (C) have $pK_a$'s less than 7
    (D) often exhibit stereoisomerism
    (E) have poor water solubility

18. Which of the following alkaloids exhibit(s) good water solubility?

    I.   morphine HCl
    II.  cocaine
    III. atropine

    (A) I only
    (B) III only
    (C) I and II only
    (D) II and III only
    (E) I, II, and III

19. Which of the following forms of the basic drug haloperidol will have good water solubility?

    I.   hydrochloride
    II.  lactate
    III. decanoate

    (A) I only
    (B) III only
    (C) I and II only
    (D) II and III only
    (E) I, II, and III

20. Which one of the following chemicals is NOT suitable as a drug excipient?

    (A) methyl paraben
    (B) starch

    (C) glycerin
    (D) benzocaine
    (E) lactose

21. Which one of the following chemicals may be included in a drug solution as a chelating agent?

    (A) ascorbic acid
    (B) hydroquinone
    (C) edetate
    (D) sodium bisulfite
    (E) fluorescein sodium

22. Which of the following ions may be effectively chelated?

    I.   sodium
    II.  lithium
    III. lead

    (A) I only
    (B) III only
    (C) I and II only
    (D) II and III only
    (E) I, II, and III

23. Solubility of a substance may be expressed in several ways. When a quantitative statement of solubility is given in the USP, it is generally expressed as

    (A) grams of solute soluble in 1 mL of solvent
    (B) grams of solute soluble in 100 mL of solvent
    (C) mL of solvent required to dissolve 1 g of solute
    (D) mL of solvent required to dissolve 100 g of solute
    (E) mL of solvent required to prepare 100 mL of saturated solution

24. Although most drugs in pharmaceutical dosage forms decompose following first-order kinetics, an exception are the drugs formulated in

    (A) capsules
    (B) oral solutions

(C) oral suspensions

(D) tablets

(E) suppositories

25. An early sign of a decomposing epinephrine solution is the presence of a

(A) brown precipitate

(B) pink color

(C) white precipitate

(D) crystal

(E) red color

26. The process of grinding a substance to a very fine powder is termed

(A) levigation

(B) sublimation

(C) trituration

(D) pulverization by intervention

(E) maceration

27. The term "impalpable" refers to a substance that is

(A) bad tasting

(B) not perceptible to the touch

(C) greasy

(D) nongreasy

(E) tasteless

28. Tartrazine may be included in drug products as a (an)

(A) antimicrobial agent

(B) coloring agent

(C) sweetener

(D) solubilizer

(E) antioxidant

29. The term "chiral" is related to a drug's

(A) chelating ability

(B) eutectic properties

(C) stereoisomerism

(D) partition coefficient

(E) complexation

30. Advantages of developing chiral forms of a drug include

I. more specific drug action

II. decreased toxicity

III. more economical product

(A) I only

(B) III only

(C) I and III

(D) II and III

(E) I, II, and III

31. Different crystalline forms (polymorphs) of the same drug exhibit different

I. metabolism rates

II. melting points

III. solubilities

(A) I only

(B) III only

(C) I and II only

(D) II and III only

(E) I, II, and III

32. An example of a nonionic surfactant would be

(A) ammonium laurate

(B) cetylpyridinium chloride

(C) docusate sodium

(D) sorbitan monopalmitate

(E) triethanolamine stearate

33. According to the Poiseuille equation, the factor that has the relatively greatest influence on the rate of flow of liquid through a capillary tube is the

(A) length of the tube

(B) viscosity of the liquid

(C) pressure differential on the tube

(D) radius of the tube

(E) temperature of the liquid

34. Patients following low-sodium diets may resort to the use of sodium-free salt substitutes such as NoSalt. The major ingredient in these products is

    (A) ammonium chloride
    (B) calcium chloride
    (C) potassium chloride
    (D) potassium iodide
    (E) none of these

35. Potassium supplements are administered in all of the following manners EXCEPT

    (A) IV infusion
    (B) IV bolus
    (C) elixirs, po
    (D) effervescent tablets
    (E) slow-release tablets, po

36. Which of the following statements concerning fluorouracil is NOT true?

    (A) Its chemical structure is a modified pyrimidine similar to uracil and idoxuridine.
    (B) It is effective only when administered by injection.
    (C) Anorexia and nausea and vomiting are very common side effects.
    (D) The drug interferes with the synthesis of ribonucleic acid.
    (E) Leukopenia is a major clinical toxic effect.

37. A pharmacist associates a "black box warning" with which of the following?

    (A) drug company disclaimers concerning a product
    (B) drug product inserts
    (C) medical devices
    (D) off-label claims
    (E) TV advertising of drugs

38. Which one of the following sequences lists the three types of cautions found in drug product inserts in the order of least serious to most serious?

    (A) contraindication, precaution, warning
    (B) precaution, warning, contraindication
    (C) warning, contraindication, precaution
    (D) warning, precaution, contraindication
    (E) contraindication, warning, precaution

39. A comparison of individual amino acids present in commercial amino acids injection solutions may be found in

    I. *Facts and Comparisons*
    II. *Trissel's Handbook on Injectable Drugs*
    III. *Remington's Pharmaceutical Sciences*

    (A) I only
    (B) III only
    (C) I and II only
    (D) II and III only
    (E) I, II, and III

40. The containers used to package drugs may consist of several components and/or be composed of several materials. The release of an ingredient from packaging components into the actual product is best described by the term

    (A) absorption
    (B) adsorption
    (C) leaching
    (D) permeation
    (E) porosity

41. The gauge numbers used to size hypodermic needles reflect the needle's

    (A) bevel size
    (B) external diameter of the cannula
    (C) internal diameter of the cannula
    (D) length of the needle
    (E) size of the lumen opening

42. The designation, "winged" needles, is most closely associated with which type of injection?

    (A) intradermal
    (B) intramuscular
    (C) intrathecal
    (D) intravenous
    (E) subcutaneous

43. Insulin preparations are usually administered by

    (A) intradermal injection
    (B) intramuscular injection
    (C) intravenous bolus
    (D) intravenous infusion
    (E) subcutaneous injection

44. Which one of the following needles is most suited for the administration of insulin solutions?

    (A) 16G 5/8"
    (B) 21G 1/2"
    (C) 21G 5/8"
    (D) 25G 5/8"
    (E) 25G 1"

45. The term "venoclysis" is most closely associated with

    (A) intravenous injections
    (B) intrathecal injections
    (C) intravenous infusions
    (D) intrapleural withdrawals
    (E) peritoneal dialysis

46. The designation "minibottles" refers to

    (A) partially filled parenteral bottles with 50- to 150-mL volumes
    (B) any parenteral bottle with a capacity of less than 1 L
    (C) 10–30 mL glass vials
    (D) prescription bottles with capacities of 4 oz or less
    (E) vials with a capacity of less than 10 mL

47. The term "piggyback" is most commonly associated with

    (A) intermittent therapy
    (B) intrathecal injections
    (C) intravenous bolus
    (D) slow intravenous infusions
    (E) total parenteral nutrition

48. Which of the following acronyms refer to parenteral nutrition?

    I. TPN
    II. TNA
    III. PMN

    (A) I only
    (B) III only
    (C) I and II only
    (D) II and III only
    (E) I, II, and III

49. What is the approximate maximum volume of fluid that should be administered daily by intravenous infusion to a stabilized patient?

    (A) 1 L
    (B) 4 L
    (C) 8 L
    (D) 12 L
    (E) 16 L

50. Although isotonicity is desirable for almost all parenterals, it is particularly critical for which injections?

    (A) intra-articular
    (B) intradermal
    (C) intramuscular
    (D) intravenous
    (E) subcutaneous

51. A suspension is NOT a suitable dosage form for what type of injection?

    (A) intra-articular
    (B) intradermal
    (C) intramuscular
    (D) intravenous
    (E) subcutaneous

52. Which one of the following designations is most appropriate for a medical order requiring an intravenous bolus injection?

    (A) per IV
    (B) IVP
    (C) IVPB
    (D) po
    (E) KVO

53. Even distribution of a drug into the blood after an IV bolus injection can be expected

    (A) instantaneously
    (B) within 4 min
    (C) in 5–10 min
    (D) within 30 min
    (E) only after a few hours

54. The quantities of all ingredients present in parenteral solutions must be specified on the label EXCEPT for

    I.   antimicrobial preservatives
    II.  isotonicity adjustors
    III. pH adjustors

    (A) I only
    (B) III only
    (C) I and II only
    (D) II and III only
    (E) I, II, and III

55. The usual expiration dating that should be placed on a parenteral admixture prepared in a hospital pharmacy is

    (A) 1 h
    (B) 24 h
    (C) 48 h
    (D) 72 h
    (E) 1 week

56. Parenteral solutions that are isotonic with human red blood cells have an osmolality of approximately how many mOsm/L?

    (A) 20
    (B) 40
    (C) 50
    (D) 150
    (E) 300

57. Which of the following injectables is (are) isotonic with human red blood cells?

    I.   $D_5W$
    II.  $D_{2.5}W/0.45NS$
    III. $D_5W/NS$

    (A) I only
    (B) III only
    (C) I and II
    (D) II and III
    (E) I, II, and III

58. The osmotic pressure of a 0.1 molar dextrose solution will be approximately how many times that of a 0.1-molar sodium chloride solution?

    (A) 0.5
    (B) 1
    (C) 2
    (D) 3
    (E) 4

59. Which one of the following parenteral solutions is considered to most closely approximate the extracellular fluid of the human body?

    (A) Dextrose 2.5% and sodium chloride 0.45% injection
    (B) Lactated Ringer's injection
    (C) Ringer's injection
    (D) Sodium chloride injection
    (E) Sodium lactate injection

60. Which of the following types of injection routes should be limited to volumes 1 mL or less?

    I.   intramuscular into gluteus maximus
    II.  intramuscular into deltoid
    III. subcutaneous

    (A) I only
    (B) III only
    (C) I and III
    (D) II and III
    (E) I, II, and III

61. Which one of the following routes of parenteral administration is suitable for injecting the smallest volume of drug solution?

    (A) intravenous
    (B) intramucular
    (C) intrathecal
    (D) intradermal
    (E) subcutaneous

62. An IM injection site suitable for a small child (<3 years of age) is the

    (A) gluteus maximus
    (B) gluteus minimal
    (C) gluteus ultima
    (D) ventrogluteal
    (E) vastus lateralis

63. Which of the following parenteral routes of administration is (are) considered suitable for heparin sodium injection USP?

    I.   continuous IV infusion
    II.  subcutaneous
    III. intramuscular

    (A) I only
    (B) III only
    (C) I and II only
    (D) II and III only
    (E) I, II, and III

64. Which of the following parenteral routes of administration is (are) commonly employed for the administration of insulin USP?

    I.   continuous IV infusion
    II.  subcutaneous
    III. intramuscular

    (A) I only
    (B) III only
    (C) I and III only
    (D) II and III only
    (E) I, II, and III

65. Which of the following facts concerning regular insulin is (are) true?

    I.   Degradation occurs only in the liver.
    II.  Product is available without a prescription.
    III. Drug has a short plasma half-life.

    (A) I only
    (B) III only
    (C) I and III only
    (D) II and III only
    (E) I, II, and III

66. The parenteral system known as "ADD-Vantage" is best described as being a

    (A) disposable needle and syringe
    (B) premixed minibag of drug solution
    (C) two-compartment container
    (D) vial attached to a minibag of diluent
    (E) burette type of administration set

67. IVAC's CRIS (controlled-release infusion system) is best described as being

    (A) a plastic disposable adaptor
    (B) a minipump
    (C) a volumetric burette
    (D) an implantable catheter
    (E) a magnetically controlled infusion device

68. An example of an implantable catheter for the administration of parenteral solutions is the

    (A) Hickman
    (B) Foley
    (C) Broviac
    (D) Port-A-Cath
    (E) Port-In-Fuse

69. Which of the descriptions of Pharmacy Bulk Packages is (are) true?

    I.   units intended for preparation of sterile parenterals
    II.  do not have an antimicrobial preservative
    III. may be used for direct infusion of drugs into patients

    (A) I only
    (B) III only
    (C) I and II only
    (D) II and III only
    (E) I, II, and III

70. Parenteral containers of potassium chloride concentrate must be packaged

    (A) as single dose units only
    (B) in vials not greater than 20 mL capacity
    (C) in vials with a capacity of 10 mL or less
    (D) with a black flip-off button
    (E) with a red flip-off button

71. What is the usual maximum volume allowed as a parenteral package for Bacteriostatic Water for Injection?

    (A) 10 mL
    (B) 20 mL
    (C) 30 mL
    (D) 50 mL
    (E) 60 mL

72. The antimicrobial agent, methylparaben, is an ester of

    (A) benzoic acid
    (B) *p*-hydroxybenzoic acid
    (C) *p*-aminosalicylic acid
    (D) propionic acid
    (E) benzyl alcohol

73. Which of the following vitamins possesses antioxidant properties?

    I. ascorbic acid
    II. ergocalciferol
    III. pantothenic acid

    (A) I only
    (B) III only
    (C) I and III only
    (D) II and III only
    (E) I, II, and III

74. Which one of the following parenteral antibiotics is the most stable in an aqueous solution?

    (A) gentamicin sulfate
    (B) amoxicillin sodium
    (C) oxacillin sodium
    (D) tetracycline hydrochloride
    (E) vancomycin hydrochloride

75. Biologicals can be used to obtain either active or passive immunity. Which one of the following pairs is NOT correct?

    (A) antiserum, passive immunity
    (B) antitoxin, passive immunity
    (C) human immune serum, active immunity
    (D) toxoid, active immunity
    (E) vaccine, active immunity

76. Which one of the following is a vaccine used for active immunization against measles (rubeola)?

    (A) Attenuvax
    (B) Fluogen
    (C) Recombivax HB
    (D) Havrix
    (E) Sabin

77. The route of administration for tuberculin USP is

    (A) intradermal
    (B) subcutaneous
    (C) intramuscular
    (D) intra-arterial
    (E) interarticular

78. The intermediate tuberculin skin test (intermediate strength PPD) contains

    (A) 2 tuberculin units
    (B) 5 tuberculin units
    (C) 25 tuberculin units
    (D) 250 tuberculin units
    (E) 500 tuberculin units

79. Tuberculin syringes are

    I. only suitable for administration of TB vaccine
    II. prefilled syringes
    III. 1 mL units with 0.05 mL accuracy

    (A) I only
    (B) III only
    (C) I and III
    (D) II and III
    (F) I, II, and III

80. Immune serum globulin (gamma globulin) is usually administered by what type of injection?

(A) intradermal
(B) intramuscular
(C) intravenous
(D) subcutaneous
(E) any of the usual methods of injection

81. Pediarix is a combination vaccine for protection against all of the following EXCEPT

(A) diphtheria
(B) hepatitis B
(C) hepatitis C
(D) pertussis
(E) polio

82. Which of the vaccines should NOT be administered to pregnant women?

I. measles
II. mumps
III. rubella

(A) I only
(B) III only
(C) I and III only
(D) II and III only
(E) I, II, and III

83. Which of the following preparations will induce passive rather than active immunity?

(A) tetanus toxoid
(B) botulism antitoxin
(C) typhoid vaccine
(D) mumps virus vaccine, attenuated
(E) cholera vaccine

84. All of the following descriptions of toxoids are true EXCEPT

(A) detoxified toxins
(B) antigens
(C) produce permanent immunity
(D) are often available in a precipitated or adsorbed form
(E) produce artificial active immunity

85. The DTP series of injections is intended for administration to

(A) infants
(B) children
(C) children 6 years and older
(D) children and adults
(E) only after puberty

86. All of the following are viral infections EXCEPT

(A) influenza
(B) measles
(C) mumps
(D) hepatitis
(E) typhoid fever

87. Which of the following populations are good candidates for the pneumonia vaccine?

I. geriatrics
II. young adults
III. infants

(A) I only
(B) III only
(C) I and II only
(D) II and III only
(E) I, II, and III

88. The usual storage condition specified for biologicals is

(A) below 2°C
(B) 2–8°C
(C) a cool place
(D) 8–15°C
((E) room temperature

89. The usual method of administering smallpox vaccine is

(A) intradermal injection
(B) intramuscular injection
(D) subcutaneous injection
(D) oral solution
(E) oral suspension

90. Techniques used in the development of "biotechnological drugs" include

    I. gene splicing
    II. preparation of monoclonal antibodies
    III. lyophilization

    (A) I only
    (B) III only
    (C) I and II only
    (D) II and III only
    (E) I, II, and III

91. Which of the following are used to prepare "targeted drug delivery systems"?

    I. liposomes
    II. nanoparticles
    III. transdermal patches

    (A) I only
    (B) III only
    (C) I and II only
    (D) II and III only
    (E) I, II, and III

92. Most of the recently developed biotechnological drugs are formulated into which dosage form?

    (A) inhalation solutions
    (B) parenteral
    (C) capsules
    (D) tablets
    (E) topicals

93. Which one of the following drugs is NOT prepared by recombinant DNA technology?

    (A) human growth hormone
    (B) epoietin alpha
    (C) Humulin
    (D) interferon
    (E) urokinase

94. Which of the following home diagnostic tests incorporates monoclonal antibodies into the testing procedure?

    I. fecal occult blood
    II. ovulation prediction
    III. pregnancy determination

    (A) I only
    (B) III only
    (C) I and II only
    (D) II and III only
    (E) I, II, and III

95. The Norplant implant system is

    I. inserted under the skin
    II. effective for only 1 year
    III. classified as a targeted delivery system

    (A) I only
    (B) III only
    (C) I and II only
    (D) II and III only
    (E) I, II, and III

96. Which one of the following descriptions best fits units such as Baxter's Intermates?

    (A) elastomeric balloons
    (B) minibags containing preset amounts of a drug
    (C) disposable prefilled plastic syringes
    (D) PCAs
    (E) multidose vials

97. Which of the following is (are) true concerning patient-controlled analgesia (PCA) devices?

    I. Unit is intended to be used only with analgesics.
    II. Patient may be ambulatory when using the unit.
    III. Bolus dosing is possible with the unit.

    (A) I only
    (B) III only
    (C) I and II only
    (D) II and III only
    (E) I, II, and III

98. Which of the following statements is (are) true concerning the elastomeric balloon pumps such as Intermate or Homepump?

    I.   Unit may be used in the home for ambulatory patient.
    II.  Unit is refillable.
    III. Bolus dosing is possible with the unit.

    (A) I only
    (B) III only
    (C) I and II only
    (D) II and III only
    (E) I, II, and III

99. Colostomy pouches are classified by

    I.   an open versus closed design
    II.  size of stoma
    III. whether for a male or female

    (A) I only
    (B) III only
    (C) I and II only
    (D) II and III only
    (E) I, II, and III

100. Which of the following is considered effective in the treatment of accidental drug poisoning?

    I.   activated charcoal
    II.  ipecac syrup
    III. universal antidote

    (A) I only
    (B) III only
    (C) I and II only
    (D) II and III only
    (E) I, II, and III

101. While most iron salts are administered orally, a commercially available parenteral product is

    (A) Chel-Iron
    (B) Feosol
    (C) Simron
    (D) DexFerrum
    (E) Troph-Iron

102. Which of the following statements concerning iron sucrose injection is (are) accurate?

    I.   Indications are similar to those for iron dextran injection.
    II.  It may be administered using Z-track injection techniques.
    III. It is indicated for treatment of iron deficiency anemia in hemodialysis patients.

    (A) I only
    (B) III only
    (C) I and II only
    (D) II and III only
    (E) I, II, and III

103. Which one of the following chemicals is an effective and safe drug in the treatment of either diarrhea or constipation?

    (A) activated charcoal
    (B) bismuth salts
    (C) kaolin
    (D) attapulgite
    (E) polycarbophil

104. Simethicone is most likely to be included in what type of OTC product?

    (A) antacid
    (B) cough product
    (C) decongestant
    (D) laxative
    (E) weight control

105. Insoluble bismuth salts are used as adsorbents and also possess useful astringent and protective properties. A commercial product containing a bismuth compound is

    (A) Bisacodyl
    (B) Donnagel
    (C) Kaopectate
    (D) Pepto-bismol
    (E) Rheaban

106. Which of the following antidiarrheal products contains the adsorbent clay attapulgite?

    I.   Donnagel
    II.  Kaopectate caplets
    III. Mitrolan

    (A) I only
    (B) III only
    (C) I and II only
    (D) II and III only
    (E) I, II, and III

107. A common building block for liposomes are the

    (A) anionic surfactants plus mineral oil
    (B) nonionic surfactants plus mineral oil
    (C) phospholipids
    (D) polyethylene glycols
    (E) straight chain hydrocarbons combined with phosphoric acid

108. Liposomal dosage forms are suited for which of the following routes of administration?

    I.   parenteral
    II.  topical
    III. oral

    (A) I only
    (B) III only
    (C) I and II only
    (D) II and III only
    (E) I, II, and III

109. Which of the following internal analgesic products contain ketoprofen?

    I.   Actron
    II.  Aleve
    III. Nuprin

    (A) I only
    (B) III only
    (C) I and II only
    (D) II and III only
    (E) I, II, and III

110. Which of the following drugs have label warnings against their use during pregnancy, especially during the last trimester?

    I.   acetaminophen
    II.  aspirin
    III. ibuprofen

    (A) I only
    (B) III only
    (C) I and II only
    (D) II and III only
    (E) I, II, and III

111. Which one of the following OTC internal analgesics contains magnesium salicylate?

    (A) Bromo-Seltzer
    (B) Doan's Original
    (C) Ecotrin
    (D) Pamprin
    (E) Sinarest

112. Characteristics of dextromethorphan as a cough suppressant include all of the following EXCEPT

    (A) as effective as codeine on a weight/weight basis
    (B) does not cause respiratory depression
    (C) is nonaddicting
    (D) doses of 10–15 mg suppress coughing for at least 4 h
    (E) maximum daily adult dose is 30 mg

113. Disadvantages of calcium carbonate as an antacid include all of the following EXCEPT

    (A) some patients may develop hypercalcemia
    (B) capacity for acid neutralization is poor
    (C) may cause constipation
    (D) may induce gastric hypersecretion
    (E) prolonged use may induce renal calculi and decreased renal function

114. Which of the following products contain calcium carbonate as the active ingredient?

I. Basaljel capsules
II. Rolaids chewable tablets
III. Titralac chewable tablets

(A) I only
(B) III only
(C) I and II only
(D) II and III only
(E) I, II, and III

115. Which one of the following antacid products is a chemical combination of aluminum and magnesium hydroxides?

(A) Gelusil
(B) Maalox
(C) Mylanta
(D) Riopan
(E) Tums

116. Which one of the following ingredients is NOT present in OTC laxative products marketed in the United States?

(A) bisacodyl
(B) docusate
(C) cellulose
(D) phenolphthalein
(E) sennosides

117. Which one of the following statements concerning bisacodyl is NOT true?

(A) Laxative action occurs within 6 h after oral administration.
(B) Action of the suppositories occurs within 1 h of insertion.
(C) Suppositories may cause rectal irritation with continued administration.
(D) Tablets should be swallowed whole.
(E) Tablets should be administered with milk to avoid gastric irritation.

118. Which one of the following OTC products does NOT contain bisacodyl as the active ingredient?

(A) Correctol
(B) ExLax, Regular Strength
(C) ExLax, Ultra
(D) Carter's Laxative
(E) Fleet Stimulant Laxative

119. Which one of the following statements concerning tablet dissolution is NOT true?

(A) Disintegration precedes dissolution.
(B) In vivo disintegration is usually a good predictor of dissolution.
(C) Changing a drug's crystalline state may change dissolution rates.
(D) Increasing tablet compression will increase dissolution rates.
(E) Micronization of drug powder will decrease dissolution times.

120. A product label indicates storage in a refrigerator. Which of the following condition is most appropriate for the product?

(A) a location held between 0°C and 4°C
(B) a cold place held between 2°C and 8°C
(C) any place with temperature between 0°C and 32°F
(D) an air-conditioned room with temperature below 32°C
(E) a freezer

121. A patient requests a container of Abreva. In which section of a pharmacy would this product most likely be stocked?

(A) cold sore remedies
(B) cough products
(C) with the prescription drugs
(D) in the refrigerator of the prescription department
(E) vitamins

122. Aspartame is included in some drug products as a (an)

(A) nutrient
(B) vitamin
(C) solubilizer
(D) sweetener
(E) stimulant

**123.** The term "circadian rhythm" refers to which of the following?

(A) irregular heart beats

(B) biological events that occur in one-month intervals

(C) normal consequential heart beat

(D) cycles of approximately 24 h

(E) breathing patterns

**124.** An antihypertensive drug product that is based on circadian rhythm is

(A) Catapres (clonidine)

(B) Covera-HS (verapamil)

(C) Aldomet (methyldopa)

(D) Monopril (fosinopril)

(E) Vasotec (enalapril)

**125.** Which of the following properties is desirable in a pharmaceutical suspension?

  I. caking

 II. pseudoplastic flow

III. thixotropy

(A) I only

(B) III only

(C) I and II only

(D) II and III only

(E) I, II, and III

**126.** Characteristics of inhalation aerosol dosage forms include

  I. avoid first-pass effect

 II. rapid onset of action

III. can administer large amounts of drug to intended site

(A) I only

(B) III only

(C) I and II only

(D) II and III only

(E) I, II, and III

**127.** Which of the following ingredients is (are) packaged as OTC MDI for asthmatics?

  I. epinephrine

 II. albuterol

III. ephedrine

(A) I only

(B) III only

(C) I and II only

(D) II and III only

(E) I,II, and III

**128.** Burns are classified according to relative severity. Characteristics of a first-degree burn are

(A) erythema, pain, no blistering

(B) erythema, pain, blistering

(C) blisters, pain, skin will regenerate

(D) no blisters, leathery appearance of skin, skin grafting necessary

(E) blackened skin, danger of deep infection

**129.** Benzocaine may be present in some OTC products as

(A) an appetite suppressant

(B) a topical antiseptic

(C) a preservative

(D) a source of nitrogen

(E) an antiasthmatic

**130.** Effective local anesthetics present in OTC burn remedies include

  I. benzocaine

 II. lidocaine

III. phenol

(A) I only

(B) III only

(C) I and II only

(D) II and III only

(E) I, II, and III

**131.** For effectiveness as a local anesthetic, the level of benzocaine in a topical preparation should be AT LEAST

(A) 0.1%

(B) 1.0%

(C) 2.0%

(D) 5.0%

(E) 25%

132. Which one of the following statements concerning dextranomer (Debrisan by Johnson & Johnson) is NOT correct?

(A) aids in the removal of wound exudates

(B) can be used to treat decubitus ulcers

(C) consists of spherical hydrophilic beads

(D) is effective in the healing of both secreting and nonsecreting wounds

(E) must be physically removed after treatment

133. A basal thermometer is

(A) used to detect neuroleptic malignant syndrome (NMS)

(B) used to estimate time of ovulation

(C) used to determine basal metabolic rate

(D) graduated only in Celsius degrees

(E) used vaginally

134. Rectal clinical thermometers differ from oral thermometers in

(A) bulb shape

(B) stem length

(C) distance between graduation marks on the stem

(D) standards for accuracy

(E) stem shape

135. Which one of the following statements concerning allergic reactions to insect bites and stings is NOT true?

(A) Cross-sensitization to bites of different insects (ants, wasps, bees, etc.) can be expected.

(B) Death may occur due to anaphylactic reaction.

(C) The initial systemic reaction will usually occur within 20 min of the time of the bite.

(D) The toxicity of the venom is the prime cause of the severe reaction or death.

(E) Subsequent sting episodes usually cause more severe reactions than the earlier stings.

136. Emergency insect sting and bite kits usually contain all of the following except

(A) antiseptic pads

(B) antihistamines

(C) epinephrine HCl injection

(D) tourniquet

(E) tweezers

137. An ileostomy differs from a colostomy in which of the following characteristics?

I. The discharge from an ileostomy is more viscous.

II. The stoma is significantly larger.

III. The discharge is more irritating to the skin.

(A) I only

(B) III only

(C) I and II only

(D) II and III only

(E) I, II, and III

138. The "French" scale is commonly used in this country for denoting the diameters of

I. urinary catheters

II. enteral feeding tubes

III. syringe needles

(A) I only

(B) III only

(C) I and II only

(D) II and III only

(E) I, II, and III

139. Pamabrom is present in certain OTC products as a (an)

(A) analgesic

(B) diuretic

(C) antirheumatic

(D) sedative

(E) mild stimulant

140. Which one of the following procedures or ingredients has been recognized by the FDA for the removal of ear cerumen?

    (A) carbamide peroxide
    (B) diluted acetic acid
    (C) cotton tips wetted with warm water
    (D) cotton tips wetted with alcohol
    (E) vinegar

141. Which one of the following procedures would NOT improve the absorption of a drug into the skin?

    (A) applying the ointment and covering the area with an occlusive bandage or Saran wrap
    (B) incorporating an oil-soluble drug in polyethylene glycol ointment rather than white ointment
    (C) applying the medicated ointment on the back of the hand rather than on the palms
    (D) increasing the concentration of the active drug in the ointment bases
    (E) using an ointment base in which the active drug has excellent solubility

142. Melatonin is available in some products as a (an)

    (A) amino acid supplement
    (B) sleep aid
    (C) digestant
    (D) noncaloric sweetener
    (E) coloring agent

143. The cosmetic lotion, Eucerin Light Moisture-Restorative, contains allantoin, which is present as a (an)

    (A) antibacterial agent
    (B) antifungal agent
    (C) antipruritic
    (D) emollient
    (E) vulnerary (healing agent)

144. Most commercial vaginal suppositories use a base of

    (A) beeswax
    (B) cocoa butter
    (C) glycerin
    (D) glycerinated gelatin
    (E) polyethylene glycols

145. Which one of the following diluents is usually used for compressed vaginal tablet formulation?

    (A) lactose
    (B) starch
    (C) sucrose
    (D) talc
    (E) glucose

146. Characteristics of rectal drug administration include all of the following EXCEPT

    (A) neutral pH of colon fluids lessens possible drug inactivation by stomach acidity
    (B) drugs may avoid first-pass hepatic inactivation
    (C) drugs intended for systemic activity can be administered
    (D) the release and absorption of drugs is predictable
    (E) irritating drugs have less effect on the rectum than on the stomach

147. Which of the following vaginal suppository products have contraceptive properties?

    I. Norforms
    II. Terazol
    III. Semicid

    (A) I only
    (B) III only
    (C) I and II only
    (D) II and III only
    (E) I, II, and III

148. Carbomers may be included in a topical product as

    (A) antimicrobial preservatives
    (B) buffers
    (C) penetration enhancers
    (D) sweeteners
    (E) thickening agents

149. Colligative properties are useful in determining

(A) tonicity
(B) pH
(C) solubility
(D) sterility
(E) stability

150. The colligative properties of a solution are related to the

(A) total number of solute particles
(B) pH
(C) number of ions
(D) number of unionized molecules
(E) the ratio of the number of ions to the number of molecules

151. Which one of the following values must be similar for a solution to be considered isotonic with blood?

(A) total salt content
(B) pH
(C) fluid pressure
(D) osmotic pressure
(E) level of sodium chloride present

152. Mixing a hypertonic solution with red blood cells may cause___of the red blood cells.

(A) bursting
(B) chelating
(C) crenation
(D) hemolysis
(E) hydrolysis

153. Sodium chloride equivalents are used to estimate the amount of sodium chloride needed to render a solution isotonic. The sodium chloride equivalent or "E" value may be defined as the

(A) amount of sodium chloride that is theoretically equivalent to 1 g of a specified chemical
(B) amount of a specified chemical theoretically equivalent to 1 g of sodium chloride
(C) milliequivalents of sodium chloride needed to render a solution isotonic

(D) weight of a specified chemical that will render a solution isotonic
(E) percent sodium chloride needed to make a solution isotonic

154. Which one of the following reference sources has the most extensive listings of sodium chloride equivalents and freezing point depression values?

(A) *Merck Manual*
(B) *Merck Index*
(C) *Remington*
(D) *USP/NF*
(E) *USP DI*

155. A second method commonly used for adjusting solutions to isotonicity is based on

(A) boiling point elevation
(B) blood coagulation time
(C) freezing point depression
(D) milliequivalent calculation
(E) refractive index

156. Evaluate the following two statements. All aqueous solutions that freeze at −0.52°C are isotonic with red blood cells. They are also iso-osmotic with each other.

(A) Both statements are true.
(B) Both statements are false.
(C) The first statement is true but the second is false.
(D) The second statement is true but the first is false.
(E) There is no correlation between freezing points and osmotic pressures of solutions.

157. The capacity of the human eye for instilled ophthalmic drops is approximately

(A) 0.01–0.05 mL
(B) 0.1 mL
(C) 0.5 mL
(D) 1.0 mL
(E) 2.0 mL

158. All of the following have been included in ophthalmic solutions as viscosity builders EXCEPT

    (A) hydroxypropylmethylcellulose
    (B) polyvinyl alcohol
    (C) polyvinylpyrrolidone
    (D) methylcellulose
    (E) Veegum

159. What is the main reason for including methylcellulose and similar agents in ophthalmic solutions?

    (A) increase drop size
    (B) increase ocular contact time
    (C) reduce inflammation of the eye
    (D) reduce tearing during instillation of the drops
    (E) reduce drop size

160. The presence of *Pseudomonas aeruginosa* would be of particular danger in an ophthalmic solution of

    (A) atropine sulfate
    (B) fluorescein sodium
    (C) pilocarpine hydrochloride
    (D) silver nitrate
    (E) zinc sulfate

161. A microorganism that has resulted in ophthalmic infections in patients using contact lens solutions is

    (A) *Acanthamoeba*
    (B) *Aspergillus*
    (C) *Escherichia*
    (D) *Helicobacter*
    (E) *Trichophyton*

162. The combination of preservatives that appears to be most effective for ophthalmic use consists of

    (A) benzalkonium chloride and edetate
    (B) benzalkonium chloride and chlorobutanol
    (C) chlorobutanol and EDTA
    (D) methyl and propyl paraben
    (E) phenylmercuric nitrate and phenylethyl alcohol

163. Which of the following ingredients may be present in soft contact lens cleaning products to remove protein buildup?

    I.   benzalkonium chloride
    II.  subtilisin
    III. papain

    (A) I only
    (B) III only
    (C) I and II only
    (D) II and III only
    (E) I, II, and III

164. The presence of sodium bisulfite in a drug solution implies that the drug

    (A) has poor water solubility
    (B) is heat labile
    (C) is susceptible to oxidation
    (D) requires an alkaline media
    (E) will sustain growth of microorganisms

165. Which one of the following side effects occurs in some individuals who are sensitive to bisulfites?

    (A) difficulty in breathing
    (B) a dry cough
    (C) diarrhea
    (D) dizziness
    (E) upset stomach

166. Which of the following descriptions is (are) correct concerning the sterilization by membrane filtration of an extemporaneously prepared solution?

    I.   suitable for heat labile drug solutions
    II.  convenient for sterilizing small volumes
    III. greater assurance of sterility than using autoclaving

    (A) I only
    (B) III only
    (C) I and II only
    (D) II and III only
    (E) I, II, and III

167. Which of the following ophthalmic solutions may be dispensed on a prescription for epinephrine borate solution?

    I. Epinal (Alcon)
    II. Epifrin (Allergan)
    III. Glaucon (Alcon)

    (A) I only
    (B) III only
    (C) I and II only
    (D) II and III only
    (E) I, II, and III

168. What is the prime reason why pharmaceutical companies will utilize a lyophilized powder in a parenteral vial?

    (A) enhance the solubility of the active drug
    (B) increase the rate of dissolution of the active drug
    (C) increase the stability of the drug
    (D) improve the bioavailability of the drug
    (E) reduce the production cost

169. Which one of the following ingredients may be included in lyophilized products as a bulking agent?

    (A) benzalkonium chloride
    (B) mannitol
    (C) magnesium oxide
    (D) aspartame
    (E) zinc chloride

170. Benzyl alcohol is present in some parenteral solutions as a (an)

    (A) antimicrobial preservative
    (B) antioxidant
    (C) chelating agent
    (D) buffering agent
    (E) tonicity adjuster

171. pH is mathematically

    (A) the log of the hydroxyl ion concentration
    (B) the negative log of the hydroxyl ion concentration
    (C) the log of the hydronium ion concentration
    (D) the negative log of the hydronium ion concentration
    (E) none of the above

172. Data required to determine the pH of a buffer system include

    I. molar concentration of the weak acid present
    II. the p$K_a$ of the weak acid
    III. the volume of solution present

    (A) I only
    (B) III only
    (C) I and II only
    (D) II and III only
    (E) I, II, and III

173. pH is equal to p$K_a$ at

    (A) pH 1
    (B) pH 7
    (C) the neutralization point
    (D) the end point
    (E) the half-neutralization point

**Answer questions 174 through 177 by referring to the following table as necessary.**

TABLE OF p$K_a$ VALUES FOR ACIDS

| Acid | p$K_a$ |
| --- | --- |
| Acetic | 4.76 |
| Acetylsalicylic | 3.49 |
| Boric | 9.24 |
| Lactic | 3.86 |
| Salicylic | 2.97 |

174. Which one of the following acids would have the greatest degree of ionization in water?

    (A) acetic
    (B) boric
    (C) hydrochloric
    (D) lactic
    (E) salicylic

175. Which one of the following acids would be considered the weakest (with the least amount of ionization) in water?

    (A) acetic
    (B) acetylsalicylic
    (C) boric
    (D) lactic
    (E) salicylic

176. To prepare a buffer system with the greatest buffer capacity at a pH of 4.0, one would use which one of the following acids?

    (A) acetic
    (B) acetylsalicylic
    (C) boric
    (D) lactic
    (E) salicylic

177. A pharmacist prepares a buffer system by mixing 1 dL of 0.005 molar boric acid with 1 dL of 0.05 molar sodium borate in sufficient water to make 1 L. What will be the approximate pH of this solution?

    (A) 8.24
    (B) 9.24
    (C) 10.24
    (D) <8.0
    (E) >10.5

178. Ibuprofen has a $pK_a$ of 5.5. If the pH of a patient's urine is 7.5, what would be the ratio of disassociated to undisassociated drug?

    (A) 2:1
    (B) 100:1
    (C) 20:1
    (D) 1:2
    (E) 1:100

179. A patient has consumed a large number of aspirin tablets. The pH of her urine is 4.5. What percentage of the aspirin is present in the un-ionized form if the $pK_a$ of aspirin is 3.5?

    (A) 10
    (B) 20

    (C) 50
    (D) 90
    (E) 100

180. Characteristics of drugs intended for formulation into sustained-release dosage forms include

    I. usually given in doses of 500 mg t.i.d.
    II. intended for treatment of chronic conditions
    III. have a high therapeutic index

    (A) I only
    (B) III only
    (C) I and II only
    (D) II and III only
    (E) I, II, and III

181. Drugs with which of the following half-lives are the best candidates for oral sustained-release formulations?

    (A) <1 h
    (B) 1–2 h
    (C) 4–8 h
    (D) 12–16 h
    (E) >16 h

182. Which of the following trademarked sustained-release systems are based on encapsulated drug particles that will dissolve at various rates?

    I. Sequels
    II. Spansules
    III. Extentabs

    (A) I only
    (B) III only
    (C) I and II only
    (D) II and III only
    (E) I, II, and III

183. Drugs that are available as sustained-release dosage forms utilizing ion-exchange resins include

    I. Ionamin
    II. Contac
    III. Fero-Gradumet

(A) I only

(B) III only

(C) I and II only

(D) II and III only

(E) I, II, and III

184. Drug products that utilize the osmotic pressure–controlled drug delivery system include

   I. Efidac/24

   II. Acutrim

   III. Contac

(A) I only

(B) III only

(C) I and II only

(D) II and III only

(E) I, II, and III

185. Which of the following drug products is (are) suitable for sprinkling the contents of the opened capsule onto applesauce before consuming?

   I. Depakote

   II. Effexor XR

   III. Ditropan XL

(A) I only

(B) III only

(C) I and II only

(D) II and III only

(E) I, II, and III

186. According to the USP, the instruction "protect from light" in a monograph indicates storage in a (an)

(A) dark place

(B) amber glass bottle

(C) light-resistant container

(D) hermetic container

(E) tight glass container

187. The label for trazodone tablets indicates the presence of yellow ferric oxide. For which one of the following reasons is this ingredient most likely to be present?

(A) prevent oxidation of the active drug

(B) keep the drug in the oxidized state

(C) increase the rate of absorption

(D) give color to the tablet

(E) provide a daily dose of iron

188. The expiration date on a pharmaceutical container states "Expires July 2007." This statement means that by that expiration date, the product may have lost

(A) up to 5% of its activity

(B) up to 10% of its activity

(C) at least 10% of its activity

(D) at least 50% of its activity

(E) sufficient activity to be outside USP monograph requirements

189. A pharmacist has reconstituted a powder dosage form to form a solution. Which of the following statement(s) concerning a beyond-use date is (are) appropriate when determining an expiration date for this product

   I. The beyond-use date is identical to the manufacturer's expiration date.

   II. The beyond-use date is never more than 10 days for reconstituted products.

   III. The beyond-use date for nonsolid dosage forms shall not be greater than 1 year from the date of dispensing.

(A) I only

(B) III only

(C) I and II only

(D) II and III only

(E) I, II, and III

190. A reconstituted drug solution assays at 1.5 mg/mL after 24 h. What is the first-order reaction rate if the original solution concentration was 2.0 mg/mL?

(A) 0.2/day

(B) 0.25/day

(C) 0.3/day

(D) 0.33/day

(E) 0.5/day

191. By storing the above-reconstituted drug solution in the refrigerator, its half-life is extended to 4 days. What will be the concentration of the drug solution (mg/mL) after 12 days?

    (A) 0.25 mg/mL
    (B) 0.5 mg/mL
    (C) 1.0 mg/mL
    (D) 1.2 mg/mL
    (E) 1.5 mg/mL

192. When reconstituted, an experimental biotech drug follows first-order kinetics and has a half-life of 24 h. If the original solution has a concentration of 10,000 units/mL, how many mL should be injected into a rabbit three days after the solution was reconstituted if a dose of 2000 units is desired?

    (A) 1.0 mL
    (B) 1.6 mL
    (C) 2.0 mL
    (D) 3.2 mL
    (E) 5.8 mL

193. For which one of the following categories of chemicals is denaturation a major stability problem?

    (A) amino acids
    (B) benzodiazepines
    (C) catecholamines
    (D) cephalosporins
    (E) proteins

194. Which one of the following chemicals is NOT suitable for use as an antioxidant?

    (A) ascorbyl palmitate
    (B) ascorbic acid
    (C) butylated hydroxytoluene
    (D) chlorobutanol
    (E) vitamin E

195. Units for expressing radioisotope decay include the

    I.  Rad
    II. Curie
    III. Becquerel

    (A) I only
    (B) III only
    (C) I and II only
    (D) II and III only
    (E) I, II, and III

196. The decay of radioactive atoms occurs

    (A) at a constant rate
    (B) as a first-order reaction
    (C) as a zero-order reaction
    (D) as a second-order reaction
    (E) at constantly increasing rates

197. Which one of the following forms of radiation has the greatest penetrating power?

    (A) alpha radiation
    (B) beta radiation
    (C) gamma radiation
    (D) x rays
    (E) ultraviolet radiation

198. Which of the following widely used radioisotopes is considered to be an almost ideal isotope for medical applications and is commercially available as a radioisotope generator?

    (A) $^{131}$I (iodine)
    (B) $^{99m}$Tc (technetium)
    (C) $^{32}$P (phosphorus)
    (D) $^{59}$Fe (iron)
    (E) $^{198}$Au (gold)

199. A radioisotope generator is a (an)

    (A) pharmaceutical product labeled with a radioactive substance
    (B) ion-exchange column on which a nuclide has been adsorbed
    (C) ionization chamber
    (D) high-energy–yielding radioactive isotope that produces one or more isotopes, emitting low-energy radiation
    (E) apparatus in which radioactive isotopes are incorporated into biologic molecules

**200.** A cough syrup is labeled as containing 20% alcohol by volume. Which of the following statements is (are) true?

    I. Each 100 mL of syrup contains exactly 20 mL alcohol USP.

    II. There is an equivalent of 20 mL of absolute alcohol present in every 100 mL of syrup.

    III. The strength of this product may be expressed as 40 proof.

    (A) I only
    (B) III only
    (C) I and II only
    (D) II and III only
    (E) I, II, and III

**201.** Which of the following chemicals is (are) included in topical formulas as sunscreens?

    I. benzophenones
    II. cinnamates
    III. methyl salicylate

    (A) I only
    (B) III only
    (C) I and II only
    (D) II and III only
    (E) I, II, and III

**202.** A fair-skinned client claims that he normally begins to sunburn in approximately 30 min when exposed to the midday sun. What maximum length of protection could he expect using a sun lotion with an SPF of 12?

    (A) 1 h
    (B) 2–3 h
    (C) 4–6 h
    (D) 10–12 h
    (E) 24 h

**203.** Vehicles for nasal medications should possess all of the following properties EXCEPT

    (A) an acid pH
    (B) isotonicity
    (C) high buffer capacity

    (D) ability to resist growth of microorganisms
    (E) all of the above are important properties; no exceptions

**DIRECTIONS (Questions 204 through 208):** For each of the following drug trade names, select the dosage strength(s) that is (are) commercially available for oral administration. Use the response key of

    (A) I only
    (B) III only
    (C) I and II only
    (D) II and III only
    (E) I, II, and III

**204.** Inderal

    I. 10 mg
    II. 20 mg
    III. 40 mg

**205.** Coumadin

    I. 5 mg
    II. 10 mg
    III. 20 mg

**206.** Prozac

    I. 5 mg
    II. 10 mg
    III. 40 mg

**207.** Zoloft

    I. 50 mg
    II. 100 mg
    III. 250 mg

**208.** Avandia

    I. 2 mg
    II. 4 mg
    III. 10 mg

**209.** Which of the following products is (are) combinations of two active ingredients?

    I.   Augmentin

    II.   Ziac

    III.   Zithromax

    (A)  I only

    (B)  III only

    (C)  I and II only

    (D)  II and III only

    (E)  I, II, and III only

**210.** The active ingredients in Percodan include

    I.   aspirin

    II.   hydrocodone

    III.   acetaminophen

    (A)  I only

    (B)  III only

    (C)  I and II only

    (D)  II and III only

    (E)  I, II, and III

**211.** Which of the following drugs for asthma is (are) NOT available as an inhalation dosage form?

    I.   Accolate

    II.   Intal

    III.   Tilade

    (A)  I only

    (B)  III only

    (C)  I and II only

    (D)  II and III only

    (E)  I, II, and III

**212.** Which one of the following products exhibits sustained- or controlled-release activity due to enteric coatings?

    (A)  Augmentin

    (B)  ERYC

    (C)  Glucotrol XL

    (D)  Oramorph SR

    (E)  Toprol-XL

**DIRECTIONS (Questions 213 through 217): SELECT the brand-name product(s) that may be substituted for the numbered brand-name product when filling a hospital medication order. Assume that a formulary system that allows same drug substitution is in effect. Use the response key of**

    (A)  I only

    (B)  III only

    (C)  I and II only

    (D)  II and III only

    (E)  I, II, and III

**213.** Micronase

    I.   DiaBeta

    II.   Glynase

    III.   Glucotrol

**214.** Proventil

    I.   Atrovent

    II.   Vanceril

    III.   Ventolin

**215.** Cardizem CD 120-mg capsule

    I.   Dilacor XR

    II.   Tiazac

    III.   Verelan

**216.** Coumadin

    I.   Hytrin

    II.   Sofarin

    III.   Panwarfin

**217.** Vicodin

    I.   Oxycontin

    II.   Tylox

    III.   Zydone

**DIRECTIONS (Questions 218 through 303): Each group of items in this section consists of lettered answers followed by numbered questions. Select the letter answer that is most closely associated with each question. A lettered answer may be selected once, more than once, or not at all.**

**Questions 218 through 224**
MATCH the lettered manufacturer with the associated numbered trade-marked dosage form.

   (A) Abbott
   (B) GlaxoSmithKline
   (C) Lilly
   (D) Schering
   (E) Alza
   (F) Pfizer
   (G) Schering

218. Filmtab

219. Pulvule

220. Diskus

221. Gradumet

222. Reditab

223. Repetab

224. Oros

**Questions 225 through 229**
MATCH the following lettered drug trade name with the associated numbered generic name.

   (A) Amerge
   (B) Imitrex
   (C) Maxalt
   (D) Relpax
   (E) Zomig

225. Sumatriptan

226. Eletriptan

227. Naratriptan

228. Zolmitriptan

229. Rezatriptan

**Questions 230 and 231**
MATCH the lettered brand name of anesthetic with the numbered nonproprietary name most closely related to it.

   (A) Marcaine
   (B) Carbocaine
   (C) Novocaine
   (D) Xylocaine
   (E) Tronothane

230. Lidocaine

231. Procaine

**Questions 232 through 235**
MATCH the lettered dosage strength with its most closely corresponding numbered drug brand name.

   (A) 10 mg
   (B) 20 mg
   (C) 50 mg
   (D) 100 mg
   (E) 250 mg

232. Glucotrol

233. Ultram

234. Sporanox

235. Ambien

**Questions 236 through 240**
MATCH the lettered dosage strength with its most closely corresponding numbered drug brand name.

   (A) 1 mg
   (B) 10 mg
   (C) 50 mg
   (D) 60 mg
   (E) 80 mg

236. Paxil

237. Prilosec

238. Kytril

239. Claritin

240. Sudafed

**Questions 241 through 249**
MATCH the lettered generic name most closely corresponding to the numbered drug brand name.

   (A)   atomoxetine
   (B)   amlodipine
   (C)   paroxetine
   (D)   oxaprozin
   (E)   triamterene
   (F)   pentoxifylline
   (G)   amphotericin B
   (H)   olanzapine
   (I)   terbinafine
   (J)   zaleplon

**241.** Daypro

**242.** Strattera

**243.** Dyazide

**244.** Paxil

**245.** AmBisome

**246.** Trental

**247.** Lamisil

**248.** Zyprexa

**249.** Sonata

**Questions 250 through 253**
MATCH the lettered trade name most closely corresponding to the numbered generic name.

   (A)   Ziac
   (B)   Serevent
   (C)   Tramadol
   (D)   Tenormin
   (E)   Toprol

**250.** Atenolol

**251.** Metoprolol

**252.** Bisoprolol

**253.** Salmeterol

**Questions 254 through 258**
MATCH the lettered generic name most closely corresponding to the numbered trade name.

   (A)   nifedipine
   (B)   enalapril
   (C)   felodipine
   (D)   ramipril
   (E)   misoprostol

**254.** Plendil

**255.** Adalat

**256.** Cytotec

**257.** Altace

**258.** Vasotec

**Questions 259 through 262**
MATCH the lettered drug brand name having the same active therapeutic ingredient as the numbered drug brand name.

   (A)   Procan SR
   (B)   Calan
   (C)   Flovent
   (D)   Sorbitrate
   (E)   Dilacor

**259.** Pronestyl

**260.** Isordil

**261.** Flonase

**262.** Covera HS

**Questions 263 through 265**
MATCH the lettered generic name with the associated numbered trade name.

   (A) celecoxib
   (B) citalopram
   (C) clonazepam
   (D) divalproex
   (E) fosphenytoin

263. Celebrex

264. Cerebyx

265. Celexa

**Questions 266 through 269**
MATCH the lettered trade name of each of the following topical decongestant products with the related numbered nonproprietary name.

   (A) Benzedrex
   (B) Afrin
   (C) Privine
   (D) Neo-Synephrine Extra
   (E) Otrivin

266. Phenylephrine

267. Xylometazoline

268. Oxymetazoline

269. Naphazoline

**Questions 270 through 274**
MATCH the lettered antacid ingredients with the corresponding numbered commercial antacid product.

   (A) aluminum hydroxide
   (B) mixture of aluminum and magnesium hydroxides
   (C) mixture of aluminum hydroxide, magnesium trisilicate, and sodium bicarbonate
   (D) calcium carbonate
   (E) sodium bicarbonate

270. Amphojel suspension

271. Gaviscon tablets

272. Tums

273. Maalox suspension

274. ALternaGEL liquid

**Questions 275 through 278**
MATCH the lettered manufacturer with the associated numbered parenteral syringe system that it markets.

   (A) Abbott
   (B) Pfizer
   (C) Roche
   (D) GlaxoSmithKline
   (E) Wyeth

275. Carpuject

276. Isoject

277. Tubex

278. STATdose

**Questions 279 through 281**
MATCH the lettered manufacturer with the associated numbered parenteral container system that it manufactures.

   (A) Abbott
   (B) Baxter
   (C) Lilly
   (D) McGaw
   (E) Wyeth

279. Excell

280. Lifecare

281. Viaflex

**Questions 282 through 285**
MATCH the lettered term concerning hypodermic needles with the associated numbered description

(A) bevel
(B) cannula
(C) hub
(D) heel of bevel
(E) lumen

282. Extension of needle that fits onto the syringe

283. Portion of needle that is ground for sharpness

284. Shaft portion of the needle

285. The hole in the needle

**Questions 286 through 289**
As a pharmacist you may be asked for advice in selecting a suitable product for a skin condition. MATCH the lettered OTC ointment with the most appropriate numbered request.

(A) calamine 10%
(B) hydrogen peroxide 2%
(C) coal tar 2%
(D) ichthammol 10%
(E) salicylic acid 17%

286. To treat inflammation and boils

287. An astringent/protective

288. To treat a wart on the finger

289. To treat a mild case of psoriasis

**DIRECTIONS (Questions 290 through 293): It is often desirable to formulate a dosage form so that its pH approximates that of the area to which it is administered. MATCH the lettered pH value that is nearest to the pH usually found in the numbered body areas. Answers may be used once, more than once, or not at all.**

(A) 4.0–4.5
(B) 5.5
(C) 6.4

(D) 7.0
(E) 7.4

290. Blood

291. Eye

292. Skin

293. Vagina

**Questions 294 through 296**
MATCH the lettered formulation design that best describes the mechanism of release for each of the following sustained-release drug delivery systems:

(A) encapsulated dissolution
(B) ion-exchange
(C) matrix diffusion
(D) matrix dissolution
(E) osmotic pump

294. Drug is bound to a resin and released due to changes in pH.

295. Drug plus a slowly soluble polymer are compressed into tablets.

296. Drug particles are microencapsulated and a mixture of the particles is placed into the dosage form.

**Questions 297 through 299**
MATCH the numbered delayed-release or sustained-action principle with the corresponding lettered drug product.

(A) Ornade
(B) Tussionex
(C) Rynatan
(D) Demazin Repetab
(E) Oramorph SR

297. Hydrophilic matrix

298. Tablet with inner core

299. Complexation with tannic acid

**Questions 300 through 303**
MATCH the lettered vitamin B numbers with the correct nonproprietary name.

   (A)  vitamin $B_1$
   (B)  vitamin $B_2$
   (C)  vitamin $B_6$
   (D)  vitamin $B_{10}$
   (E)  vitamin $B_{12}$

300.  Cyanocobalamin

301.  Pyridoxine

302.  Riboflavin

303.  Thiamine

304.  Advantages of transdermal drug delivery systems include

   I.  avoids first-pass effect
   II.  improves patient compliance
   III.  suitable for drugs with relatively short half-lives

   (A)  I only
   (B)  III only
   (C)  I and II only
   (D)  II and III only
   (E)  I, II, and III

305.  All of the following drugs are available as transdermal drug dosage forms EXCEPT

   (A)  scopolamine
   (B)  estradiol
   (C)  bupropion
   (D)  fentanyl
   (E)  testosterone

306.  Which one of the following ranges of pH is most suitable for an extemporaneously prepared nasal solution?

   (A)  <4.0
   (B)  4.0–5.5
   (C)  5.5–7.5
   (D)  7.5–8.0
   (E)  >8.0

307.  Which one of the following practices would NOT be classified as "alternative medicine" in the United States?

   (A)  allopathy
   (B)  chiropractic
   (C)  naturopathy
   (D)  nutraceutical
   (E)  reflexology

308.  An alternative medical practice that stresses the use of extremely small doses of drugs is known as

   (A)  folk medicine
   (B)  holistic medicine
   (C)  homeopathic medicine
   (D)  orthomolecular medicine
   (E)  faith healing

**Questions 309 through 313**
MATCH the numbered herb with its most appropriate lettered therapeutic use.

   (A)  mild sedative
   (B)  improve memory
   (C)  reduce severity of a cold or virus infection
   (D)  improve urinary flow
   (E)  reduce GI spasms

309.  Echinacea

310.  Ginkgo biloba

311.  St. John's wort

312.  Saw palmetto

313.  Valerian

314.  Ginger root has been shown to be effective in

   (A)  the treatment of nausea or motion sickness
   (B)  reducing bronchial spasms
   (C)  treating constipation
   (D)  treating diarrhea
   (E)  reducing blood pressure

315. Which one of the following herbals should the pharmacist definitely discourage a patient from using?

(A) garlic
(B) comfrey
(C) ginger
(D) milk thistle
(E) hawthorn

316. Which one of the following herbals is believed to possess hepatoprotective effects?

(A) garlic
(B) ginger
(C) milk thistle
(D) ginkgo biloba
(E) peppermint

317. Which one of the following herbals exhibits the LEAST effect on blood coagulation?

(A) echinacea
(B) garlic
(C) ginseng
(D) ginkgo
(E) St. John's wort

318. Which of the following are standard methods for extracting active ingredients from crude herbals?

I. maceration
II. percolation
III. reverse osmosis

(A) I only
(B) III only
(C) I and II only
(D) II and III only
(E) I, II, and III

319. A customer purchasing a nonprescription drug combination containing glucosamine is probably using the product to prevent/treat

(A) joint pain
(B) malnutrition
(C) mild hypertension
(D) obesity
(E) high cholesterol values

320. Which one of the following herbals is most likely to interfere with the activity of oral birth control tablets?

(A) garlic
(B) ginger
(C) ginseng
(D) ginkgo biloba
(E) St. John's wort

# Answers and Explanations

1. **(A)** Official standards in the form of drug monographs are presented in the United States Pharmacopeia/National Formulary (USP/NF). These monographs may describe therapeutically active drugs or other ingredients, known as excipients, that are essential for formulating a stable drug product. *(24)*

2. **(D)** The United States Adopted Names (USAN) Council establishes nonproprietary drug names. The Council is jointly sponsored by the AMA, United States Pharmacopoeial Convention, and the APhA. Because the USAN is not an official government agency, the chosen names are not formally recognized until they are published in the Federal Register. *(24)*

3. **(C)** Federal drug laws and regulations are described in the USP Dispensing Information (DI), Volume III, which also contains listings of therapeutic equivalent drugs and drugs that are biologically inequivalent. The latter information is from the FDA's Orange Book. *(18c section:VI)*

4. **(B)** Volume II of the USP DI contains drug monographs written for the layperson. Pharmacists have permission to photocopy individual drug descriptions for distribution to the patient when dispensing the drug. Volume I of the USP DI contains drug information for health professionals. It includes more detailed and more scientific information than Volume II. *(18b; 18c)*

5. **(D)** The compressed tablet is the most commonly manufactured dosage form for several reasons. It is the most economical product for a manufacturer to produce, package, and ship. The tablet is easy for the pharmacist to dispense, and it is very convenient for most patients to consume. *(1; 24)*

6. **(B)** Almost all drugs must be in solution before they are absorbed through the walls of the gastro-intestinal tract. Since drugs are at the molecular level when present in solutions, they are more readily absorbed. Tablets and capsules must disintegrate before the drug will dissolve. Suspensions contain the drug in a form that is not readily soluble, and enteric-coated tablets are specifically formulated not to dissolve in the stomach. *(1; 24).*

7 **(D)** The speed at which tablets disintegrate usually correlates with the drug dissolution rate and speed at which drug action will occur. Sublingual tablets are intended to provide fairly fast activity which is accelerated by fast disintegration and dissolution under the tongue. While tablet compression is an important factor, uncoated compressed tablets usually disintegrate faster than coated tablets. *(1; 17)*

8. **(D)** Both film and sugar coats are water soluble and most will readily disintegrate in the stomach. However, the smooth tablet surface makes the tablet easier to dissolve with less chance of bitter drug powder remaining in the mouth or throat. Enteric coats are intended to prevent the disintegration of the tablet until it reaches the small intestine. *(1; 24)*

9. **(E)** The application of film coat, usually by spray techniques, on to large batches of tablets

is much easier and faster than sugar coating, which usually involves several steps. The film coat usually adds only 2 to 3% of weight to each tablet and is less likely to chip during handling. *(1; 24)*

10. **(A)** Magnesium stearate (as well as other stearates) is included in tablet formulations as a lubricant. *(1; 24)*

11. **(C)** Tablet lubricants are characterized by lubricity, as they are usually water insoluble and difficult to wet. The waterproofing property might retard disintegration and dissolution. *(1)*

12. **(B)** Products such as Potassium Chloride Enseals are enteric coated to protect the stomach from irritating substances or to prevent drug decomposition in the stomach. *(1; 10)*
    (A—incorrect) Endurets are sustained-release tablets. Preludin is an example.
    (C—incorrect) Extentabs are prolonged-action tablets (e.g., Dimetapp Extentabs).
    (D—incorrect) Filmtabs are tablets coated with a transparent protective coating (e.g., Eutron Filmtabs).

13. **(D)** Mannitol possesses characteristics that make it an almost ideal sweetener for chewable tablets. Although not as sweet as sucrose, it has good body, leaves a cool taste in the mouth, and is not hygroscopic. Mannitol is also easily compressed by wet granulation. *(24)*

14. **(C)** When moistened, starch will swell, thus aiding in the disintegration of a tablet. Corn starch in the form of a paste will bind powders during the formation of granules suitable for compression into tablets. *(1)*

15. **(E)** The disintegration times for uncoated tablets may vary and will be specified in the official monographs. The usual time is 30 min. For sugar coated tablets, the time may be as much as 2 h. Enteric coated tablets are first placed in gastric fluid then transferred to a simulated intestinal fluid. Buccal tablets may need four hours to disintegrate while sublingual tablets such as nitroglycerin have a limit of only a few minutes. *(1; 24)*

16. **(D)** Colloidal silicon dioxide, usually under the trade name of Cab-O-Sil, is included in some tablet formulas as a glidant. This adjuvant improves the flow characteristics of a powder being introduced into tablet dies. A second glidant is talc. *(1; 24)*

17. **(C)** Most alkaloids have a $pK_a$ above 7; therefore, they are weak bases that will form salts with an acid (e.g. pilocarpine hydrochloride, morphine sulfate). *(1)*
    (D—incorrect) Stereoisomerism is common in alkaloid structures; large differences in therapeutic activity can be expected among isomers

18. **(A)** Naturally occurring alkaloids which are weak organic bases have relatively poor water solubility but are soluble in alcohol. Most pharmaceutical products use the alkaloid salts such as morphine HCl, cocaine HCl, and atropine sulfate to increase the drugs' water solubility. *(1)*

19. **(C)** Haloperidol is a butyrophenone derivative and the base form has very poor water solubility (1 g in more than 10,000 mL). The hydrochloride salt is water soluble, as is the lactate salt, which is utilized in preparing the aqueous injection of haloperidol. Haloperidol decanoate is the ester form that is dissolved in an oil vehicle. This injection product is injected intramuscularly and has a half-life of approximately three weeks. *(1)*

20. **(D)** Pharmaceutical excipients are selected for specific characteristics that will improve the drug formulation. This includes solvents (glycerin), ointment bases (petrolatum), tablet diluents (lactose), antioxidants (sodium bisulfite), and antimicrobial preservatives (the parabens). Because they must be relatively pharmacologically inert, the local anesthetic benzocaine would not be suitable. *(24)*

21. **(C)** A chelating agent forms a compound by the combination of an electron donor with a metal ion to form a ring structure. The molecule that forms the ring structure is called a ligand or chelating agent. The metals that may be chelated must have valences of two or more.

A major pharmaceutical use for chelating agents is to bind trace metals such as iron and copper that would otherwise catalyze oxidation of active drugs. Edetate (ethylenediamine tetraacetic acid) is commonly used in parenteral solutions. *(24)*

22. **(B)** Edetate calcium disodium (Versenate) is usually administered by intramuscular parenteral injection to reduce blood levels and depot stores of lead in acute and chronic lead poisoning and lead encephalopathy. The chelate formed with lead is stable, water-soluble, and readily excreted by the kidneys. The other choices, lithium and sodium, are monovalent ions and will not complex with EDTA. *(1)*

23. **(C)** For example, boric acid solubility in water is expressed as 1:18. This indicates that 1 g of boric acid added to exactly 18 mL of purified water will result in a saturated solution. When compounding, it is advisable to use excess solvent because saturated solutions are difficult to prepare and may precipitate if there are changes in temperature. *(1)*

24. **(C)** Drugs in suspensions are likely to follow zero-order kinetics because the limiting factor is the amount of drug actually in solution. The classic example is aspirin suspension. *(12)*

25. **(B)** Epinephrine, a catecholamine, is very sensitive to oxidation, which results in biologically inactive products. The first indication of oxidation is the development of a pink color that darkens to form a brown precipitate. *(1; 24)*

26. **(C)** The term trituration usually refers to reducing the particle size of powders, often in a mortar and pestle. However, trituration has also been used to describe the simple mixing of two or more powders in the mortar. *(24)*

(A—incorrect) Levigation is the process of reducing the particle size of solids by adding a small amount of a liquid or an ointment base to make a paste, which is then rubbed with a spatula on an ointment tile. *(1)*

(B—incorrect) Sublimation is the conversion of a solid to a vapor without passing through a liquid phase. *(1)*

(D—incorrect) Pulverization by intervention is a process for reducing particle size by using a second agent that can then be readily removed. For example, camphor is reduced by the intervention of alcohol. *(1:)*

(E—incorrect) Maceration is an extraction process in which the ground drug is soaked in a solvent until the cellular structure is penetrated and the soluble constituents have been dissolved. *(1)*

27. **(B)** Powders that are either directly applied to the skin or are incorporated into topical products should be extremely fine or impalpable. Trituration is often needed to reduce particles to an extremely fine size so that the patient will not discern individual particles when the product is rubbed on the skin. Usually a particle size of 50 µm or smaller is desired. *(1; 4; 24)*

28. **(B)** Tartrazine (F D & C Yellow 5) is a popular coloring agent in both oral tablets and solutions. There are reported cases of individuals being sensitive to this dye. *(1; 14)*

29. **(C)** Chiral relates to the optical activity of a molecule. Stereoisomers of a specific drug may exhibit distinctly different degrees of therapeutic activity. For some drugs, the activity or major side effects may be due to only one of the isomers present. *(1)*

30. **(C)** A specific stereoisomer may possess greater desired activity than its mixture. If the more active form is isolated and used exclusively in a dosage form, there will usually be less toxicity and side effects. The actual synthesis, formulation, and manufacturing of the purified isomer into a commercial dosage form will not significantly result in a more economical drug than by using a mixture. *(1)*

31. **(D)** Polymorphs differ in their melting points, x-ray diffractions, infrared spectra, and dissolution rates. For example, riboflavin has three polymorphs, each with significantly different solubilities. Theobroma oil (cocoa butter) can exist in four forms, each differing in melting point. Gentle heating of cocoa butter will favor the formation of the stable beta polymorph.

This crystalline form is desired because it melts at 34.5°C, which is close to, but lower than body temperature. Metabolic rates of a drug's polymorphs will not vary because once the drug has dissolved, the polymorphs no longer exist. *(1)*

32. **(D)** Sorbitan monopalmitate is a sorbitan fatty acid ester, commercially available as Span 40. It is classified as nonionic because the molecules do not have the tendency to migrate to either pole in an electric field. *(1)*

   (A—incorrect) (C—incorrect) (E—incorrect) These compounds are anionic surfactants. This designation implies that the large active portion of the surfactant molecule bears a negative charge and, therefore, migrates to the anode in an electric field. For example, the stearate portion of triethanolamine stearate is considered the active ion.

   (B—incorrect) Cetylpyridinium chloride is a cationic surfactant. The active surfactant portion, cetylpyridinium, has a positive charge and migrates to the cathode.

33. **(D)** The equation may be expressed as

$$V = \frac{r^4 \times t \times \Delta P}{8 \times l \times n}$$

The volume of liquid (*V*) passing during a unit of time (*t*) is directly proportional to the radius of the tube (*r*) and the pressure differential (Δ*P*) at each end of the tube and inversely proportional to the length of the tube (*l*) and the viscosity of the liquid (*n*). Because the radius is raised to the fourth power, doubling the radius would cause a 16-fold change in the flow provided all other factors remained constant. The capillary can be envisioned as a simple glass tube or a human blood vessel. *(1; 12)*

34. **(C)** Potassium chloride is an obvious substitute for sodium chloride because it has a similar salty taste, is crystalline, and is an electrolyte already present in the body. However, the use of this salt substitute is contraindicated in patients with severe kidney disease or oliguria. Symptoms such as weakness, nausea, and muscle cramps indicate excessive sodium depletion. Increased sodium intake is warranted. *(10)*

35. **(B)** IV injection of high concentrations of potassium may cause cardiac arrest. Intravenous administration must be by slow infusion to allow dilution of the potassium to occur. When plasma potassium levels are above 2.5 mEq/L, rates up to 10 mEq/h (total of 100 to 200 mEq/day) may be set. In more serious conditions, with plasma levels below 2 mEq/L, rates of 40 mEq/h (total of 400 mEq/day) have been employed. Available injection forms contain 10 to 80 mEq per vial. IV admixtures are prepared by diluting these solutions to 250–1000 mL. Oral dosage forms include Kay Ciel elixir, Kaon tablets, K-Lor, and K-Lyte packets. Slow–K tablets have a wax matrix from which the KCl slowly dissolves in the GI tract. *(1)*

36. **(B)** Topical dosage forms are used. For example, both creams and solutions are available under the trade names of Efudex and Fluoroplex. In fact, however, fluorouracil is usually administered by IV injection. It is not given orally because of irregular absorption from the GI tract. *(3; 6)*

37. **(B)** The product inserts for many drug products contain various categories of statements including drug description, pharmacokinetics, warnings, precautions, indications for use, dosage and administration. Both the prescriber and the pharmacist carefully review any black box warnings since these are of extreme importance. The boxed material is usually located at the beginning of the product insert so that it is readily visible. *(1; 24)*

38. **(B)** A precaution is intended to advise the physician of possible problems that may occur with the use of a drug. For example, the use of tetracycline may result in overgrowth of nonsusceptible microorganisms. A warning signifies a more serious problem with greater potential for harm to a patient. For example, renal impairment may require reduction in the drug dose. A contraindication is the most restrictive limitation because it refers to an absolute prohibition against the use of a drug

under certain conditions. For example, the use of penicillin derivatives is prohibited in patients known to be sensitive to penicillin. *(24)*

39. **(C)** Both *Facts and Comparisons* and the *Handbook on Injectable Drugs* present tables comparing the commercial amino acid injections. *(21; 10)*

40. **(C)** The term leaching is used specifically to designate the release of a container ingredient into the product itself. For example, zinc and accelerators may be leached from rubber closures into a parenteral vial. *(24)*

    (A—incorrect) Adsorption would refer to the binding of a substance onto the surface of the container wall.

    (B—incorrect) Diffusion is the passage of a substance through a second substance. For example, volatile oil or dye may diffuse from a solution through the walls of a plastic container.

    (D—incorrect) Permeation would denote the solution of a substance in the cell wall followed by passage through the wall.

    (E—incorrect) Porosity indicates small holes, or passages through which a substance could pass.

41. **(B)** Hypodermic needle sizes are expressed by a gauge system based on the external diameter of the cannula: the larger the number, the smaller the diameter of the needle. For example, the 21–gauge needle is smaller in diameter than the 19–gauge needle. Generally, the length of the cannula is also specified. This measurement, expressed in inches, represents the distance from the needle tip to the junction with the hub. *(13)*

42. **(D)** The winged (scalp–vein, scalp, or butterfly) needle consists of a stainless steel needle with two flexible plastic wing-like projections. The wings serve two purposes: They ease manipulation of the needle during insertion into the vein and then allow the needle to be anchored with tape to the skin. *(13)*

43. **(E)** Insulin is usually administered by subcutaneous injection into the abdomen, arm or thigh. Absorption of the insulin is good, and this route is both convenient and safe for self-administration of the drug. Some studies indicate that the absorption rate from the arm is 50% faster than from the thigh. *(13)*

44. **(D)** Insulin solutions have low viscosities, and only small volumes are injected. Therefore, small-bore needles (25 G up to 30 G) may be used. Short-length (3/8 to 5/8 in) needles are usually adequate for the usual subcutaneous route of insulin administration. *(13)*

45. **(C)** The term venoclysis is synonymous with intravenous infusion. *(13)*

46. **(A)** Partially filled glass containers (minibottles) usually consist of 250-mL bottles containing 50, 100, or 150 mL of either $D_5W$ or NS. To these bottles one can easily add drug solutions, taking advantage of the vacuum present in the minibottle. Plastic bags are also employed for preparing parenteral admixtures. The plastic units do not have a vacuum but are flexible enough to accommodate additional liquids. *(1)*

47. **(A)** Intermittent therapy refers to administration of parenteral drugs at spaced intervals. One of the most convenient methods of administration for the pharmacist, is to prepare a minibottle containing active drug solution such as an antibiotic added to a diluent. This unit is attached to the tubing of a large-volume parenteral (LVP) bottle already hanging on the patient. This piggyback concept saves the patient from multiple injections and assures high blood levels of the additive drug, because the minibottle solution is infused in a short period of time. *(1; 13)*

48. **(C)** TPN (total parenteral nutrition) and TNA (total nutritional admixture) refer to solutions administered parenterally to provide calories, amino acids, and other nutrients by parenteral infusion. PMN is an abbreviation sometimes used for phenylmercuric nitrate, an antimicrobial preservative. *(4)*

49. **(B)** Although the maximum volume will vary depending on the condition of the patient, the

normal daily water requirement is approximately 25 to 40 mL/kg of body weight. Daily volumes greater than 3 to 4 L in normal (non-dehydrated) patients may cause a fluid overload. A dehydrated patient will require larger quantities. Water replacement therapy (hydration therapy) in an adult may be 70 mL/kg. Thus, a 50 kg patient will need 3500 mL (replacement) plus 2400 mL (maintenance). *(24)*

50. **(E)** A subcutaneous injection will come into contact with a large number of nerve endings and may remain at the injection site for a long period of time. Pain will be experienced if the solution is not isotonic. The potential effects of hypotonic or hypertonic intravenous solutions are offset by their dilution in the large volume of blood into which they are injected, provided the volume injected is not excessive and the rate of injection is slow. *(1; 24)*

51. **(D)** There is the potential danger of suspension particles blocking blood vessels. Also, relatively insoluble particles of suspension may dissolve faster than desired if injected intravenously into a relatively large volume of patient's blood, thus giving immediate therapeutic activity, when a sustained release activity was desired. For example, only insulin solution is administered by the IV route while the various suspension dosage forms are intended for subcutaneous injection. *(1; 24)*

52. **(B)** The abbreviation of IVP represents intravenous push (bolus) administration indicating fast injection (usually < 1 min) of the parenteral solution. IVPB requires a minibottle or minibag setup known as the piggyback arrangement. These bottles are usually infused over a time span of 20 min to 1 h. KVO means to keep the vein open, by setting up a large volume parenteral (LVP) of 5% dextrose or 0.9% sodium chloride injection for very slow infusion. The intent is to allow the quick hookup of additional drug solutions without having to enter the vein several times. *(13)*

53. **(B)** Factors affecting the distribution of a drug in the blood after an IV bolus include the blood volume, heart rate, and injection rate. Assuming

that even distribution occurs within 4 min, drug sampling may be initiated after that time. *(1)*

54. **(D)** The pH of solutions is often adjusted during the manufacturing procedure by the addition of either acid (hydrochloric acid) or alkali (sodium hydroxide). The amount needed may vary from batch to batch. Therefore, the label cannot specify an exact quantity. Also, isotonicity adjusters may be listed by name only with a statement as to their purpose. *(18c)*

55. **(B)** Although many of the parenteral admixtures are chemically stable for long periods of time, potential contamination of the products during preparation by the pharmacist is of prime concern. Usually no significant microbial growth will occur until after 24 to 36 h. Therefore, an expiration date of 24 h is safest unless the solution is known to be less stable chemically. Some hospitals use a 28 h expiration date. Refrigeration also helps to retard microbial growth. *(13)*

56. **(E)** Osmolarity, expressed as mOsm/L, is included on the labels of large volume parenteral (LVPs). Those injections with a value of approximately 300 mOsm/L will be isoosmotic and presumably isotonic with the blood. For example, 5% dextrose injection has a value of 280 mOsm/L, whereas 0.9% sodium chloride injection has a value of 308 mOsm/L. One calculates the osmolarity of a solution by first determining the millimoles of chemical present, then multiplying by the number of ions formed from one molecule. One liter of 0.9% sodium chloride solution contains 9 g of sodium chloride (mol wt = 58.4). The millimole concentration will be

$$9 \text{ g}/58.4 = 0.154 \text{ mol or } 154 \text{ mM}$$

The milliosmole (mOsm) concentration will be

$$154 \text{ mM} \times 2 \text{ (ions present in NaCl)}$$
$$= 308 \text{ mOsm} \qquad (1)$$

57. **(C)** Dextrose 5% injection ($D_5W$) has an osmolarity of approximately 300 mOsm/L, as does 0.9% sodium chloride injection (NS). If 1 L of

solution contains both 5% dextrose and 0.9% sodium chloride, its osmolarity will be approximately 600 mOsm/L and will be hypertonic. Fortunately, infusing hypertonic solutions such as $D_5W/NS$ is not dangerous, since the solution is rapidly diluted by the blood with no significant damage to the red blood cells. One formula often used for infusion is $D_{2.5}W/0.45NS$, which is isotonic. *(1; 23)*

58. **(A)** The osmotic pressure of the dextrose solution will be approximately one-half that of an equimolar sodium chloride solution. The osmotic pressure of a substance in solution is an example of a colligative property. Equimolar concentrations of nonelectrolytes will have similar osmotic pressures. However, electrolytes ionize to form particles that quantitatively increase the magnitude of the colligative property. Because sodium chloride ionizes into two particles, a 0.1 molar solution has twice the osmotic pressure of a 0.1 molar solution of a nonelectrolyte such as dextrose. Deviations from this simple theory arise from interionic attractions, solvation, and other factors. *(1)*

59. **(B)** Except for the lactate concentration and the absence of sodium bicarbonate, lactated Ringer's (Hartmann's) solution closely approximates the extracellular fluid. Although the injection has a pH of 6 to 7.5, it has an alkalinizing effect because the lactate is metabolized to bicarbonate. *(1)*

60. **(B)** To avoid pain at the injection site, solutions injected into subcutaneous sites should be limited to not more than 1 mL. The usual limit suggested for deltoid IM injections is up to 2 mL, while IM injections into the gluteal medial muscle may be up to 5 mL. *(4)*

61. **(D)** Intradermal injections are usually limited to diagnostic determinations, densitization, or immunization into the forearm. Usually, only 0.1 mL volumes are used. *(24)*

62. **(E)** The vastus lateralis is the largest developed muscle in young children and is free of major nerves and veins. The volume limitation should be 1 mL. *(4)*

63. **(C)** Heparin sodium is given by both IV bolus and infusion as well as by subcutaneous injection. The IM route is not used since it may be painful and also cause a localized hematoma. *(1)*

64 **(C)** Self-administration of insulin is most readily accomplished by subcutaneous injection into the abdomen or thigh. Intravenous infusion is used in institutional settings and, in emergencies, IV bolus doses may be given. The development of portable infusion pumps and other devices is expanding the methods for insulin administration. *(1; 13)*

65. **(D)** There are two main sites of degradation for insulin—the liver and the kidneys. Insulin is filtered through the glomeruli and reabsorbed by the tubules, where some degradation occurs. When injected by the IV route, the half life is estimated to be 5 to 6 min. Approximately, 50% of the insulin that reaches the liver through the portal vein is destroyed. U-100 insulin is available over-the-counter. *(10)*

66. **(D)** The ADD-Vantage system consists of a vial usually containing a powder which is already attached to a minibag. The health professional simply has to engage the vial into the bag thus allowing reconstitution of the powder and subsequent mixing with the main body of diluent. *(1; 24)*

67. **(A)** The CRIS unit is a plastic disposable adaptor which allows the quick transfer of a drug solution into an infusion container. A vial is hooked to the adaptor, the valve device is turned, and the vial contents will enter the infusion line mixing with the infusion solution flowing into the patient. The unit avoids the need to initially mix the additive with the primary infusion solution. *(1)*

68. **(D)** Pharmacia's Port-A-Cath is a stainless steel unit with a self-sealing septum through which drug solutions may be injected over 100 times. The unit is implanted under the skin in a location allowing the patient to self-administer solutions. A similar unit is Infusaid's Infuse-A-Port. Answers A and C are incorrect. These two catheters are classified as central catheters

and are mainly used for infusing hypertonic TPN solutions. *(1; 13; 22)*

69. **(C)** Pharmacy bulk packages are intended to provide the compounding pharmacist with a unit, the contents of which may be aseptically subdivided into several parenteral admixtures. The package is pierced only once, and used within a short period of time, therefore it does not contain an antimicrobial preservative. Bulk packages are ideal when reconstituting an antibiotic powder for transfer into several mini-bottles or bags. *(4; 13)*

70. **(D)** Potassium chloride concentrate solutions are potentially very dangerous if infused undiluted. Because of numerous fatalities in hospitals, the FDA specifies that it is the only product that must be packaged in vials with black flip-off buttons. There is no color code for other parenteral solutions that are packaged in vials. *(18c)*

71. **(C)** The inclusion of an antimicrobial preservative in parenteral solutions is intended only for multidose containers from which fairly small volumes of solution are used at one time. When large volumes of solution are infused, the presence of an antimicrobial preservative may increase potential toxicity of the product. *(24)*

72. **(B)** Esters of *p*-hydroxybenzoic acid are used as preservatives to protect against mold and yeast growth in pharmaceuticals. Toxicity, preservative effect, and lipid solubility all increase as the molecular weight increases. Of the four esters—methyl, ethyl, propyl, and butyl—the latter two are more suitable for oils and fats. They are often used in combination with each other, but these chemicals are slow acting and are now unacceptable as ophthalmic antimicrobial preservatives. *(1)*

73. **(A)** Although vitamin C's main attribute is in the prevention and cure of scurvy, it has been advocated for the prevention and alleviation of symptoms of the common cold, to facilitate absorption of iron by maintaining iron in the ferrous state, and as an antioxidant in both pharmaceuticals and foods. The fat-soluble

vitamin E also possesses antioxidant properties, and is sometimes employed as a preservative in lipid pharmaceutical and cosmetic products. *(1)*

Ergocalciferol (Vitamin D$_2$) prevents or treats rickets and is used in the management of hypoparathyroidism and hypocalcemia. *(1)*

Pantothenic acid is biologically important as a component in coenzyme A (CoA). *(1)*

74. **(A)** Gentamicin sulfate (Garamycin) is stable for two years at room temperature. Of the five antibiotics listed, it is the only one marketed as an aqueous solution, ready for injection. The others are packaged as powders for reconstitution. *(21)*

75. **(C)** Human immune serum is obtained from human blood. It contains specific antibodies reflecting the diseases contracted by the donor. The immunity is passive because the recipient's body does not actively develop either antibodies or sensitized lymphocytes in response to a foreign antigen. Passive immunity does not last long; usually not more than two or three weeks of protection are achieved. Active immunity implies that the recipient of the biological will develop specific immunity due to an active response to the introduction of antigenic substances. *(24)*

76. **(A)** Protection against measles is recommended for persons 15 months and older. Usually, the vaccine is administered as part of the measles, mumps, and rubella virus mixture. However, all individuals born after 1956 are considered susceptible to natural measles and should be revaccinated if they are unable to show immunity to measles. Fluogen protects against influenza. Havrix against hepatitis A, Recombivax HB against hepatitis B and Sabin against poliomyelitis. *(1; 25)*

77. **(A)** Tuberculin is a solution of soluble products of tubercle bacillus. The solution is used as a diagnostic aid for exposure to the bacillus. It is administered intradermally. *(24)*

78. **(B)** The tuberculin skin test is based on skin hypersensitivity to a specific bacterial protein

antigen. Tuberculin can be administered intracutaneously (Mantoux test) or by the multiple puncture method (Tine test). The intracutaneous method using purified protein derivative (PPD) is more reliable. Generally, the intermediate strength (5 U/0.1 mL) is used. The first strength (1 U) is generally used for individuals suspected of being highly sensitive, and the second strength (250 U) is exclusively for those who did not react to previous injections of either 1 or 5 units. *(1; 9)*

79. **(B)** Tuberculin syringes are made of either plastic or glass with a total capacity of 1 mL. Despite their  name, they are suitable for measuring small volumes of any liquid. *(13)*

80. **(B)** The immune gamma globulin is used to prevent or modify several diseases, including measles, infectious  hepatitis, German measles, and chickenpox. The immunity is passive, lasting for one to two months. There are also special forms for individuals exposed to mumps, pertussis, tetanus, vaccinia, and rabies. *(1; 24)*

81. **(C)** Pediarix vaccine is a vaccine offering protection against diphtheria, tetanus, acellular pertussis, hepatitis B, and poliovirus. However, it does not protect against hepatitis C. *(3; 25)*

82. **(E)** There may be some danger to both mother and fetus if live attenuated vaccines are administered. While the evidence is  not conclusive, neither the individual or combination MMR (measles, mumps, and rubella vaccine) should be administered during pregnancy or during the previous three months, for women considering pregnancy. *(24)*

83. **(B)** Passive immunizations are usually accomplished by the administration of purified and concentrated antibody solutions (antitoxins) derived from humans or animals that have been actively immunized against a live antigen. Active immunizations are usually accomplished by the administration of one of the following: (1) toxoids (e.g., A—incorrect), (2) inactivated (killed) vaccines (e.g., choices C and E—incorrect), (3) live attenuated vaccines (e.g., choice D—incorrect). *(1; 24)*

84. **(C)** Booster doses of the common toxoids are required to sustain immunity. For example, a 0.5 mL dose of tetanus toxoid should be administered as a routine booster about every 10 years or, as a booster in the management of minor clean wounds, not more frequently than every six years. *(1)*

85. **(A)** Diphtheria, tetanus toxoid, and pertussis vaccine (DTP) is administered as a series of four injections starting when the baby is six weeks to two months of age. Two additional injections are given at six-week intervals, with a final dose given one year later. If needed, a booster injection can be given when the child is four to six years old. DTP must never be given to children older than six years because of serious reactions that may occur. *(1; 24)*

86. **(E)** Typhoid fever is a bacterial infection. *(1)*

87. **(C)** All people over the age of two are appropriate candidates for  pneumonia vaccinations. There are several products on the market such as Merck's Pneumovax and Wyeth's Pnu-Imune. The vaccine is given by either intramuscular or subcutaneous injection and provides active immunization. *(24)*

88. **(B)** The labeling on biologicals is required to specify the recommended storage temperature. With few exceptions, biologicals are stored in a refrigerator at 2 to 8°C *(24)*

89. **(A)** Smallpox vaccine is administered by intradermal (pinprick) injection. The dried, live virus provides active immunization. *(1; 14 )*

90. **(C)** Monoclonal antibodies (MAb) are antibodies derived from single hybrid cells. The resulting product has enhanced selectivity, making it invaluable as a specific diagnostic agent or drug. Gene splicing refers to those procedures resulting in alterations of the DNA make-up of a microorganism. Using recombinant DNA technology, specific antibodies useful for medical and agricultural applications can be developed. *(1; 24)*

**91.** **(C)** Liposomes consist of phospholipids that when dispersed in water form multilamellar vesicles. These liposomes can be utilized as drug carriers delivering drugs to specific body sites. Nanoparticles refer to a dispersed drug consisting of colloidal size particles with diameters between 200 and 500 nm. After IV injection, the nanoparticles are taken up by the reticuloendothelial system and localized in the liver. Transdermal delivery systems allow diffusion of a drug through the skin into the general circulation. They do not target specific sites for drug delivery. *(1; 24)*

**92.** **(B)** Most biotechnological drugs consist of amino acid sequences. Because these proteins have relatively poor stability in the GI tract and have erratic absorption, most of the drugs are intended for parenteral administration. *(13; 24)*

**93.** **(E)** The thrombolytic agent urokinase is an enzyme isolated from cultures of human kidney tissue. *(1)*

(A—incorrect)  Human growth hormone (Protropin) is intended for the long-term treatment of children with growth failure due to insufficient endogenous hormone. A similar product is Lilly's Humatrope. *(24)*

(B—incorrect) Epoietin alpha (Epogen, Procrit) is used in dialysis, anemia, and chronic renal failure to promote red blood cell formation. *(24)*

(C—incorrect) Humulin is Lilly's human insulin. *(24)*

(D—incorrect) The interferons are used in numerous diseases including AIDS-related Kaposi's sarcoma and multiple sclerosis. *(24)*

**94** **(D)** The increased sensitivity of both types of tests is due to the use of monoclonal antibodies (MAb), which allow earlier determination of the specific hormones involved. Ovulation prediction tests detect surges in luteinizing hormone (LH), which indicate that ovulation is about to occur. Pregnancy determination tests detect an increased level of human chorionic gonadotropin (HCG) hormone that occurs when the egg is fertilized. The fecal occult blood tests are based on the colorimetric detection

of hemoglobin. Various chemicals, such as guaiac, tetramethylbenzidine, etc., are used to elicit a characteristic color. The occult blood tests are not very selective or sensitive. *(2)*

**95.** **(A)** Wyeth's Norplant system consists of levonorgestrel in a silastic polymer. The silastic rods are inserted under the skin of the upper arm and slowly release the drug for up to five years. It is considered a reversible contraceptive system. However, it is not classified as a targeted delivery system, which would imply the delivery of the drug only to a specific organ or area. *(1)*

**96.** **(A)** Intermates are transparent plastic units containing an elastic balloon which may be aseptically filled with sterile solutions. The unusual characteristic of the balloon is that it collapses at a constant rate when the administration set is opened thus giving a constant flow rate. For example, the Intermate 100 will deliver 100 mL in a one hour period. The pharmacist may control the amount of drug received by the patient by either changing the fill volume or the concentration of drug present. However, the flow rate is preset and can not be changed. A similar unit is provided by Block Medical as the Homepump. *(22)*

**97.** **(D)** PCA devices such as Pharmacia's CADD models allow the slow infusion of drug solutions into the patient. Not only can small volumes be infused, the units may be programmed to vary flow at different intervals and also provide bolus doses when desired. There is also a lock-out device which prevents too frequent bolus doses. The PCA units are very convenient for delivery of analgesics but also may be used for other drug solutions. *(22)*

**98.** **(A)** The elastomeric balloon pumps flow by pressure not gravity. Thus, the patient may store the unit in his pocket or backpack even while infusing the solution. The individual units are not intended to be refilled, i.e., they are considered disposable. Because the infusion is at a constant rate, there is no mechanism for obtaining a bolus dose. This curtails the use of these units for pain management. Instead the units are used for such purposes as home infusion of antibiotics. *(22)*

99. **(C)** Colostomy pouches are available in several sizes based on the opening that will surround the stoma on the body. These sizes are designated in inches of diameter. Pouches are designed as either open end, in which the effluent may be drained while the pouch is on the patient, or closed end, for which the pouch must be removed to be either emptied or discarded. There is no difference between pouches worn by males or females but there are pediatric pouches with a smaller capacity. *(1; 2)*

100. **(C)** Both ipecac syrup and activated charcoal have proved effective in the treatment of many types of drug poisoning. However, they must not be used concurrently because the charcoal will adsorb the active alkaloids present in ipecac syrup. Thus the desired emetic effect may be lost. If both agents are to be administered, it is best to induce vomiting first with the ipecac, then administer the charcoal to absorb remnants of the poison. Activated charcoal is usually administered as a water slurry of 60 to 100 g. Often a mild cathartic such as magnesium sulfate is administered after the charcoal. Some charcoal products already contain either sorbitol or methylcellulose as a laxative. (2) (E—incorrect) The universal antidote is a mixture of activated charcoal, magnesium oxide, and tannic acid. Only the charcoal in this combination is effective, and its activity is probably reduced by the other two ingredients. *(2)*

101. **(D)** DexFerrum and InFeD are parenteral products containing iron dextran. They are colloidal solutions of ferric hydroxide complexed with partially hydrolyzed dextran. Because of incidences of fatal anaphylactic-type reactions, their use should be limited to the treatment of confirmed cases of iron-deficiency anemia, particularly among those patients who cannot tolerate, or who fail to respond to oral administration of iron. *(1; 3)*

102. **(B)** Iron sucrose injections are available under the trade name of Venofer. It is intended for treating iron-deficiency anemia in patients undergoing chromin hemodialysis and are receiving erythropoietin therapy. The solution is administered only intravenously into the dialysis line. The Z–track technique used to prevent skin discoloration which may occur when administering IM iron dextran is not used for iron sucrose since this drug solution is given IV. *(1; 3)*

103. **(E)** Polycarbophil absorbs large quantities of water, allowing the formation of stools. There does not appear to be any effect on the action of digestive enzymes or nutrients. The drug itself is not absorbed systemically. Polycarbophil is present in Mitrolan and FiberCon. *(1; 2)*
   (A—incorrect) Activated charcoal possesses good adsorption properties but is seldom used as an antidiarrheal.
   (C—incorrect) (D—incorrect) Kaolin and attapulgite are typical examples of adsorbent clays. Attapulgite is a colloidal hydrated magnesium aluminum silicate clay. Studies have indicated that it is an effective adsorbent for alkaloids, toxins, bacteria, and strains of human enteroviruses. However, attapulgite and kaolin are not selective and will also adsorb nutrients and digestive enzymes. Probably their greatest efficacy is in the treatment of mild functional diarrhea. *(2; 11)*

104. **(A)** Simethicone is a mixture of inert silicon polymers that may be used as a defoaming agent to relieve GI tract gas. This antiflatulent ingredient is present in Mylicon drops and Phazyme tablets. Simethicone is included in a number of combination antacid products (Mylanta, Riopan, and Gelusil). A newer antiflatulent agent is alpha-galactosidase, an enzyme that breaks down oligosaccharides before they form intestinal gas. A commercial product containing this compound is Beano. *(2)*

105. **(D)** Pepto-Bismol contains bismuth subsalicylate. The subsalicylate salt is the preferred insoluble form because the subnitrate may form the nitrite ion in the gut. Absorption of this ion could cause hypotension and possibly methemoglobinemia. Bismuth salicylate is safe

when taken orally but should not be consumed by patients sensitive to aspirin. Patients should be counseled that black-stained stools, that may occur with bismuth intake, are harmless. *(2; 11)*

106. **(C)** Both Donnagel and Kaopectate caplets contain the clay attapulgite, which has been proven to be a more effective adsorbent than kaolin. Another ingredient in Kaopectate and Donnagel is pectin, which is classified as an intestinal absorbent, adsorbent, and protective. The belladonna alkaloids formerly present in Donnagel as antispasmodics have been removed because of the lack of proof of efficacy. Kaopectate Liquid contains bismuth subsalicylate, and Mitrolan contains the absorbent calcium polycarbophil. *(2; 3)*

107. **(C)** Liposomes are small vesicles of a bilayer of phospholipid encapsulating an aqueous compartment. Since phospholipids have both hydrophilic and hydrophobic portions, either lipophilic or hydrophilic drugs may be incorporated into the structure. Liposomes may vary in shape, usually with sizes between 0.5 and 100 μm. *(17; 24)*

108 **(E)** Liposomal dosage forms may be developed for any route of administration, but their parenteral use is exciting. Liposomal forms of amphotericin B have activity targeted fungi localized in tissue, thus allowing lower doses and fewer side effects. The chemotherapeutic agent, doxorubicin, has been formulated into parenteral liposomes with reduced cardiotoxicity when compared to the conventional product. *(17; 24)*

109. **(A)** Actron contains 12.5 mg of ketoprofen. Aleve contains 225 mg naproxyn sodium, and Nuprin has 200 mg ibuprofen. *(2; 3)*

110. **(D)** Of the three analgesics, acetaminophen appears the safest for use during pregnancy. Aspirin, as well as all other salicylates, is especially dangerous during the last trimester and when breastfeeding mainly due to increased fetal and maternal morbidity. Ibuprofen may also cause postpartum bleeding and prolonged labor. *(2; 11)*

111. **(B)** Magnesium salicylate is similar to sodium salicylate in its analgesic activity, but there is the danger of systemic magnesium toxicity, especially in the renal-impaired patient. *(2)*

112. **(E)** The usual adult dose of dextromethorphan is 30 mg every 8 h, with a maximum daily dose of 120 mg. Individual doses of 30 mg or higher do not appreciably increase antitussive activity. *(2; 11)*

113. **(B)** Calcium carbonate is a rapid, prolonged, potent neutralizer of gastric acid. Some scientists and consumer groups have advocated its use because of its high effectiveness and low cost. However, the listed side effects should warrant curtailment of its use, particularly for chronic therapy. *(2)*

(A—incorrect) Some of the insoluble calcium carbonate is converted to soluble calcium chloride, which is absorbed. Significant amounts of calcium may be absorbed after a few days of antacid therapy.

(D—incorrect) Gastric hypersecretion is believed to be caused by the local effect of calcium on the gastrin-producing cells.

114. **(D)** Calcium carbonate appears to be the antacid of choice when formulating chewable tablets. Although both the Titralac and Rolaids products contain calcium carbonate, Rolaids chewable tablets also contain magnesium hydroxide. Basaljel capsules contain only aluminum hydroxide. Other antacids containing only aluminum hydroxide include Amphojel and ALternaGEL. *(2; 11)*

115. **(D)** The generic name for Riopan is magaldrate. The product is a chemical rather than a physical combination of aluminum and magnesium hydroxides. Although this chemical form has a lower neutralizing capacity, it is still considered to be an effective antacid with a low sodium level and does not cause electrolyte imbalance in the body. *(1; 2)*

116. **(D)** Historically, phenolphthalein was a very popular stimulant laxative in a number of OTC products. However, because of some evidence that phenolphthalein may be carcinogenic,

companies have reformulated their products by using other laxatives. For example, the sennosides have properties similar to phenolphthalein. *(2; 3)*

117. **(E)** The tablets are enteric coated to avoid gastric irritation. They should not be taken within 1 h of ingestion of milk or antacids because the enteric coating may be dissolved prematurely. *(4)*

118. **(B)** Since companies have a degree of latitude in changing their OTC formulas, it is difficult for health professionals and laypersons to be certain of specific active ingredients in a specific product. The best procedure is to read recent labels. All of the products mentioned in the question contain 5 mg of biscodyl per tablet except Regular Strength ExLax which contains 15 mg of sennosides. There is also an ExLax Maximum Strength which contains 25 mg of sennosides per tablet. Another active ingredient, docusate, is present in Correctol Gentle Laxative. *(2)*

119. **(D)** Excessive tablet compression may hinder tablet disintegration into aggregates, thus slowing the dissolution process. Other factors that affect dissolution include drug solubility, particle size, and crystalline structure; though these factors may not influence the disintegration rate. However, there is usually a fairly good correlation between tablet disintegration characteristics and dissolution, and disintegration times are a convenient in-house manufacturing control. Increasing drug particle surface area by micronization of drugs such as griseofulvin, chloramphenicol, and sulfadiazine have increased their dissolution rates (decreased dissolution times) and improved absorption. *(1)*

120. **(B)** The USP/NF has established official storage conditions which the pharmacist should follow for all pharmaceutical products. Temperatures within a refrigerator are described as being between 2 and 8°C. *(1; 24)*

121. **(A)** Abreva is a nonprescription topical preparation intended to be placed on cold sores to speed healing time. Present in the formula are moisturizers which relieve dryness and prevent painful cracking, thus reducing pain, burning, and itching of the sore. *(2; 3)*

122. **(D)** Aspartame is a dipeptide that is approximately 200 times sweeter than sucrose. Because it provides less than 1 calorie per dose and does not impart the bitter aftertaste experienced by some people after consuming saccharin, it is a popular sweetening agent in drug products and foods. Its tendency to disintegrate on heating limits potential uses. Patients with phenylketonuria should avoid aspartame because one breakdown ingredient is phenylalanine. *(2)*

123. **(D)** Circadian refers to rhythmic cycles that recur in approximately 24 h intervals. *(1; 14)*

124. **(B)** Searle's Covera-HS is formulated into a COFR-24 delivery system. The 180 or 240 mg tablets are intended for bedtime dosing to insure maximum plasma levels in the early morning. This time factor design is intended to take advantage of the body's circadian rhythm because blood pressures tend to be higher when the patient arises in the morning. *(10)*

125. **(D)** Thickening a suspension will slow its sedimentation, but it is still necessary to get the product out of the bottle. A pseudoplastic flow is desirable because it is characterized by a greater flow rate after the system has been agitated. Thixotropy refers to a reversible sol-gel system; it is characterized by a gel that forms a flowable sol when shaken. On standing, the reformation of the gel will slow particle settling. Caking is undesirable because settling particles form a dense pack at the bottom of the container. It is very difficult to break this cake and to reconstitute the original suspension. *(1)*

126. **(C)** Inhalation aerosol products may be intended for either localized activity (bronchodilators for asthma) or systemic action (ergotamine for migraine). In either situation, the onset of action will be rapid. When the drug is absorbed through the alveolar–capillary membrane, the first-pass metabolism in the

liver is avoided. Because of the limited capacity of aerosol units, especially in the small-chamber metered valves only a limited amount of drug can be administered. *(1)*

127. **(A)** The acronym MDI refers to metered dose inhaler which is a pressurized aerosol unit that dispense accurate metered doses. Epinephrine is the active bronchodilator in such OTC products as Bronkaid Mist and Primatene Mist. Ephedrine is available OTC only in tablet and syrup dosage forms. Its future status may change because of deaths attributed to ephedra's misuse. Albuterol aerosol products are by prescription only. *(2; 11)*

128. **(A)** The first-degree burn is the mildest injury because only the epidermis is affected.

   (C—incorrect) These are characteristics of a second-degree burn, which affects the epidermis and portions of the dermis.

   (D—incorrect) A third-degree burn penetrates through the entire skin. Damage may be permanent.

   (E—incorrect) These are characteristics of the fourth-degree or char burn. Both the skin and underlying tissues are affected. *(2)*

129. **(A)** Benzocaine is included in some dietary aid products at levels of 3 to 15 mg. The products are formulated as lozenges, gum, or candies. The benzocaine is believed to decrease the person's ability to detect sweetness, thus reducing appetite. *(2; 11)*

130. **(C)** Benzocaine is widely used for surface anesthesia of the skin and mucous membranes. It remains on the skin for a long period of time because of its poor water solubility and because it is poorly absorbed. Systemic toxicity is rare. Although the possibility of local sensitization should be considered, the incidence is low considering the frequent use of benzocaine. Although the incidence of hypersensitivity to lidocaine is lower than that of benzocaine, prolonged administration of lidocaine to a large skin area may result in systemic side effects. Lidocaine is present in Medi-Quik Aerosol, Bactine, and Unguentine Plus. *(1)*

Although phenol (carbolic acid) possesses both antiseptic and local anesthetic effects, there is the possibility that it may accentuate tissue damage because of its caustic properties. *(1; 2)*

131. **(D)** A topical preparation should contain a minimum of 5% benzocaine. Some studies have indicated that 10 to 20% of the drug is needed. *(2; 11)*

132. **(D)** Debrisan is not useful in the treatment of nonsecreting wounds. Its action appears to be absorption of fluids and particles that impede tissue repair. The product is available as 0.1- to 0.3-mm spherical beads (4 g packets) that are sprinkled onto secreting wounds. The hydrophilic nature of the beads creates a strong suction force; each gram absorbs about 4 mL of fluid. The beads become grayish yellow when they are saturated with fluid; they should then be washed away by irrigating with sterile water or saline. *(1)*

133. **(B)** Because fertilization can occur within only a few hours (perhaps 24 h) after ovulation, accurate knowledge of this event could permit timing of intercourse to either increase or decrease the possibility of conception. Basal temperature (the lowest temperature of the body during waking hours) typically passes through a biphasic cycle over the course of the menstrual cycle. From an initially low temperature, a midcycle thermal shift occurs to a high level, where it remains until it again becomes low premenstrually. The temperature rise roughly corresponds to the time of ovulation. The thermometer is used orally or rectally once daily, immediately on awakening in the morning and before getting out of bed. *(1)*

   (D—incorrect) The scale may be either Fahrenheit or Celsius. The temperature rise is only about 0.5°F, which would be difficult to measure on the usual clinical thermometer. The basal thermometer scale ranges only from 96 to 100°F and is graduated to 0.1°F.

134. **(A)** The rectal thermometer bulb has a strong, blunt shape that facilitates insertion into the

rectum and retention by sphincter muscles. The oral bulb is cylindrical, elongated, and thin walled for quick registration of temperature. Rectal thermometers can be used orally. The oral bulb is too easily broken and is not suitable for rectal use. The short, sturdy security bulb represents a compromise intermediate shape. *(1)*

135. **(D)** Although the venoms of some insects are potent, the amounts injected are too small to be toxic. The severity of the sting reaction in some individuals is due to their hypersensitivity to certain proteins in the venom. This results in the anaphylactic shock. *(2; 11)*

136. **(D)** Persons who experience severe anaphylactic reactions to insect sting or bites should carry emergency kits. These kits usually contain antiseptic pads (to clean and disinfect the area), both an antihistamine and epinephrine injection (to counteract the anaphylactic reaction), and tweezers (to remove the stingers). A tourniquet would be of little value because the amount of venom is very small. Self-injectable units of epinephrine, such as EpiPen, are also available for individuals known to be susceptible to stings. *(3; 10)*

137. **(B)** An ileostomy results when the entire colon (large intestine) and a portion of the small intestine are removed, and the remaining end of the small intestine is attached to the abdominal wall. Because of the narrow diameter of the small intestine, the wall opening (stoma) is not as large when compared to colostomy stomas. The fecal discharge is watery because there has been limited opportunity for water reabsorption. Also there are higher concentrations of enzymes present that may irritate the skin. *(1; 22)*

138. **(C)** The French system is used for designating sizes of both urinary catheters and tubing used for enteral feedings. One French unit equals 1 mm on the outside circumference. Thus, a catheter with an outside circumference of 20 mm is identified as a 20F or 20Fr size. Syringe needles are sized by another system—the Stubbs numbers in which the number designation increases as the diameter of the needle shaft decreases. *(1; 2)*

139. **(B)** Pamabrom, a xanthine derivative is present in several OTC products for the prevention of premenstrual syndrome (PMS), specifically bloating. Its diuretic activity is obtained with a dose of 25 to 50 mg four times a day. Examples of products containing pamabrom include Midol PMS and Pamprin. *(2; 11)*

140. **(A)** The carbamide peroxide will effervesce, thereby softening the waxy material. An example of an OTC product is Debrox which also contains glycerin and propylene glycol that act as solvents. *(2: 11)*

141. **(E)** Diffusion of a drug from a vehicle into the skin is often related to the solubility of the drug in the vehicle relative to the solubility in the skin, i.e., the partition coefficient. Drugs that are very soluble in a vehicle will tend to remain in the vehicle, and will penetrate more slowly than drugs with poorer solubility in the vehicle. *(1)*

(A—incorrect) Covering the area to which a topical drug product has been applied will often enhance the rate of drug absorption. Sweat accumulation at the skin–vehicle interface induces hydration of the skin, a condition that facilitates penetration of drugs.

(B—incorrect) Poorer solubility of the drug in PEG ointment than in white ointment may lead to faster diffusion. This is the converse of choice E.

(C—incorrect) The thicker epidermis of the palms results in slower drug penetration than that which occurs on the backs of the hands.

(D—incorrect) Higher drug concentrations will increase the rate of diffusion and penetration. *(1; 24)*

142. **(B)** Melatonin is an endogenous hormone produced by the human pineal gland. It appears to shift the circadian rhythm and serves as a sleep aid when taken 1 to 2 h before bedtime. *(2)*

143. **(E)** Allantoin is included in many topical formulations as a vulnerary (healing agent), which is a substance that stimulates tissue repair. *(1)*

144. **(E)** Selected combinations of the polyethylene glycols (PEGs) can be formulated into

water-miscible suppositories with a range of consistency. They are easy to insert and do not require refrigeration. *(24)*

145. **(A)** Lactose is a readily compressible and water-soluble inert ingredient. It also encourages the growth of Doderlein's bacilli, a microorganism present in the healthy vagina. *(24)*

146. **(D)** The extent of drug release and absorption will vary depending upon the properties of the drug, the suppository base, and the condition of the colon. Oil-soluble drugs will be poorly released from a cocoa-butter base because of their high lipid/water solubility. *(24)*

    (A—incorrect) The rectal fluid pH is essentially neutral and has a low buffer capacity. Therefore, drugs that can be destroyed by the acidity of the stomach may be successfully administered rectally.

    (B—incorrect) Drugs that are absorbed through the colon pass into the lower hemorrhoidal veins and into the general systematic circulation. Avoidance of first-pass exposure to the liver may enhance the effect of those drugs inactivated by the liver. Drugs that are absorbed from the upper intestinal tract pass directly through the portal vein into the liver, where metabolism may occur.

    (E—incorrect) The lesser dose frequency and lower propensity for irritation are the reasons certain drugs can be administered rectally but not orally.

147. **(B)** Semicid inserts contain 100 mg of the spermicide nonoxynol-9. The active ingredient in Norforms vaginal suppositories is the quaternary ammonium germicide, benzethonium chloride, which decreases odor-producing microorganisms. Terazole contains terconazole for the treatment of moniliasis. *(2; 24)*

148. **(E)** Carbomers (Goodrich's Carbopols) are polymers with a number of carboxy groups present. When the pH of a solution containing the carbomer is increased, there will be a significant increase in viscosity. *(1)*

149. **(A)** Solutions with equal osmotic pressure are iso-osmotic; they also will be isotonic if separated

by a membrane permeable to the solvent but impermeable to the solute. Any of the colligative properties can be used to determine tonicity of solutions. Freezing-point depression values are used most frequently. The freezing point of a 0.9% sodium chloride aqueous solution is −0.52°C; the same as that of human blood and tears. Saline solutions of this concentration are isotonic with these body fluids. More concentrated solutions are hypertonic; less concentrated are hypotonic. *(1)*

150. **(A)** Properties of a solution that depend on the number of particles of the solute and are independent of the chemical nature of the solute are termed colligative properties. The magnitude of vapor pressure, freezing-point reduction, boiling-point elevation, and osmotic pressure are all related to the number of particles in solution. *(1)*

151. **(D)** Solutions with the same osmotic pressure as blood are usually isotonic with blood. Solutions that have a higher osmotic pressure (i.e., hypertonic) will cause water to pass out of the red blood cells. Solutions that have a lower osmotic pressure (i.e., hypotonic) will allow water to pass into the cells. This causes them to swell and rupture with a release of hemoglobin (hemolysis). *(1; 24)*

152. **(C)** A hypertonic solution will draw water from within the cell until an equilibrium is reached with equal pressure on each side of the cell membrane. Because of the loss of volume, the cell will shrink and take on a wrinkled appearance (crenation). *(1; 24)*

153. **(A)** A sodium chloride equivalent is the weight of sodium chloride that will produce the same osmotic effect as 1 g of the specified chemical. For example, morphine hydrochloride has an E value of 0.15. This indicates that 1 g of morphine hydrochloride produces the same osmotic pressure (and depression of freezing point) in solutions, as 0.15 g of sodium chloride. *(1; 12)*

154. **(C)** *The Remington: The Science and Practice of Pharmacy* presents extensive tables of sodium

chloride equivalents (E) and freezing point depression (D) values. *(1)*

155. **(C)** Any two solutions that have the same freezing points will have the same osmotic pressure and should be isotonic. Because blood freezes at −0.52°C, any aqueous solution that freezes at this temperature will be iso-osmotic. The use of freezing-point data for isotonicity adjustment for both ophthalmic and parenteral solutions is common in the pharmaceutical industry because freezing points can be measured easily. *(1; 12)*

156. **(D)** Aqueous solutions that freeze at the same temperature as blood have the same osmotic pressure as blood (i.e., are iso-osmotic with blood and each other). However, to be isotonic a solution must maintain a certain pressure, or tone, with the red blood cells. If the chemical in a solution passes freely through the red blood cell membrane, equalized pressure on both sides of the membrane is not possible without changes in the cell volume. Tone will not be maintained, and the solution will not be isotonic, though it might be iso-osmotic with blood. *(1; 12)*

157. **(A)** The capacity of the cul-de-sac is estimated to be not more than 0.03 mL, with a normal tear volume of approximately 0.007 mL. Probably less than 0.02 mL of an ophthalmic solution can be placed successfully in an eye at one time. This volume is less than the nominal 0.05 mL (1 drop) usually requested in prescription directions. This implies that a portion of the dose is lost through drainage or overflow onto the cheek. *(1)*

158. **(E)** In spite of its name, Veegum is not an organic gum but is an inorganic clay. It is water insoluble and would probably be unsuitable for ophthalmic administration since insoluble particles could be deposited in the ocular areas. *(1)*

159. **(B)** Increasing the contact time between a drug and the cornea will often increase the amount of drug absorption that will occur. *(1; 4)*

160. **(B)** Fluorescein sodium is an ophthalmic diagnostic agent. It is instilled into the eye to delineate scratches and corneal lesions. It would be very dangerous to place a contaminated solution on a damaged cornea through which microorganisms may easily pass. If *Pseudomonas aeruginosa* enters the interior of the eyeball, blindness may occur quickly. Pharmacists should not prepare fluorescein sodium solutions extemporaneously unless sterility can be guaranteed. Pharmaceutical manufacturers supply fluorescein as unit-dose solutions or individual paper strips. *(1)*

161. **(A)** *Acanthamoeba* keratitis has been identified in solutions used by contact lens wearers. These solutions were either home-made or commercial solutions that were recycled. Thermal disinfection is effective in eliminating microbial contamination including *Acanthamoeba*. *(2)*

162. **(A)** The combination of benzalkonium chloride and edetate (0.01% of each) is effective against those microorganisms likely to contaminate ophthalmic solutions. These include some strains of *Pseudomonas aeruginosa* that are resistant to benzalkonium chloride alone. *(4; 24)*

163. **(D)** Papain and subtilisin are proteolytic enzymes that aid in the removal of proteinaceous residues that slowly build up on soft lenses during wear. Allergan markets Enzymatic Contact Lens Cleaner as tablets containing papain. Subtilisin is present in Bausch & Lomb's ReNu series of products. A third enzyme that has been used is pancreatin. Once weekly, the soft lenses are soaked overnight in solutions prepared from the previously mentioned products. Hydrogen peroxide is the active ingredient in a number of soft lens disinfecting products. *(2)*

164. **(C)** Sodium bisulfite and sodium metabisulfite are included in pharmaceutical solutions as antioxidants. For example, the oxidation of epinephrine may be retarded by the presence of sodium bisulfite, which is preferentially oxidized. Unfortunately, some individuals are

sensitive to the bisulfites and must avoid products containing them. The labels of many wines caution about the presence of bisulfites. *(1; 4)*

165  **(A)** One of the first signs of sensitivity to bisulfites is difficulty in breathing. Also, the patient may experience hives, abdominal pain, and wheezing. Bisulfites are one of the few ingredients that must be included on the labels of wines. *(24)*

166.  **(C)** Because membrane filtration does not involve heat, it is suitable for drug solutions that either are sensitive to heat or have not been studied sufficiently concerning their heat stability. The pharmacist may purchase presterilized filter units such as Millipore's Millex through which 15 to 100 mL of solution can be filtered. However, autoclaving is still considered the most reliable sterilization procedure. *(13)*

167.  **(A)** Epinal contains epinephrine borate while the other two products (Epifrin and Glaucon) contain the hydrochloride salt of epinephrine. There may be a distinct advantage in using the borate salt since the pH of the solution will be higher, thus causing less irritation when placed in the eye. *(3)*

168.  **(C)** Lyophilization or freeze-drying is a procedure by which water is sublimed from a frozen product. The remaining drug powder (cake) is more stable than the original solution. Although a second advantage is that the powder will dissolve quickly when diluent is added for reconstitution, that is not the main purpose for the procedure. The process of freeze-drying is relatively expensive and is usually reserved for drugs that have limited stability in aqueous solutions. *(1)*

169.  **(B)** Often the weight of active drug in a lyophilized powder is very low and difficult to observe by the pharmacist attempting to reconstitute the dry powder. To obtain a larger, more visible cake, a bulking agent such as mannitol may be included in the formula so that the pharmacist may more readily ascertain when dissolution is completed. *(1)*

170.  **(A)** Benzyl alcohol is used in many parenterals, especially in Bacteriostatic Sterile Water for Injection as an antimicrobial agent. Although its relative toxicity is low, there are a few reports of hypersensitivity. Also, it is contraindicated for use in premature infants because of reports of fetal toxic syndrome. *(13)*

171.  **(D)** By definition. *(1; 12)*

172.  **(C)** The Henderson-Hasselbalch equation, or buffer equation for a weak acid and its corresponding salt, is represented by

$$pH = pK_a + \log\left(\frac{[salt]}{[acid]}\right)$$

where $pK_a$ is the negative log of the dissociation constant of the weak acid and salt/acid is the ratio of the molar concentrations of salt and acid in the system. The volume of the solution is not critical because the chemical concentrations are already expressed in terms of molar concentration. *(12)*

173.  **(E)** According to the Henderson-Hasselbalch equation, pH will equal $pK_a$ when the expression $\log([salt]/[acid])$ is equal to zero. This can occur only when the salt/acid ratio equals 1, because the log of 1 is 0. The point at which the salt concentration equals the acid concentration is the half-neutralization point. It is also the pH at which a buffer system, based upon the weak acid's $pK_a$, has the best buffering capacity. *(12)*

174.  **(C)** Hydrochloric acid is classified as a strong acid. Strong acids ionize almost completely into hydronium ions and the corresponding anions. Other strong acids are sulfuric and nitric. These acids do not have $pK_a$ values listed because the values would be close to 0. The fact that all of the other acids listed in the question have $pK_a$s indicate that they are weaker acids (with less ionization) than hydrochloric acid. *(12)*

175.  **(C)** Strong acids have larger ionization constants than weak acids. Because the $pK_a$ is the reciprocal of the log of the ionization constant, stronger acids have lower $pK_a$s than weaker acids. Of the acids listed, boric acid has the

highest $pK_a$; thus, it is the weakest of these acids. Salicylic acid, which has the lowest $pK_a$ on the list, is the strongest. *(12)*

176. **(D)** A buffer system consists of a weak acid or base and its corresponding strong salt. In preparing a buffer system, one should choose an acid or a base with a $pK_a$ close to the desired pH. For example, lactic acid and sodium lactate can be combined to obtain a pH of exactly 4.0. The needed molar concentration of each may be calculated by using the Henderson-Hasselbalch equation. *(1; 12)*

177. **(C)** This problem may be solved using the Henderson-Hasselbalch equation knowing that the $pK_a$ of boric acid is 9.24.

$$pH = pK_a + \log\left(\frac{salt}{acid}\right)$$

$$pH = 9.24 + \log\left(\frac{0.05 \text{ mol/dL}}{0.005 \text{ mol/dL}}\right)$$

$$pH = 9.24 + \log 10$$

$$pH = 9.24 + 1 = 10.24 \qquad (23)$$

178. **(B)** For determining the ratio of a weak acid to its salt present at a given pH, the Henderson-Hasselbalch equation is used.

$$pH = pK_a + \log\left(\frac{dissociated}{undissociated}\right)$$

or

$$pH = pK_a + \log(B/A)$$

[B = ibuprofen salt; A = ibuprofen]

Substituting the $pK_a$ of ibuprofen (5.5) and the pH of the urine of 7.5

$$7.5 = 5.5 + \log(B/A) \qquad \log(B/A) = 2.0$$

Thus, the ratio of the dissociated form of the drug (B) to the undissociated form (A) will be the antilog of 2, a numeric value of 100. *(24)*

179. **(A)** This problem is solved using the same thought process as for question 178.

$$pH = pK_a + \log\left(\frac{dissociated}{undissociated}\right)$$

or

$$pH = pK_a + \log(B/A)$$

[B = salt of aspirin; A = aspirin]

Substituting the $pK_a$ of aspirin (3.5) and the pH of the urine of 4.5

$$4.5 = 3.5 + \log(B/A) \qquad \log(B/A) = 1.0$$

Thus, the ratio of the dissociated form of the drug (B) to the undissociated form (A) will be the antilog of 1, a numeric value of 10 or 10/1. Since (A) represents the aspirin, only 1 of every 11 molecules will be aspirin (a percentage of 9%) and 10 molecules will be the salt of aspirin (a percentage of 91%). *(24)*

180. **(D)** Because of individual patient biologic variation and the technologic limitations of the precise control of drug release, drugs with either short half-lives or low therapeutic indexes are not suited for sustained-release products. A drug which requires a dosage of 500 mg t.i.d. is usually not suitable since 1500 mg would be needed in the sustained release dosage form. Almost all sustained-release products are designed for the treatment of chronic conditions in which acute dosing adjustments are not necessary. Hopefully, sustained-release products will improve patient compliance by requiring less frequent dosing. *(24)*

181. **(C)** Sustained-release dosage forms are intended to reduce dosing frequency while maintaining relatively consistent blood levels of the drug. The duration of activity of drugs with half-lives between 2 and 8 h can be extended to obtain convenient once- or twice-daily dosing. Although it would be desirable to increase the therapeutic duration of those drugs with half-lives of less than 2 h, the required high drug-release rates and high drug concentration in the dosage form reservoir usually preclude sustained-release dosage formulation. Also, individual biologic variation could result in either sub- or hypertherapeutic blood levels.

Drugs with half-lives greater than 8 h usually have long intervals between doses, making sustained-release formulations unnecessary. (1)

182. **(C)** GlaxoSmithKline's Spansule formulation consists of medicated pellets in a capsule dosage form. Some pellets are uncoated to give almost immediate drug release, whereas other pellets have lipid coatings of various thicknesses. Thus, the initial dose is reinforced with additional drug release over a period of time. Examples of Spansule products include Compazine and Thorazine, Another group of products based on the same principle are Lederle's Sequels including Diamox, and Ferro-sequels. (1; 24)

183. **(A)** Pennwalt's Ionamin capsules contain phentermine, an agent used for dieting. (1)

184. **(C)** The OTC product Efidac/24 contains pseudoephedrine for use as an oral nasal decongestant. Other osmotic tablets include Procardia XL (nifedipine) and Volmax (albuterol). Because the rate-limiting factor in these tablets is the osmotic pressure, drug release is not affected by GI tract pH. (1; 10; 24)

185. **(C)** Effexor XR (venlafaxine) is an extended release product for treatment of depression. It is available in a capsule dosage form suitable to be either swallowed or sprinkled onto food. Depakote (divalproex sodium) is also available as sprinkle capsules and is used in epilepsy therapy. Ditropan XL (oxybutynin chloride) is an extended release tablet formula which must be swallowed whole. Its mechanism is the osmotic pressure-controlled delivery. (3; 10)

186. **(C)** A container that reduces light transmission in the range of 290 to 450 nm to the level specified in the USP may be considered light resistant and affords suitable protection from light. The container may be constructed of glass or plastic. Although amber units are most common, other colored or opaque containers may meet the official requirements. (4; 18c; 24)

187. **(D)** Yellow ferric oxide is included in some tablet formulas as a coloring agent. The amount of iron present is a subtherapeutic dose. Red ferric oxide is mixed with white zinc oxide to prepare calamine which has a pink color. (1; 4)

188. **(E)** The expiration date for a pharmaceutical is based on the length of time during which the product continues to meet the specified monograph requirements. Requirements are stated in terms of amount of active ingredient that is present as determined by suitable assay. Most drug products are considered usable until approximately 10% of the drug or drug activity has been lost. However, some monographs specify other ranges. For example, digoxin tablets must assay between 92 and 108% of label claim. (1)

189. **(B)** Pharmacists are using beyond-use dating quite often as guidelines when dispensing prescriptions to limit prolonged use of the drug by the patient. This date is usually a shorter time span than the manufacturer's expiration date found on the original package. The beyond-use date shall be not later than either the expiration date on the manufacturer's container or one year from the date of dispensing, whichever is earlier. For reconstituted products, the beyond-use date will be of a significantly shorter duration and is based upon the manufacturer's recommendation in the package insert or on the package. (4)

190. **(B)** The drug solution lost 0.5 mg of its 2.0 mg/mL concentration in 24 h. This represents a loss of

$$\frac{0.5}{2.0} = 0.25 \text{ or } 25\%$$

Since first order reaction rates are expressed as fraction per unit of time, the value will be 0.25/day. (24)

191. **(A)** This problem may be solved either by using an equation or by the simple relationship of

| | |
|---|---|
| Original concentration | = 2.0 mg/mL |
| After one half-life (4 days) | = 1.0 mg/mL |
| After two half-lives (8 days) | = 0.5 mg/mL |
| After three half-lives (12 days) | = 0.25 mg/mL |

(24)

192. **(B)** First determine the concentration after three days.

Original concentration = 10,000 units/mL
After one half-life (1 day) = 5000 units
After two half-lives (2 days) = 2500 units
After three half-lives (3 days) = 1250 units

Next determine the mL of the final solution that contains the required dose of 2000 units.

$$\frac{1250 \text{ units}}{1 \text{ mL}} = \frac{2000 \text{ units}}{x \text{ mL}}$$

$$x = 1.6 \text{ mL} \qquad (24)$$

193. **(E)** Not only do drugs that consist of proteins undergo the normally expected decomposition due to heat, they also are susceptible to denaturation. This process may occur during excessive or vigorous shaking of the protein solutions. *(1; 10)*

194. **(D)** Chlorobutanol is included in some ophthalmic and parenteral solutions as an antimicrobial preservative. All of the other chemicals listed may serve as antioxidants. Ascorbyl palmitate, butylated hydroxytoluene, and vitamin E are oil soluble, thus limiting their use to lipophilic systems. Ascorbic acid is a water-soluble antioxidant. *(4)*

195. **(D)** For many years, the Curie (Ci) has been the basic unit for expressing radioisotope decay. Now the Becquerel is recognized as the official unit. One Becquerel equals one decay per second (dps).

$$1 \text{ curie} = 3.7 \times 10^{10} \text{ Bq (dps)}$$

The rad is a quantitative measure of radioactivity. *(24)*

196. **(B)** Decay rate is the rate at which atoms undergo radioactive disintegration. The rate of decay $(-dn/dt)$ is proportional to the number of atoms $(n)$ present at any time $(t)$; thus, radioactive decay is a first-order process. *(1)*

197. **(C)** Gamma radiation, x rays, and ultraviolet radiation are forms of electromagnetic radiation and are radiated as photons or quanta of energy. These forms of radiation differ only in wave length and are the most penetrating types of radiation. Gamma rays are the most penetrating of all and can easily penetrate more than a foot of tissue and several inches of lead. *(1; 13)*

(A—incorrect) Alpha radiation is particulate radiation consisting of two protons and two neutrons. The range of alpha particles is about 5 cm in the air and less than 100 μm in tissue.

(B—incorrect) Beta radiation is also particulate radiation, but exists as two types, the negative electron (negatron) and the positive electron (positron). Both may have a range of over 10 feet in the air and up to about 1 mm in the tissue.

198. **(B)** $^{90m}$Tc is available commercially as a technetium generator from various manufacturers in which molybdenum $^{99}$Mo is the parent nuclide. The half-life of technetium (6 h) is long enough to allow completion of usual diagnostic procedures for which it is used, yet short enough to minimize the radiation dose to the patient. Lack of a beta component in its radiation further decreases the dose delivered to the patient. The gamma energy is weak enough to achieve good collimation, yet strong enough to penetrate tissue sufficiently to permit deep-organ scanning. *(1; 13)*

199. **(B)** Although it is desirable to use isotopes with short half lives to minimize the radiation dose received by the patient, it is evident that the shorter the half life, the greater the problem of supply. Radioisotope generators, or cows, have been developed to deal with this problem. A radioisotope generator is an ion-exchange column containing a resin of alumina on which a long-lived parent nuclide is absorbed. Radioactive decay of the long-lived parent results in the production of a short-lived daughter nuclide that is eluted or milked from the column by means of an appropriate solvent such as sterile, pyrogen-free saline. *(1)*

200. **(D)** Although Alcohol USP (95% v/v ethanol) is usually used in the production of pharmaceuticals, labels stating alcohol concentration are based on 100% v/v ethanol (absolute alcohol).

Proof strengths of products are easily calculated by simply doubling the %v/v ethanol concentration. *(1; 23)*

**201.** **(C)** The benzophenones are effective in screening out the harmful (skin burning) UVB wavelengths as well as some of the UVA spectra. The cinnamates will screen the UVB wavelengths and a combination of the two categories of sunscreens are often incorporated into commercial formulas. Methyl salicylate (oil of wintergreen) is included in topical products mainly for its pleasant odor. It does not possess sunscreening properties. However, homomenthyl salicylate (homosalate) is a sunscreen. *(2; 11)*

**202.** **(C)** The SPF (sun protection factor) is a numeric value that indicates the multiple length of time an individual may be exposed to the sun with minimum erythema as compared to the exposure time without any protection. In this example, 30 min × 12 = 6 h is the maximum protection that may be expected. Obviously there are many variables that affect the quantity of radiation received on any day. *(2; 11)*

**203.** **(C)** Both ophthalmic and nasal preparations should have only a mild buffer capacity so that the organ's natural buffer system can overcome any pH differences. Otherwise, irritation might result. *(1)*

(A—incorrect) Nasal preparations usually have a pH in the range of 5.5 to 6.5. Often, phosphate buffers are used.

(B—incorrect) Rendering the nasal solution isotonic will decrease potential for damage to the local tissue.

(D—incorrect) The presence of an antimicrobial preservative is important because there may be accidental contamination of the dropper or nasal spray tip.

**204.** **(D)** Inderal (propranolol) is available as 20, 40, and 60 mg tablets; long-acting capsules (Inderal LA at 80, 120, and 160 mg); and an injection (1 mL ampules containing 1 mg of drug). *(25)*

**205.** **(C)** Coumadin is DuPont's brand of warfarin sodium and is available in several strengths

for convenient dosage adjustments. Tablets containing 2, 2.5, 5, 7.5, and 10 mg are marketed. *(25)*

**206.** **(D)** The antidepressant, Prozac (fluoxetine) is available in several strengths and dosage forms including Pulvules (10, 20, and 40 mg), a 10 mg tablet, a liquid (20 mg/5 mL), and a 90 mg tablet intended for once a week dosing. *(3)*

**207.** **(C)** Zoloft (sertraline) is an antidepressant available as both 50 and 100 mg tablets. *(25)*

**208.** **(C)** The antidiabetic drug, rosiglitazone, is available under the trade name of Avandia. Dosage strengths of the tablets include 2, 4, and 8 mg. *(3)*

**209.** **(C)** Augmentin consists of amoxicillin and clavulanate potassium. Ziac contains bisoprolol plus hydrochlorothiazide. Zithromax has only azithromycin as an active ingredient. *(3: 25)*

**210.** **(A)** Percodan contains aspirin plus oxycodone. *(3; 10)*

**211.** **(A)** Accolate (zafirlukast), a leukotriene receptor antagonist, is available as a 20 mg tablet, not in an inhalation dosage form. Tilade inhaler (nedocromil) is used in maintenance therapy in patients with mild to moderate bronchial asthma. Intal inhaler (cromolyn sodium) is a mast cell stabilizer which prevents acute bronchospasms. *(24)*

**212** **(B)** ERYC capsules are formulated with enteric coated pellets to delay the release of erythromycin. A somewhat similar product is E-Mycin Delayed Release tablets which are enteric coated tablets. *(10; 24)*

**213.** **(C)** *(10)*

**214.** **(B)** Although all three products are available as inhalation aerosols, Vanceril contains beclomethasone and Atrovent contains ipratropium. *(10)*

215. **(C)** Dilacor XR and Tiazac are available as extended-release forms of diltiazem. Verelan contains verapamil. *(10)*

216. **(D)** Sofarin and Panwarfin are brands of warfarin. Hytrin is an antihypertensive agent, terazosin. *(10)*

217. **(B)** Zydone contains hydrocodone plus acetaminophen. Oxycontin contains only oxycodone while Tylox contains a mixture of oxycodone and acetaminophen. *(10)*

218. **(A)** *(25)*

219. **(C)** *(25)*

220. **(B)** *(25)*

221. **(A)** *(25)*

222. **(G)** *(25)*

223. **(G)** *(25)*

224. **(E)** *(25)*

225. **(B)** *(25)*

226. **(D)** *(25)*

227. **(A)** *(25)*

228. **(E)** *(25)*

229. **(C)** *(25)*

230. **(D)** Lidocaine (Xylocaine) is a (local) anesthetic available as a cream, an ointment, and an oral spray. Lidocaine HCl is administered by injection as well as topically. *(3; 25)*

231. **(C)** Procaine (Novocain) is available only for parenteral use. *(1; 6)*

232. **(A)** The antihyperglycemic drug Glucotrol (glipizide) is also available as a 5 mg tablet. *(10)*

233. **(C)** Ultram (tramadol) is classified as a central analgesic. *(10)*

234. **(D)** Sporanox (itraconazole) is an oral antifungal agent. *(10)*

235. **(A)** The nonbenzodiazepine, zolpidem (Ambien) may be classified as a hypnotic, sedative, or tranquilizer. *(10)*

236. **(B)** The antidepressant Paxil (paroxetine) is available as 10-, 20-, 30-, and 40-mg tablets. *(10)*

237. **(B)** Prilosec (omeprazole) is available as both a 10- and 20-mg delayed-release capsule. It is intended for the short-term treatment of active duodenal ulcers. *(10)*

238 **(A)** Kytril (granisetron) is marketed as a 1 mg tablet and an injection solution (1 mg/mL) for the prevention of nausea and vomiting. *(10)*

239. **(B)** Claritin (loratadine) is available as a nonprescription drug antihistamine. There are several dosage forms including a regular 10 mg tablet and as Claritin Reditabs which contain 10 mg of micronized drug for faster dissolution by placement on the tongue. Claritin-D contains 5 mg loratadine + 120 mg of pseudoephedrine. *(10)*

240. **(D)** *(10)*

241. **(D)** *(10)*

242. **(A)** *(10)*

243. **(E)** *(10)*

244. **(C)** *(10)*

245. **(G)** *(10)*

246. **(F)** *(10)*

247. **(I)** *(10)*

248. **(H)** *(10)*

249. **(J)** *(10)*

250. **(D)** *(10)*

251. **(E)** *(10)*

252. **(A)** *(10)*

253. **(B)** *(10)*

254. **(C)** *(10)*

255. **(A)** *(10)*

256. **(E)** *(10)*

257. **(D)** *(10)*

258. **(B)** *(10)*

259. **(A)** Procainamide *(10)*

260. **(D)** Isosorbide dinitrate *(10)*

261. **(C)** Fluticasone propionate *(10)*

262. **(B)** Verapamil HCl *(10)*

263. **(A)** Celebrex is available as 100 and 200 mg capsules for either once daily or twice a day dosing. It is intended for treatment of rheumatoid arthritis and osteoarthritis. *(10)*

264. **(E)** Cerebyx injection is intended as a replacement for parenteral Dilantin for both the prevention and treatment of seizures. *(10)*

265. **(B)** Celexa is available as 20- and 40-mg tablets for depression and is given once a day. *(10)*

266. **(D)** *(2; 11)*

267. **(E)** *(2; 11)*

268. **(B)** Besides Afrin, both Dristan 12-h and Neosynephrine 12-h sprays contain 0.05% oxymetazoline. *(2; 11)*

269. **(C)** *(2; 11)*

270. **(A)** Aluminum hydroxide is a commonly used antacid because of its nonabsorbability, demulcent activity, and ability to adsorb pepsin. It is somewhat slow in respect to the onset of action.

A second antacid product with just aluminum hydroxide is Basaljel. *(2; 11)*

271. **(C)** Magnesium trisilicate appears to be longer acting than aluminum hydroxide. When it reacts with hydrochloric acid in the stomach, hydrated silicon dioxide, which may coat ulcers, is formed. Gaviscon and Gaviscon-2 contain alginic acid, which forms a viscous solution, thereby prolonging the contact time. The product is claimed to be effective in the relief of gastroesophageal reflux. All of the other Gaviscon products (Extra Strength and Liquid) contain aluminum hydroxide and magnesium carbonate but no magnesium silicate. *(1; 2; 11)*

272. **(D)** Calcium carbonate is often considered the antacid of choice because of the rapid onset of action, high neutralizing capacity, and relatively prolonged action. Side effects include constipation, which may be prevented by combining calcium carbonate with either magnesium carbonate or magnesium oxide. Prolonged use of calcium carbonate may result in the formation of urinary calculi. Also, increased blood levels of calcium have been reported. *(2; 11)*

273. **(B)** Magnesium hydroxide is mixed with aluminum hydroxide in order to reduce the incidence of constipation attributed to the aluminum ion, and to reduce the incidence of diarrhea due to the magnesium ion. Most antacid products on the market consist of this combination. *(2; 11)*

274. **(A)** *(2; 11)*

275. **(A)** *(13)*

276. **(B)** *(13)*

277. **(E)** *(13)*

278. **(D)** *(25)*

279. **(D)** *(1)*

280. **(A)** *(1)*

281. **(B)** *(1)*

282. **(C)** The needle hub can be made of plastic or metal. It is fitted onto the syringe body either by a locking system such as the Luer-Lok or by a simple friction fit. *(13)*

283. **(A)** The bevel is ground to sharpness, but the back portion (heel) of the bevel is left dull. A dull heel has been shown to decrease the incidence of coring of the rubber closure and the skin. *(13)*

284. **(B)** Needle cannula are made of various grades of steel. Both shaft strength and flexibility are needed. *(13)*

285. **(E)** The hole in the shaft is also called the bore. *(13)*

286. **(D)** *(1)*

287. **(A)** *(1)*

288. **(E)** Many OTC products intended for assisting in the removal of warts contain the keratolytic agent, 17% salicylic acid, in a collodion vehicle. Examples of products include Compound W, Duofilm, and Clear-Away. *(11)*

289. **(C)** Coal tar, at levels of 0.5 to 5%, may help relieve mild attacks of psoriasis. *(11)*

290. **(E)** The normal pH range for the blood is 7.36 to 7.40 for venous samples and 7.38 to 7.42 for arterial samples. It is essential that the blood pH remains within the range of 7.35 to 7.45. Normal acid–base balance is generally maintained by three homeostatic mechanisms using endogenous chemical buffers (e.g., bicarbonate and carbonic acid), respiratory control, and renal function. An impairment in any of these mechanisms can result in either acidosis or alkalosis. *(1; 24)*

291. **(E)** The pH of the lacrimal fluid is approximately 7.4 but varies with certain ailments. The eye can tolerate a pH of 6 to 8 with a minimum of discomfort. The buffering system of the lacrimal fluid is efficient enough to adjust the pH of most ophthalmic solutions. However, some solutions, particularly those containing strongly acidic drugs, will cause discomfort. *(24)*

292. **(B)** The pH of the skin is usually based on measurements of the lipid film that covers the epidermis. Although the value varies greatly between individuals and in various areas of the body, the average value is reported to be 5.5, with a range of 4.0 to 6.5. *(1)*

293. **(A)** The acidic pH (3.5 to 4.2) of the vagina discourages the growth of pathogenic microorganisms while providing a suitable environment for the growth of acid-producing bacilli. *(24)*

294. **(B)** (1)

295. **(D)** (1)

296. **(A)** *(1)*

297. **(E)** Oramorph SR tablets consist of morphine sulfate in a hydrophilic matrix which protects the interior of the tablet from disintegrating too rapidly. *(1; 24)*

298. **(D)** Repetabs are designed to release an initial dose, followed by a second dose, from the inner core at a later time. This type of product reduces the number of doses the patient must take during the day. *(1; 24)*

299. **(C)** The Durabond principle consists of complexing amine drugs with tannic acid to form the corresponding tannates. These relatively insoluble drug forms are released slowly over a 12-h period. *(10; 24)*

300. **(E)**

301. **(C)**

302. **(B)**

303. **(A)**

304. **(E)** Transdermal drug delivery systems deliver drugs at an optimal rate through the skin and avoid the hepatic first-pass effect. Since the

patch needs replacement only once daily or up to once a week depending upon the drug involved, patient compliance improves. Since most of the drug is in the patch reservoir, relatively large amounts of drugs with short half-lives can be formulated into transdermal patches. One criteria is the ability of the drug to diffuse through the skin. *(24)*

305. **(C)** Bupropion (Zyban) is used to aid in smoking cessation. It is available as 100 and 150 mg sustained release tablets but not as a dermal patch. However, there are a number of nicotine patches on the market for smoking cessation. Scopolamine (Transderm Scop) is used to prevent motion sickness. Estradiol (Estraderm, Vivelle, and Climara) patches reduce post-menopausal symptoms. Also, there is an estrogen + progestin combination (Evra) for use as a contraceptive patch. Fentanyl (Duragesic) reduces chronic pain. Testosterone patches (Testoderm and Androderm) are used when there is a deficiency of testosterone. *(24)*

306. **(C)** Most nasal solutions are mildly buffered at pHs between 5.5 and 7.5 to prevent interference with normal cilia motion. The solutions should also be isotonic if possible. *(19)*

307. **(A)** Allopathy is the treatment of disease by using remedies that produce effects on the body that differ from those produced by the disease. This new set of conditions is incompatible with or antagonistic to the original symptoms of the disease. The term is now used when referring to standard or orthodox medical practice. *(1; 14)*

   (C–incorrect) Naturopathy indicates healing by the exclusive use of natural remedies (heat, light, vegetables, fruits, etc.) but no surgery or drugs.

   (D) Nutraceutical practice is one in which foods are used to promote healing and health.

308. **(C)** Homeopathy involves the use of substances that produce symptoms similar to the symptoms of the disease (the law of similarity). The drugs used, mainly herbals, are administered as very high dilutions, that is, in extremely low doses. *(1; 27)*

   (B—incorrect) Holistic medicine refers to therapies that treat the whole person—both mind and body. *(1)*

309. **(C)** Echinacea is believed to stimulate the immune system thus, reducing the severity of cold and flu symptoms especially if consumed during the early stages of the exposure. *(1; 2; 11)*

310. **(B)** Some studies have indicated that gingko extracts improve blood perfusion. There is hope that the herb will improve memory. A problem may occur if gingko is taken by individuals being treated with the anticoagulants. *(2; 11)*

311. **(A)** St. John's wort may help cases of mild depression. Its active ingredient, hypericin, is believed to cause photodermatitis if light-skinned clients are exposed to direct sunlight. *(2; 11)*

312. **(D)** Saw palmetto may be useful in treating symptoms of BPH (benign prostatic hyperplasia). It appears to improve urinary flow in men with enlarged prostates. *(2; 11)*

313. **(A)** Health authorities have accepted valerian as an effective treatment for restlessness and sleep disturbances. Some classify the herb as a mild tranquilizer. *(1)*

314. **(A)** Controlled studies of ginger root in the form of capsules indicate its ability to counteract mild cases of nausea and vomiting and also to prevent motion sickness. *(2; 11)*

315 **(B)** Comfrey has been advocated for the treatment of topical wounds. However, it has been shown to be hepatotoxic and would be particularly dangerous if placed on large areas of burns or open wounds. The USP does not recommend its use. *(1)*

316. **(C)** Milk thistle contains a group of compounds known as the silymarins. The herb appears to provide protection to the liver that has been exposed to chemicals such as carbon tetrachloride, and drugs such as acetaminophen. *(1)*

**317.** **(A)** Echinacea has not been reported as having significant effects on blood coagulation times, perhaps because it is not intended for long term use. Its main use is to prevent or reduce the severity of the common cold and other upper respiratory infections. Its efficacy depends upon consumption when the symptoms of the cold first appear. All of the other herbs in the question may affect blood coagulation and the patient taking warfarin should be informed of potential problems. *(2)*

**318.** **(C)** There are numerous chemical types of ingredients in crude drugs which make extraction of the actives an exacting science. The use of alcohol as a solvent (menstruum) is common since many actives such as alkaloids are readily soluble and evaporation of some of the alcohol allows a standardization of the product. Extraction may be accomplished by soaking (macerating) the crude plant in the menstruum or by slowly passing the menstruum through the crude plant; a process known as percolation. Historically, pharmacists prepared extracts and fluid extracts as final dosage forms. Today pharmaceutical companies perform extractions with more accurate assays and standardization. Reverse osmosis is not used for crude drug extraction. Instead the process is used for purification of liquids such as water. *(1; 24)*

**319.** **(A)** The dietary supplement, glucosamine is a natural building block of cartilage. Pure glucosamine is available in products such as Aflexa tablets. However, the most popular type of product is combinations with chondroitin which have been found effective in providing symptomatic relief from osteoarthritis. *(1; 2)*

**320.** **(E)** St. John's wort contains several active ingredients and is usually labeled based upon its concentration of hypericin or hyperforin. The herb is used for the treatment of mild depression. However, patients consuming oral contraceptive tablets should be informed of a potential reduction in the effectiveness of the birth control tablets. The herb also tends to cause a photosensitivity reaction in fair-skinned people. *(1; 2)*

# CHAPTER 4

# Pharmaceutical Compounding

Compounding is considered an intrinsic skill of the pharmacist. Although the number of extemporaneously compounded prescriptions is steadily declining, some pharmacists have experienced professional satisfaction in their ability to prepare products that would otherwise not be available to the patient. Pharmacists in institutional settings are expected to prepare parenteral admixtures, reconstitute parenteral powders, and advise other health professionals in the handling, storage, administration, and potential incompatibilities of sterile products. The emerging field of home health care has called on both community and institutional pharmacists to prepare sterile chemotherapeutic, analgesic, and nutritional formulations.

This chapter reviews some of the compounding techniques, ingredients, and calculations that the practicing pharmacist may need to use.

# Questions

**DIRECTIONS (Questions 1 through 106): Each of the numbered items or incomplete statements in this section is followed by answers or by completions of the statement. Select the ONE lettered answer or completion that is BEST in each case.**

1. The prescription balance needed for weighing chemicals is currently designated as a Class —— balance by the NBS.

    (A) I
    (B) II
    (C) III
    (D) P
    (E) Q

2. Which one of the following statements concerning single-pan electronic balances as replacements for the Class III balance is true?

    (A) They cannot be used since they are too accurate for routine weighings.
    (B) They are not suitable since the official shift and rider balance tests cannot be performed.
    (C) They may be used if they have a sensitivity requirement of 6 mg or better.
    (D) They are not recommended since their total weight capacity is often less than 120 g.
    (E) They may be used if their total weight capacity is not greater than 120 g.

3. Pharmacists performing extemporaneous compounding should select chemical grades that meet specifications found in which of the following references?

    I. *Remington Science and Practice of Pharmacy*
    II. *USP/DI*
    III. *USP/NF*

    (A) I only
    (B) III only
    (C) I and II only
    (D) II and III only
    (E) I, II, and III

4. How many grams of ferrous gluconate dihydrate are needed to obtain 100 g of pure ferrous gluconate? [mol wt of anhydrous ferrous gluconate = 446; formula wt of ferrous gluconate dihydrate = 482; valence of iron +2 and +3]

    (A) 46
    (B) 54
    (C) 100
    (D) 108
    (E) 162

5. A bottle of morphine sulfate labeled "Anhydrous Morphine Sulfate" also indicates the presence of 2% unbound water. How many mg of this powder is needed to prepare 120 mL of a solution containing 20 mg/mL of anhydrous morphine sulfate? [mol wt anhydrous morphine sulfate = 669; hydrated morphine sulfate = 759]

    (A) 2350
    (B) 2720
    (C) 2115
    (D) 2400
    (E) 2450

**Questions 6 through 9 relate to the following prescription:**

For: James Latimer                                  Age: 3

**Rx**
  Sodium fluoride                                   500 µg
  M & Ft Cap DTD # LX

Sig: one cap QD

6. How many mg of sodium fluoride are required to prepare this prescription?

(A) 0.5
(B) 30
(C) 50
(D) 300
(E) 500

7. Problem(s) that the pharmacist should anticipate in preparing this prescription include

I. caustic nature of sodium fluoride
II. poor water solubility of sodium fluoride
III. difficulty in weighing a small quantity of powder

(A) I only
(B) III only
(C) I and II only
(D) II and III only
(E) I, II, and III

8. The best choice of a diluent for stock powders, especially when preparing capsules, is

(A) ascorbic acid
(B) lactose
(C) sodium chloride
(D) starch
(E) talc

9. The pharmacist fills a #2 capsule and finds that the net weight of the powder is 40 mg less than needed. She may elect to

I. use a #1 capsule
II. place additional powder into the head of the capsule
III. use a #3 capsule

(A) I only
(B) III only
(C) I and II only
(D) II and III only
(E) I, II, and III

**Questions 10 through 12 refer to the following prescription:**

For: Daniel Cummins                                 Age: 16

**Rx**
  Codeine sulfate                                   210 mg
  Dimenhydrinate                                    1000 mg
  ASA                                               3000 mg
  M & Ft cap #20

Sig: i cap q.i.d. p.r.n. for pain

**NOTE:** The pharmacist has 50-mg dimenhydrinate tablets, each weighing 200 mg, and 30-mg codeine sulfate tablets, each weighing 100 mg. Aspirin is available as a powder.

10. Which of the following statements concerning the prescription is (are) true?

I. The amount of codeine being consumed per day is an overdose.
II. There is a chemical incompatibility between dimenhydrinate and codeine.
III. The patient should be cautioned about the possibility of drowsiness from the capsules.

(A) I only
(B) III only
(C) I and II only
(D) II and III only
(E) I, II, and III

11. When compounding this prescription, the pharmacist must

    I. use a rubber spatula rather than a stainless steel spatula
    II. add lactose to the formula
    III. take into consideration the weight of the excipients in the codeine and dimenhydrinate tablets

    (A) I only
    (B) III only
    (C) I and II only
    (D) II and III only
    (E) I, II, and III

12. The final weight of each capsule will be approximately

    (A) 150 mg
    (B) 210 mg
    (C) 235 mg
    (D) 360 mg
    (E) 385 mg

**Answer questions 13 through 15 based on the following prescription:**

| | |
|---|---|
| Name: James McMaster | Age: 4 |
| | Wt: 44 lb |

**Rx**

| | |
|---|---|
| Ondansetron HCl | 0.15 mg/kg/tsp |
| Cherry syrup | qs 60 mL |

Sig: 1 tsp before therapy

13. How many 4-mg commercial tablets are needed to prepare this order?

    (A) 3
    (B) 6
    (C) 9
    (D) 12
    (E) 15

14. Which of the following statements concerning compounding this prescription is (are) true?

    I. It is necessary to dissolve the crushed tablets in alcohol before adding to the syrup.
    II. The pH of the final product should be adjusted to a neutral pH.
    III. It is possible to use ondansetron injectable solution in place of the tablets.

    (A) I only
    (B) III only
    (C) I and II only
    (D) II and III only
    (E) I, II, and III

15. When preparing a liquid oral dosage form, elixirs may be preferred over syrups because elixirs have better solvent properties for

    I. weak organic acids
    II. weak organic bases
    III. flavoring oils

    (A) I only
    (B) III only
    (C) I and II only
    (D) II and III only
    (E) I, II, and III

**Questions 16 through 22 relate to the following parenteral admixture order as received in a hospital pharmacy:**

| | |
|---|---|
| Patient: Ronald Hazelton | Room no. 614 |
| | DOB: 4/28/44 |
| Aminophylline | 400 mg |
| KCl | 20 mEq |
| Thiamine HCl | 100 mg |
| Heparin | 2000 units |
| $D_5W$ | 500 mL |

Infuse over 4 h at 1000, 1400, and 1800

16. Which ingredient in the above parenteral admixture may present a compatibility problem?

    (A) aminophylline
    (B) potassium chloride
    (C) thiamine HCl

(D) heparin

(E) dextrose

17. Aminophylline is available in 20-mL ampules (25 mg/mL). How many ampules are needed daily for this order?

(A) 1

(B) 2

(C) 3

(D) 4

(E) 5

18. When reviewing this order, the pharmacist should

(A) suggest that the heparin be given subcutaneously

(B) inform the prescriber that the dose of aminophylline is too high

(C) plan on sending the finished product in a light protecting bag

(D) recognize that the flow rate is too high

(E) fill the order as written

19. Correct method(s) for preparing the previously shown admixture include

   I. adding the potassium chloride solution to the $D_5W$, followed by the aminophylline solution

   II. adding the aminophylline solution to the $D_5W$ first, then add the potassium chloride solution

   III. mixing the aminophylline solution and the potassium chloride solution, then add this mixture to the $D_5W$

(A) I only

(B) III only

(C) I and II only

(D) II and III only

(E) I, II, and III

20. The total amount (mg) of potassium administered in each admixture bottle is (K = 39.1, Cl = 35.5)

(A) 780

(B) 1180

(C) 2340

(D) 4480

(E) 2240

21. After removing the aminophylline solution from the ampule, the pharmacist should pass the solution through a device such as a filter needle. The filter needle is intended for the removal of

   I. particulate matter

   II. microorganisms

   III. pyrogens

(A) I only

(B) III only

(C) I and II only

(D) II and III only

(E) I, II, and III

22. Which of the following laminar flow hoods is (are) considered a suitable working area for preparing the previously mentioned admixture order?

   I. convergent

   II. horizontal

   III. vertical

(A) I only

(B) III only

(C) I and II only

(D) II and III only

(E) I, II, and III

23. Which of the following are appropriate techniques when preparing most parenteral admixtures?

   I. Work within 6 in of the HEPA filter.

   II. Use a vertical laminar flow hood.

   III. Work in an area at least 6 in from the edge of the benchtop.

(A) I only

(B) III only

(C) I and II only

(D) II and III only

(E) I, II, and III

**24.** Which of the following would the pharmacist consider as suitable agents for disinfecting a laminar flow hood?

   I.   alcohol 70%
  II.   acetone
 III.   betadine

(A) I only
(B) III only
(C) I and II only
(D) II and III only
(E) I, II, and III

**25.** The American Society of Health-System Pharmacists (ASHP) has developed a risk level classification with the strictest controls designated as

(A) risk level 1
(B) risk level 3
(C) risk level X
(D) risk level A
(E) risk level F

**Questions 26 through 28 relate to the following medication order:**

> Patient: Constance Morehead
>
>                          Age: 57
>                       Room: CCU
>
> Morphine sulfate 15 mg + Hydroxyzine HCl 25 mg STAT

**26.** Which of the following consultations between the pharmacist and the nurse is (are) appropriate?

   I.   The two solutions may be mixed together in a syringe in order to administer a single injection.
  II.   The morphine injection may be administered by either the IM or SC route.
 III.   A precipitate may occur if either drug solution is injected into a heparinized scalp vein infusion set.

(A) I only
(B) III only
(C) I and II only

(D) II and III only
(E) I, II, and III

**27.** Which of the following steps is INCORRECT when the pharmacist removes 1.5 mL of solution from a 30-mL multidose vial of morphine sulfate injection (10 mg/mL)?

(A) Draw up 1.5 mL of air into the syringe.
(B) Place point of syringe needle onto the vial's rubber closure at a 45° angle.
(C) Rotate needle so that the bevel opening is facing upwards.
(D) Raise the needle angle to 90° and insert needle through the rubber closure.
(E) After injecting the air, remove 2 mL of solution and aspirate excess solution into an alcohol swab.

**28.** When obtaining a 3-mL dose from a 5-mL ampule, which one of the following steps is INCORRECT?

(A) Draw up 3 mL of air into the syringe.
(B) Disinfect the neck of the ampule using an alcohol swab.
(C) Break ampule neck by snapping neck toward the side of the laminar flow hood.
(D) Place needle tip into solution while holding the ampule almost horizontally.
(E) After drawing up approximately 4 mL of solution, aspirate excess solution into the alcohol swab.

**Answer questions 29 through 31 in reference to the following medication order:**

> Medication Order—Carefree Hospital
>
> Patient: James Gardner        Room 314
>
> Potassium Pen G 2 Megaunits in 100 mL minibottles q6h ATC for 4 days

**NOTE:** The pharmacy has vials containing 5 million units of potassium penicillin G that, when reconstituted with diluent, will contain 750,000 units/mL. The label on the vial states that the powder contains a citrate buffer to maintain a pH of 6 to 6.5.

29. The total number of minibottles needed for Mr. Gardner's therapy will be

(A) 3
(B) 4
(C) 10
(D) 12
(E) 16

30. Which of the following vehicles is (are) suitable for the above order?

I. $D_5W$ (pH = 4.5)
II. N/S (pH = 6.0)
III. $D_{2.5}W/0.45NS$ (pH = 5.0)

(A) I only
(B) III only
(C) I and II only
(D) II and III only
(E) I, II, and III

31. Which of the following procedures should the pharmacist use in preparing the minibottles?

(A) Remove 2.7 mL of vehicle from the minibottle, then inject 2.7 mL of penicillin solution.
(B) Inject 2.7 mL of penicillin solution directly into the minibottle.
(C) Remove 6.7 mL of vehicle from the minibottle, then inject 6.7 mL of penicillin solution.
(D) Inject 6.7 mL of penicillin solution directly into the minibottle.
(E) Inject 4 mL of penicillin solution directly into the minibottle.

**Questions 32 through 34**
Alcohol has many pharmaceutical uses and is available in several concentrations. MATCH the lettered concentration (% v/v) with the associated numbered official product.

(A) 49%
(B) 70%
(C) 92%
(D) 95%
(E) 100%

32. Alcohol  95

33. Diluted alcohol   49

34. Rubbing alcohol   70

**Questions 35 through 37 refer to the following prescription:**

| Rx | |
|---|---|
| Calamine | |
| Zinc oxide | aa qs 15 g |
| Resorcinol | 2 g |
| Glycerin | 15 mL |
| Alcohol 70% | 30 mL |
| Pur. water ad | 120 mL |
| | |
| Sig: Use as directed t.i.d. | |

35. The final dosage form of this prescription is best described as a (an)

(A) colloidal solution
(B) elixir
(C) O/W emulsion
(D) W/O emulsion
(E) suspension

36. When preparing the prescription, the pharmacist will

I. use 15 g of calamine
II. dissolve the resorcinol in the alcohol
III. triturate calamine and zinc oxide together and wet with glycerin

(A) I only
(B) III only
(C) I and II only
(D) II and III only
(E) I, II, and III

37. Which of the following auxiliary labels should the pharmacist attach to the container when dispensing the previously mentioned product?

   I. for external use only
   II. shake well
   III. keep in a cool place

   (A) I only
   (B) III only
   (C) I and II only
   (D) II and III only
   (E) I, II, and III

38. The following prescription is received:

---

**Rx**

| | |
|---|---|
| Itraconazole | 1% |
| Propylene glycol | 10 mL |
| MC 1500 | 1.5% |
| Purified water | qs 60 mL |

Sig: Apply to nail bed b.i.d. ut dict

---

When preparing this prescription, the pharmacist should

   I. disperse 0.9 g of methylcellulose 1500 in hot water
   II. use the contents from six 100-mg Sporanox capsules
   III. wet the capsule powder with the propylene glycol

   (A) I only
   (B) III only
   (C) I and II only
   (D) II and III only
   (E) I, II, and III

**DIRECTIONS (Questions 39 through 45): Each group of items in this section consists of lettered headings followed by a set of numbered words or phrases. For each numbered word or phrase, select the ONE lettered heading that is most closely associated with it. Each lettered heading may be selected once, more than once, or not at all.**

**Questions 39 through 45**

   (A) hydrocarbon (oleaginous)
   (B) absorption (anhydrous)
   (C) emulsion (W/O type)
   (D) emulsion (O/W type)
   (E) water soluble

39. Cold cream

40. Hydrophilic petrolatum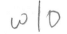

41. Lanolin

42. Petrolatum

43. Polyethylene glycol ointment

44. Hydrophilic ointment

45. Aquaphor

**Questions 46 through 48 relate to the following prescription:**

---

**Rx**

| | |
|---|---|
| Burow's solution | |
| Propylene glycol | aa 15 mL |
| White petrolatum | 60 g |

---

46. The active ingredient in Burow's solution is

   (A) acetic acid
   (B) aluminum acetate
   (C) aluminum chloride
   (D) alcohol
   (E) hydrogen peroxide

47. Assuming that the pharmacist does not use an excess of each ingredient and there is no loss during compounding, the weight of the final preparation will be

   (A) less than 60 g
   (B) 60 g
   (C) 75 g
   (D) 90 g
   (E) greater than 90 g

48. When preparing this prescription, the pharmacist may wish to include

    I.   Aquaphor
    II.  Alcohol USP
    III. Tween 80

    (A) I only
    (B) III only
    (C) I and II only
    (D) II and III only
    (E) I, II, and III

49. A prescription calls for 10% urea in Aquaphor base. Which of the following is the best technique to make a pharmaceutically elegant product?

    (A) Dissolve urea in water then incorporate into the Aquaphor.
    (B) Dissolve urea in alcohol then incorporate into the Aquaphor.
    (C) Finely powder the urea and incorporate directly into the Aquaphor.
    (D) Dissolve urea in small amount of mineral oil and incorporate into the Aquaphor.
    (E) Melt the Aquaphor and dissolve the urea in the hot liquid.

50. When being incorporated into ointment bases, fine powders such as calamine and zinc oxide are often wetted and smoothed with mineral oil. What name is given to this process?

    (A) attrition
    (B) levigation
    (C) milling
    (D) pulverization by intervention
    (E) trituration

**Questions 51 through 53 refer to the following prescription:**

| Rx | |
|---|---|
| Retinoic acid | 0.02% |
| Ac. Sal. | 2% |
| Emulsion base | qs 60 g |
| | |
| Sig: Apply small amount onto spots hs | |

51. Which of the following statements concerning this prescription is (are) true?

    I.   Another name for retinoic acid is tretinoin.
    II.  The amount of aspirin needed is 1.2 g.
    III. The term "emulsion base" refers to a brand of ointment base.

    (A) I only
    (B) III only
    (C) I and II only
    (D) II and III only
    (E) I, II, and III

52. How many grams of 0.05% Retin-A cream may be used to supply the retinoic acid?

    (A) 0.012
    (B) 1.2
    (C) 2.4
    (D) 15
    (E) 24

53. Which of the following should the pharmacist use when compounding this prescription?

    I.   pill tile for mixing
    II.  rubber spatulas for weighing and incorporating the ingredients
    III. alcohol to dissolve the salicylic acid

    (A) I only
    (B) III only
    (C) I and II only
    (D) II and III only
    (E) I, II, and III

54. A prescription reads "Dilute a 0.25% steroidal cream to 0.1% strength using a vanishing cream base." How many grams of diluent should the pharmacist add to 30 g of the 0.25% cream?

    (A) 6.5 g
    (B) 12 g
    (C) 30 g
    (D) 45 g
    (E) 75 g

**55.** The request for a "vanishing cream" base is best fulfilled using which of the following bases?

(A) cold cream
(B) hydrophilic ointment
(C) lanolin
(D) Vaseline
(E) PEG ointment

**Questions 56 through 59: From the lettered list, select the most appropriate official topical base that the pharmacist should select for the desired characteristic in the numbered list. Each letter heading may be selected once, more than once, or not at all.**

(A) cold cream
(B) hydrophilic ointment
(C) hydrophilic petrolatum
(D) PEG ointment
(E) white petrolatum

**56.** For an ophthalmic drug

**57.** For an antibiotic with limited stability

**58.** For absorbing a large quantity of water

**59.** To aid in hydrating the skin

**60.** Which of the following types of topical bases require the inclusion of an antimicrobial preservative?

  I.   aqueous gels
  II.  water in oil (W/O) emulsions
  III. oil in water (O/W) emulsion

(A) I only
(B) III only
(C) I and II only
(D) II and III only
(E) I, II, and III

**61.** Which one of the following ingredients is most likely to be utilized in the formulation of a topical gel?

(A) carbomer
(B) edetate
(C) lanolin

(D) mineral oil
(E) vegetable oil

**62.** Alcohol is suitable as a solvent for menthol or salicylic acid when preparing which of the following dosage forms?

  I.   lotions
  II.  ointments
  III. suppositories

(A) I only
(B) III only
(C) I and II only
(D) II and III only
(E) I, II, and III

**63.** A lotion formula calls for coal tar solution. Which of the following statements concerning coal tar solution is NOT true?

(A) Alcohol is used as the solvent.
(B) LCD is another name for the solution.
(C) The solution is for external use only.
(D) The solution is usually diluted 1:9 with water or ointment base.
(E) The solution contains only coal tar and a volatile solvent.

**Answer questions 64 through 67 based on the following prescription:**

| Rx | |
|---|---|
| Ephedrine sulfate | 2% |
| Menthol | 0.5% |
| Camphor | |
| Methyl salicylate | aa 0.2% |
| Mineral oil | qs 30 mL |
| Sig: gtt ii both sides t.i.d. | |

**64.** This prescription may be administered into the

  I.   nose
  II.  eyes
  III. ears

(A) I only
(B) III only
(C) I and II only

(D)  II and III only

(E)  I, II, and III

65.  Which of the following ingredients will NOT dissolve in the prescribed solvent?

I.  ephedrine sulfate

II.  menthol

III.  methyl salicylate

(A)  I only

(B)  III only

(C)  I and II only

(D)  II and III only

(E)  I, II, and III

66.  Which of the following statements is (are) NOT true for camphor?

I.  It forms an eutectic mixture with menthol.

II.  It can be powdered by rubbing with a small amount of alcohol or ether.

III.  It dissolves readily in water.

(A)  I only

(B)  III only

(C)  I and II only

(D)  II and III only

(E)  I, II, and III

67.  Methyl salicylate is also known as

(A)  camphorated oil

(B)  peppermint oil

(C)  salicylamide

(D)  oil of wintergreen

(E)  sweet oil

**Questions 68 through 71 are based on the following order received from a hospital outpatient EENT clinic:**

| | |
|---|---|
| Tetracaine | 1.0% |
| Boric acid | 0.5% |
| Purified water | qs 100% |

Dispense 60 mL
Make sterile and label as
          "Ophthalmic Solution TET 1%"

68.  Which of the following characteristics concerning tetracaine in the previously mentioned formula is (are) true?

I.  poor water solubility

II.  chemically incompatible with boric acid

III.  not effective as a local anesthetic

(A)  I only

(B)  III only

(C)  I and II only

(D)  II and III only

(E)  I, II, and III

69.  Boric acid is present in the formula as a (an)

I.  antioxidant

II.  antimicrobial preservative

III.  buffering agent

(A)  I only

(B)  III only

(C)  I and II only

(D)  II and III only

(E)  I, II, and III

70.  How many mg of sodium chloride are needed to adjust the tonicity of the formula? The following "E" values are available: tetracaine HCl = 0.18; boric acid = 0.50; sodium borate = 0.42

(A)  260

(B)  280

(C)  440

(D)  540

(E)  640

71.  The most practical method for sterilizing the previous ophthalmic solution is

(A)  autoclaving for 15 min

(B)  autoclaving for 30 min

(C)  membrane filtration through 0.2-μm filter

(D)  membrane filtration through 5-μm filter

(E)  the use of ethylene oxide gas

**Questions 72 through 74 refer to the following formula:**

| | |
|---|---|
| Progesterone | 20 mg |
| PEG 400 | 60% |
| PEG 6000 | 40% |
| | |
| To make one vaginal suppository | |

72. Which of the following statements is (are) true with respect to this formula?

    I.  The weight of the individual suppository must be determined experimentally.
    II. A mold must be used to prepare this formula.
    III. The bulk density of the progesterone must be calculated.

    (A) I only
    (B) III only
    (C) I and II only
    (D) II and III only
    (E) I, II, and III

73. The ideal weight for a vaginal suppository will be approximately

    (A) 1 g
    (B) 2 g
    (C) 5 g
    (D) 10 g
    (E) 15 g

74. Which of the following suppository bases melt rather than dissolve when inserted into the rectum?

    I.   Cocoa butter
    II.  Fattibase
    III. PEGs

    (A) I only
    (B) III only
    (C) I and II only
    (D) II and III only
    (E) I, II, and III only

75. An order in a nursing home calls for 30 g of ointment to contain 15,000 units of polymyxin B

sulfate per gram. The pharmacist has 10 mL parenteral vials labeled as containing 500,000 units of polymyxin B sulfate. Which of the following statements is (are) accurate?

    I.   The pharmacist will use 9 mL of the polymyxin B sulfate solution.
    II.  It will be best to incorporate the solution into an absorption type base.
    III. The solution should be incorporated into 30 g of ointment base.

    (A) I only
    (B) III only
    (C) I and II only
    (D) II and III only
    (E) I, II, and III

76. Which one of the following diluents is LEAST suitable for reconstituting a sterile powder packaged in single-dose vials?

    (A) bacteriostatic sterile water for injection (BSWFI)
    (B) $D_5W$ injection
    (C) N/S injection
    (D) 1/2 N/S injection
    (E) sterile water for injection (SWFI)

77. Which of the following authors are associated with reference sources that contain compilations of data describing compatibilities between various parenteral drug products?

    I.   Trissel
    II.  King
    III. Remington

    (A) I only
    (B) III only
    (C) I and II only
    (D) II and III only
    (E) I, II, and III

78. A physician is seeking a commercial parenteral amino acids solution that contains a specific amount of two amino acids. Which one of the following books presents direct comparisons of such products from different companies?

(A) *Drug Facts and Comparisons*

(B) *Merck Index*

(C) *Physicians' Drug Reference*

(D) *Remington: The Science and Practice of Pharmacy*

(E) *USP/NF*

79. Which one of the following injectable solutions may result in a precipitate if added to 50 mL of D$_5$W or NS?

(A) diazepam (Valium) 20 mg

(B) folic acid (Folvite) 1 mg

(C) furosemide (Lasix) 40 mg

(D) gentamicin sulfate (Garamycin) 20 mg

(E) succinylcholine chloride (Anectine) 100 mg

80. When reviewing the amino acids present in various amino acids injection formulas, the pharmacist will note which of the following?

I. Some of the formulas do not contain the nonessential amino acids.

II. Formulas with the same overall concentrations of amino acids may vary in the relative amounts of a specific amino acid present.

III. Some of the formulas contain higher amounts of the branched chain amino acids.

(A) I only

(B) III only

(C) I and II only

(D) II and III only

(E) I, II, and III

81. When dispensing amphotericin, which of the following statements is (are) true?

I. The original powder may be reconstituted only with SWFI.

II. The resulting liquid is a colloidal solution.

III. The solution is intended to be infused into a patient within 60 min.

82. Which of the following are liposomal formulations of amphotericin?

I. Abelcet injection

II. Amphocil injection

III. Docil injection

(A) I only

(B) III only

(C) I and II only

(D) II and III only

(E) I, II, and III

83. Which of the following cautions must be considered when dispensing most parenteral liposomal products?

I. Do not reconstitute with sodium chloride injection.

II. Dosing may differ from that of the conventional drug solutions.

III. Infuse only through administration sets that have an in-line filter.

(A) I only

(B) III only

(C) I and II only

(D) II and III only

(E) I, II, and III

84. Which of the following statements concerning the development of TPN solutions is (are) true?

I. The total daily caloric density of the solution should not exceed the BEE of the patient.

II. It is desirable to avoid EFAD in the patient.

III. The final solutions may have osmolarities greater than 300 mOsm/L.

(A) I only

(B) III only

(C) I and II only

(D) II and III only

(E) I, II, and III

85. Other names given to TPN solutions that contain the intravenous fat emulsions include

    I. MCIs
    II. TNA
    III. 3 in 1s

    (A) I only
    (B) III only
    (C) I and II only
    (D) II and III only
    (E) I, II, and III

86. What caloric density value (kcal/g) should be used when calculating the contribution of dextrose in infusion solutions?

    (A) 3.4
    (B) 4.0
    (C) 5.5
    (D) 6.0
    (E) 10

87. What is the average weight in grams of nitrogen present in every 100 mL of a 10% amino acids injection?

    (A) 1.0 g
    (B) 1.6 g
    (C) 10 g
    (D) 16 g
    (E) 50 g

**Questions 88 through 102: Answer the following series of questions based on the availability of the following parenteral solutions and hospital medication order:**

| Patient: Danielle Howell | Room: Main 218 |
|---|---|
| Aminosyn II 8.5% | |
| $D_{50}W$ | aa 500 mL |
| Potassium chloride | 40 mEq |
| Sodium chloride | 20 mEq |
| Potassium phosphate | 40 mEq |
| MVI-12 | 1 vial |
| Zinc chloride | 2 mg |
| Insulin | 40 units |
| Calcium gluconate | 10 mL |

Infuse above t.i.d. for 6 days.
Add 500 mL Liposyn III 10% once daily.

**Available to the pharmacist are the following parenteral solutions:**

| Aminosyn II 8.5% | 500-mL full bts |
|---|---|
| Dextrose 50% injection | 500-mL full bts |
| Calcium chloride 10% | 10-mL vials |
| Calcium gluconate 10% | 10-mL vials |
| Intralipid 10% | 250-mL bottles |
| Magnesium sulfate | 20-mL vials |
| Sodium chloride injection | 30-mL vials |
| MTE-4 | 10-mL vials |
| Potassium chloride injection | 20-mL vials |
| Potassium phosphate | 10-mL vials |

88. The TPN formula is best prepared by

    (A) adding the $D_{50}W$ to the Aminosyn bottle
    (B) adding the Aminosyn to the $D_{50}W$ bottle
    (C) transferring both the Aminosyn and the $D_{50}W$ to an empty, sterile infusion bag
    (D) hanging the Aminosyn and the $D_{50}W$ solutions separately on the patient
    (E) piggybacking the $D_{50}W$ into the Y-tubing of the Aminosyn administration set

89. How many nonprotein kcalories are present in every liter of the TPN solution?

    (A) 850
    (B) 1000
    (C) 1250
    (D) 1700
    (E) 2000

90. Which of the following options are available to the pharmacist if $D_{50}W$ solutions were out of stock?

    I. Use 360 mL of $D_{70}W$.
    II. Increase the amount of amino acids solution to obtain the same calories.
    III. Use 200 mL of $D_{70}W$, and 300 mL of $D_{20}W$.

    (A) I only
    (B) III only
    (C) I and II only
    (D) II and III only
    (E) I, II, and III

91. The pharmacist must be cognizant of potential incompatibilities between

    (A) potassium chloride and calcium gluconate
    (B) potassium chloride and insulin
    (C) potassium phosphate and calcium gluconate
    (D) potassium phosphate and zinc chloride
    (E) insulin and zinc chloride

92. To avoid the possibility of a precipitate, the pharmacist may choose to

    I. place the calcium gluconate and potassium phosphate into separate, alternate containers
    II. use sodium phosphate rather than potassium phosphate
    III. use calcium chloride rather than calcium gluconate

    (A) I only
    (B) III only
    (C) I and II only
    (D) II and III only
    (E) I, II, and III

93. What is the prime reason for including potassium phosphate in the formula?

    (A) source of phosphorus
    (B) source of potassium
    (C) buffer
    (D) antioxidant
    (E) stabilizer

94. The prescribing physician should be encouraged to order the potassium phosphate using concentration expressions of

    (A) milliequivalents
    (B) milligrams
    (C) milliliters
    (D) millimoles
    (E) milliosmoles

95. It is convenient and accurate for the pharmacist to measure the insulin required for this order by using a

    I. tuberculin syringe
    II. low-dose insulin syringe
    III. a 10-mL regular syringe

    (A) I only
    (B) III only
    (C) I and II only
    (D) II and III only
    (E) I, II, and III

96. The pharmacist may consider contacting the physician to inform him that

    I. approximately half of the insulin will be adsorbed onto the walls of the glass container
    II. a strength of insulin is needed
    III. insulin is available as both a solution and a suspension

    (A) I only
    (B) III only
    (C) I and II only
    (D) II and III only
    (E) I, II, and III

97. The addition of Liposyn to the TPN

    I.   causes the final solution to be cloudy
    II.  is intended to prevent EFAD
    III. will adversely affect the osmolarity of the already hypertonic solution

    (A) I only
    (B) III only
    (C) I and II only
    (D) II and III only
    (E) I, II, and III

98. Before placing a patient onto IV fat emulsions, the pharmacist should confirm that the patient does not have

    (A) egg allergies
    (B) sensitivities to bisulfate
    (C) milk intolerance
    (D) lactose intolerance
    (E) sensitivities to tartrazine

99. Approximately how many additional kcal is the patient receiving when a 500-mL bottle of Liposyn 10% is included in the TPN?

    (A) 500
    (B) 1000
    (C) 1500
    (D) 1700
    (E) 2000

100. What is Ms. Howell's daily intake of nitrogen from the amino acids solution?

    (A) 7 g
    (B) 20 g
    (C) 42 g
    (D) 60 g
    (E) 130 g

101. A trace metal that the physician is likely to include in the TPN formula is

    (A) lithium
    (B) sodium
    (C) selenium
    (D) silicon
    (E) fluoride

102. Which of the following metals is NOT present in the MTE-4 or in other multiple trace element solutions?

    (A) chromium
    (B) copper
    (C) iron
    (D) manganese
    (E) zinc

103. To reduce the amount of chloride ion being consumed, the physician requests that the acetate salts of potassium and sodium be used. What information must the pharmacist utilize when making these changes?

    I.   the molecular weights of both acetate salts
    II.  the valences of the ions
    III. the concentrations of the salt solutions in mEq/mL

    (A) I only
    (B) III only
    (C) I and II only
    (D) II and III only
    (E) I, II, and III

104. A nurse reports that a previously clear TPN solution now appears to be slightly cloudy. The pharmacist should advise the nurse to

    (A) discontinue the infusion
    (B) gently warm the solution
    (C) slow the infusion rate
    (D) continue with the infusion
    (E) use an administration set that has an in-line filter

105. Infusion of morphine sulfate solutions to an ambulatory hospice patient in a home setting is best accomplished by the use of a device known as the

    (A) CADD
    (B) PVP
    (C) Homepump
    (D) Implant
    (E) Viadex

106. A home infusion pharmacy receives an order for 5-Fluorouracil 400 mg in a disposable infusion pump for 1 h delivery. Which of the following equipment would the pharmacist use in compounding this order?

    I.   primary administration set
   II.   volumetric burette
  III.  plastic syringe

(A) I only
(B) III only
(C) I and II only
(D) II and III only
(E) I, II, and III

# Answers and Explanations

1. **(C)** The prescription torsion balance designated by NBS as Class III must have a sensitivity requirement (SR) of not greater than 10 mg. This SR allowance is greater than the 6 mg requirement for the former Class A balance. Most Class III balances have a maximum capacity of 60 g rather than the usual 120 g for the Class A. The pharmacist should check the serial plate on the back of the balance to ascertain the limits of the balance. Obviously a balance with a SR of 6 mg is more accurate than one with a SR of 10 mg. The USP/NF specifies that more accurate balances, such as certain electronic balances, may be used. *(1; 4)*

2. **(C)** While free swinging pan balances based upon the torsion principle are traditional in pharmacy, the more sophisticated electronic balances are suitable provided that they meet USP/NF standards of a sensitivity requirement of 6 mg or less (better). While the usual largest quantity to be weighed on the torsion balance without causing damage was 120 g, this is not an absolute quantity. The most important value for compounding is the allowable error which should be not more than ±5%. *(19)*

3. **(B)** The primary designation that the pharmacist seeks when selecting a chemical for compounding is USP/NF grade. This indicates that the chemical meets standards described in official monographs which are recognized by the FDA. If there is no official monograph for a specific chemical, the pharmacist must carefully evaluate available grades and select one that is of high quality. For example, ACS (American Chemical Society) grade or AR (analytical reagent) grade may be suitable. It is important to consider the quantity of active moiety present since some official chemical designations do not indicate 100% pure chemical. For example, waters of hydration, a certain amount of moisture, or other impurities must be taken into consideration. *(4; 19)*

4. **(D)**

$$\frac{100 \text{ g}}{446 \text{ (Anhydrous)}} = \frac{x \text{ g}}{482 \text{ (Hydrous)}}$$

$x = 108$ g of ferrous gluconate dihydrate *(23)*

5. **(E)** Amount of anhydrous morphine sulfate needed = 120 mL × 20 mg/mL = 2400 mg

   The powder available contains 2% absorbed water thus is 98% pure.

$$Q_1 \times C_1 = Q_2 \times C_2$$

$$[2400 \text{ mg}] [100\%] = [x \text{ mg}] [98\%]$$

$$x = 2450 \text{ mg}$$

While the differences between 2400 and 2450 mg do not appear significant, the principle of correcting for either waters of hydration or unbound water is important. Drugs such as magnesium sulfate, citric acid, theophylline, and iron salts often have waters of hydration. The pharmacist must ascertain which form is present in a given formula. In this problem, the anhydrous morphine was being used but it appears to have absorbed water thus changing its strength. *(1; 4; 23)*

6. **(B)** 500 μg is equivalent to 0.5 mg, and 60 capsules were requested

$$0.5 \text{ mg} \times 60 \text{ capsules} = 30 \text{ mg} \quad (23)$$

7.  **(B)** The minimum quantity that can be weighed accurately on the Class III (Class A) prescription balance with an error of not more than 5% is 120 mg (assuming a SR of 6 mg). In order to weigh the required 30 mg of sodium fluoride, a stock powder of NaF is needed. In this problem, mixing 120 mg of NaF with 360 mg of diluent and using 120 mg of this stock powder will deliver the required 30 mg of sodium fluoride. Because of its strong ionic bonds, sodium fluoride is not caustic. A stainless steel spatula can be used for the weighing procedure. Sodium fluoride has good water solubility. *(1; 23)*

8.  **(B)** Lactose is a relatively inert water-soluble substance that also packs well into capsules. An alternative would be the use of starch. For the sodium fluoride prescription, the pharmacist will have to include additional lactose to raise the content of the capsule to a quantity that is weighable and convenient to pack into capsules. For example, a net weight of 300 mg may be selected arbitrarily. *(24)*

9.  **(A)** Empty capsules are sized by a numbering system, the largest being a #000 and the smallest a #5. If the #2 capsule is too small, the pharmacist should try the next largest, the #1. The correct capsule filling procedure is to place powder only into the body or base of the empty capsule. It is not good technique to place powder into the head of the cap because the fit of the head onto the body may not be tight. *(1; 24)*

10. **(B)** Both codeine and dimenhydrinate have a tendency to produce drowsiness as a side effect. Codeine is a weak organic base whereas dimenhydrinate is a combination of diphenhydramine and 8-chlorotheophylline. No chemical reaction between the two drugs would be expected. The amount of codeine consumed per dose is 10 mg or 40 mg daily. This is within the therapeutic dosage range for a 10-year-old child. *(1)*

11. **(B)** If only pure chemicals were available, the weight of powder in each capsule would be 210 mg (4210 mg divided by 20 capsules).

However, if the pharmacist has to use commercial tablets when preparing this prescription, the contributory weight of the additional ingredients (excipients) present in the tablets must be included in the calculations. Although lactose is a popular diluent when making capsules, the high weight of each capsule precludes its use. Weighing the aspirin with a rubber spatula is not necessary because aspirin is not as reactive as salicylic acid. *(4)*

12. **(E)** The total amount of ingredients may be calculated as follows:

| Drug | Total Weight of Powder | |
| --- | --- | --- |
| Codeine | 7 tablets each weighing 100 mg | = 700 mg |
| Dimen-hydrinate | 20 tablets each weighing 200 mg | = 4000 mg |
| Aspirin | powder weighing | 3000 mg |
| Total weight | | = 7700 mg |

7700 mg divided into 20 capsules = 385 mg each *(4)*

13. **(C)** The weight of the child in kg is

$$44 \text{ lb} \times \frac{1 \text{ kg}}{2.2 \text{ lb}} = 20 \text{ kg}$$

Each teaspoon dose will contain 0.15 mg × 20 kg = 3 mg; number of doses = 60 divided by 5 mL = 12 doses (12 doses = 3 mg/dose = 36 mg); therefore nine tablets are needed. *(23)*

14. **(B)** Ondansetron HCl injection is available in vials containing 2 mg/mL. The solution contains both methyl and propyl paraben preservatives that will protect the prescription from microbial growth. Because ondansetron HCl has good water solubility, it is inadvisable to include alcohol in the prescription. As the pH of solutions of the drug is increased, a precipitate may occur. It is best to use acidic vehicles such as orange juice, Coca-Cola, or cherry syrup. *(3; 20)*

15. **(E)** Elixirs may be defined as clear, sweetened, usually flavored, hydroalcoholic solutions

intended for oral use. Ethanol, commonly at a 20 to 25% v/v concentration is included and serves as a good solvent for most weak organic acids and bases. The water in the elixir is a good solvent of the salts of weak organic acids and bases. Although water will keep the ionized drug in solution, alcohol will dissolve any un-ionized drug formed if there is a change in solution pH. Problems caused by sucrose competing for water molecules in either syrups or elixirs have been solved by using the newer artificial sweeteners. Flavoring oils, which are usually mixtures of terpenes, possess good alcohol solubility. *(1; 4)*

16. **(C)** Alkaline pH's may cause either a fine precipitation or decrease the vitamin activity of thiamine hydrochloride solutions which have a pH of 2.5 to 4.5. Aminophylline injection has a very high pH of 8.5 to 9. Heparin sodium solutions have approximately a neutral pH (5–8) as do potassium chloride solutions. Although dextrose 5% injections have pH ranges of 4.0 to 5, they have virtually no buffering capacity. Thus, their pH values will quickly adjust to the pH of the aminophylline solution. *(21)*

17. **(C)** Each 20-mL ampule of aminophylline contains 500 mg of drug. Because the individual admixture order requires 400 mg, the pharmacist will have to open an ampule for each admixture and remove 16 mL of solution. Even if the pharmacist is preparing all three admixtures at one time, three ampules (48 mL total) will still be needed for the order. *(23)*

18. **(E)** There are no additional problems with the order once the thiamine HCl has been eliminated. Heparin may be either infused intravenously or injected subcutaneously. The dose of aminophylline is appropriate and none of the ingredients are sensitive to light. *(21)*

19. **(C)** Because no incompatibilities exist between the aminophylline and the potassium chloride, either could be added first to the D$_5$W container. It would be impractical and time consuming to mix the two solutions first in a syringe and then add them to the D$_5$W. Also there would be an increased possibility of

inaccurate measurements. For example, if only 9 mL of KCl solution was drawn up instead of the correct 10 mL, 17 mL rather than 16 mL of aminophylline solution may be drawn into a syringe to make the desired volume of 26 mL. *(21)*

20. **(A)** Each admixture container will contain 20 mEq of KCl or 20 mEq each of potassium and chloride ion. To determine the mg of potassium present, use the relationship

$$\text{mg (potassium)} = \frac{(20 \text{ mEq})(39.1)}{1}$$

$$x = 780 \text{ mg}$$

The above calculation is based upon the atomic wt of potassium being 39.1 with a valence of +1. *(23)*

21. **(A)** The pore size of filter needles is approximately 5 μm, which is too coarse for removing either pyrogens or bacteria. Instead, the filter needle is intended to remove larger particulate matter such as glass fragments that may have fallen into the ampule during the breaking of the ampule's neck. *(13)*

22. **(C)** Air in the horizontal laminar flow hood flows directly toward the operator, thereby preventing contaminants from entering the admixtures being prepared. This hood provides maximum protection for the parenteral admixture. Vertical hoods have downward air flow, which increases the risk of product contamination but protects the operator from droplets of product solution. These hoods should be used only for the preparation of products that pose a significant risk to the operator; for example, carcinogenic or mutagenic chemotherapeutic drugs. The newest concept for hood design is the convergent flow, which combines both vertical and horizontal flow. *(13)*

23. **(B)** As the air passing through the HEPA filter nears the edge of the benchtop, it becomes more turbulent, thus defeating the purpose of the horizontal or convergent laminar flow hood. For this reason, many horizontal laminar flow hoods have a line drawn 6 in from the edge as a reminder to work further inside the hood.

Usually hoods are left running 24 h a day or are turned on and left running throughout the workday. Work should not commence until the hood has been running for at least 15 to 30 min. It is inadvisable to work within 6 in of the HEPA filter because air flow may be partially blocked. *(13)*

24. **(A)** Alcohol (70%) or isopropyl alcohol (70%) are the two disinfectant solutions usually used to disinfect laminar flow hoods before compounding admixtures. Both are effective antimicrobial agents and will evaporate within a few minutes. Acetone is never used because it is flammable and dangerous if inhaled. Betadine is an effective antimicrobial agent as a skin antiseptic or hand wash but would leave a residual build-up if used in hoods. It also is not very volatile. *(1)*

25. **(B)** Improvements in quality control for the preparation of sterile products by pharmacies have been advocated by several health groups including the ASHP and FDA. The ASHP "Risk Level Classification" describes compounding, storage, and stability standards that should be followed. Of the three risk levels, level 3 is the strictest. Clean room standards have also been proposed to assure tight standards, especially when manipulating unsterile ingredients. *(24)*

26. **(E)** Both morphine sulfate and hydroxyzine HCl solutions will have acidic pHs and are therefore expected to be compatible when mixed together in a syringe. However, if either solution is placed directly into a heparinized lock or infusion set, there may be a precipitate because heparin sodium has a higher pH. *(21)*

27. **(E)** It is preferable to aspirate excessive solution and air bubbles while the needle is still in the vial. This prevents accidental contamination of the hood and personnel. Also, it is inadvisable to waste 0.5 mL of drug solution, especially a controlled substance. It is necessary to inject a volume of air equal to the volume of solution to be withdrawn. Otherwise, a vacuum would occur in the vial, making it difficult to remove liquid. *(13)*

28. **(A)** There is no reason to inject air into the opened ampule because no vacuum will form when an ampule is opened and solution is removed. All ampules are intended as single-dose units and should be discarded after opening. *(13)*

29. **(E)** The direction of q6h ATC indicates that a minibottle will be hung every 6 h around the clock. Therefore, 4 bottles daily × 4 days = 16 bottles. *(23)*

30. **(E)** The citrate buffer system is intended to readily adjust the pH of each listed vehicle to a pH range in which the penicillin is stable. Although the dextrose 5% injection has a pH of 4.5, it has virtually no buffering capacity and does not influence the pH of admixtures. Some hospitals prefer to use dextrose solutions as the vehicle for most admixtures to limit the sodium intake by patients. Other hospitals use normal saline (NS) injection to avoid supplying the calories present in dextrose solutions. *(13; 21)*

31. **(B)** There is no need to remove vehicle solution when adding small volumes of drug additives. The final volume will always vary because the manufacturer places some excess of solution into each unit. To calculate the mL of penicillin, solution required:

$$\frac{750{,}000 \text{ units}}{1 \text{ mL}} = \frac{2{,}000{,}000 \text{ units}}{x \text{ mL}}$$

$$x \text{ mL} = 2.7 \text{ mL} \qquad (23)$$

32. **(D)** Alcohol USP, sometimes known as grain alcohol, contains 94.9% v/v or 92.3% w/w of $C_2H_5OH$. The remaining portion is water. It may be used as a solvent and as a source of alcohol for oral dosage forms. *(1; 24)*

33. **(A)** Diluted Alcohol is prepared by mixing equal volumes of Alcohol USP and purified water with the final strength being 49%. Some volume shrinkage occurs because of hydrogen bonding. This attractive force between hydrogen atoms and electronegative atoms such as oxygen, fluorine, and nitrogen results in the miscibility of certain solvents and increases the

solubility of certain chemicals. The shrinkage phenomenon that occurs when mixing equal volumes of Alcohol USP (95%) and purified water results in approximately 3% shrinkage from the theoretical volume. If one wishes to prepare 100 mL of Diluted Alcohol USP, a solution that contains 49% v/v ethanol plus purified water, equal volumes of each are used. However, one must also remember to use an excess of at least 3% of both liquids to assure obtaining the required volume. *(1; 12)*

34. **(B)** Rubbing alcohol is a form of denatured alcohol containing approximately 70% of absolute alcohol. This product is used as a germicide and as an external rubefacient. *(1; 24)*

35. **(E)** A suspension must be prepared because there are water-insoluble powders present in the prescription. An emulsion is not possible because there is no oil indicated in the formula. *(1)*

36. **(D)** The designation "aa qs 15 g" translates as "of each enough to make 15 g." Therefore, 7.5 g of calamine and 7.5 g of zinc oxide are needed. The water-insoluble powders, calamine and zinc oxide, should be triturated together using a mortar and pestle, then wetted with the glycerin. Resorcinol is soluble in both water and alcohol, but it is more convenient to dissolve it in the alcohol and dilute the powder paste with the liquid. Finally, add portions of purified water to rinse out the mortar while placing the suspension into a precalibrated wide-mouth bottle. *(1)*

37. **(C)** Most of the ingredients in this preparation are intended for topical use only. Although the suspension may not separate or settle immediately, it may do so after a few days. It is standard procedure to place "shake well" labels on all suspension formulas. None of the ingredients decompose in the presence of moderate heat; therefore, a "store in a cool place" label is not required. *(24)*

38. **(E)** The easiest way to hydrate methylcellulose is to add the powder to hot water and allow the powder to hydrate for 10 to 15 min before adding cold water. Six itraconazole

(Sporanox) capsules may be opened and the powder wetted by the propylene glycol. The thickened methylcellulose solution can then be added to the powder followed by sufficient purified water to make 100 mL. *(1; 19)*

39. **(C)** Cold cream is a W/O emulsion base with good emollient properties. *(4)*

40. **(B)** Hydrophilic petrolatum is an anhydrous preparation that will absorb significant amounts of water forming a W/O emulsion. It contains cholesterol as the emulsifying agent. *(1; 24)*

41. **(C)** *(1; 4; 24)*

42. **(A)** *(1; 24)*

43. **(E)** *(1; 24)*

44. **(D)** *(1; 24)*

45. **(B)** Large quantities of liquids may be incorporated into Aquaphor. The characteristics of this ointment base are similar to hydrophilic petrolatum. *(1; 4; 19)*

46. **(B)** Burow's solution is officially known as Aluminum Acetate Topical Solution. It is classified as a topical astringent dressing. *(1; 24)*

47. **(E)** The prescription calls for 15 mL each of Burow's solution and Diluted Alcohol. Burow's solution consists mainly of water therefore 15 mL equals 15 g. However, propylene glycol has a specific gravity of 1.25 and 15 mL will weigh approximately 18.75 g. The total weight of the ointment will be 15 g + 18.75 g + 60 g = 93.75 g *(1; 23)*

48. **(A)** Aqueous solutions such as Burow's solution cannot be incorporated directly into oleaginous bases such as petrolatum or white petrolatum. Aquaphor is an adjuvant that will absorb aqueous solutions and is miscible with petrolatum. Although smaller amounts could be used, 15 g of Aquaphor will readily pick up the required amount of Burow's solution. The amount of white petrolatum must be decreased

by 15 g to assure the correct concentration of Burow's solution in the final preparation. Alcohol is seldom included in semisolid ointments or creams because it is likely to evaporate slowly. It is more likely to be included in lotion formulas. *(20)*

49. **(A)** Urea has good solubility in water. The resulting solution can readily be incorporated into the Aquaphor. *(4; 24)*

50. **(B)** Incorporating powders into ointment bases may be eased by first wetting the powders with a small amount of liquid that is miscible with the main vehicle. The wetted powder is rubbed with a spatula on an ointment tile to form a paste. Usually, mineral oil is employed when the vehicle is oleaginous. Glycerin or propylene glycol may be used for more hydrophilic bases. *(1; 4; 24)*

51. **(A)** Tretinoin is the official name for retinoic acid. The drug is commercially available under the tradename of Retin-A. The designation of Ac. Sal. refers to salicylic acid, not aspirin (acetylsalicylic acid). The term emulsion base is nondescript. It could refer to a number of ointment bases, including those with either W/O or O/W characteristics. Clarification of the type of ointment base desired should be made. Before compounding this prescription, the pharmacist should contact the prescriber concerning the inclusion of a keratolytic agent such as salicylic acid in a topical preparation containing tretinoin, a compound that exhibits keratolytic activity as a side effect. *(1; 19; 20)*

52. **(E)** An easy method for determining the amount of 0.05% cream is

60 g × 0.02% = 0.012 g of pure retinoic acid

$$\frac{0.012 \text{ g}}{x \text{ g}} = \frac{0.05 \text{ g}}{100 \text{ g}}$$

$$0.05x = 1.2$$

$$x = 24 \text{ g of } 0.05\%$$ *(23)*

53. **(C)** Incorporating powders or liquids into relatively small amounts of ointment base is best accomplished on a pill tile (also known as an ointment tile). Because of the caustic nature of salicylic acid, rubber spatulas should be used rather than stainless steel, which would be discolored by the acid. While salicylic acid is soluble in alcohol, the use of alcohol as a levigating agent is discouraged since crystals of salicylic acid may form on the surface of the product when the alcohol evaporates. *(1; 4)*

54. **(D)** Let $Q_1$ and $C_1$ represent the quantity and concentration of new product desired and $Q_2$ and $C_2$ represent the original quantity and strength:

$$Q_1 \times C_1 = Q_2 \times C_2$$

$$[x \text{ g}] [0.1\%] = [30 \text{ g}] [0.25\%]$$

$$x = 75 \text{ g (total amount of ointment that can be prepared)}$$

Therefore, 75 g − the original 30 g = 45 g of diluent needed. *(1)*

55. **(B)** Hydrophilic ointment is an O/W emulsion base containing sodium lauryl sulfate, petrolatum, and stearyl alcohol. Of the listed bases, it is closest to a vanishing cream base because such a system is characterized by the presence of an O/W stearate emulsion. When placed on the skin, the ointment appears to "disappear" but a very thin layer of stearate remains. *(24)*

56. **(E)** White petrolatum is a bland base with a very low incidence of irritation to the eye. Also, because of the absence of water, it has low susceptibility to microbial growth. *(24)*

57. **(E)** Many antibiotics undergo decomposition by hydrolysis in the presence of water. White petrolatum is anhydrous and is relatively inert. *(1; 4)*

58. **(C)** Of all the bases listed, hydrophilic petrolatum will absorb the greatest quantity of water. An alternative would be Aquaphor. *(1)*

59. **(E)** The occlusive characteristics of petrolatum will prevent further water loss through the stratum corneum. Thus, the skin will remain more hydrated and pliable. *(1)*

60. **(E)** Any product containing water will be susceptible to the growth of microorganisms and should include an antimicrobial agent. *(4; 24)*

61. **(A)** Carbomer is a high molecular weight copolymer of acrylic acid. An aqueous solution of this thickening agent will have a low viscosity and low pH. However, when the pH is raised, the viscosity will increase due to cross linkages of the molecules. Depending upon the concentration of carbomer present, a thick lotion or a semisolid gel can be formed. *(4; 24)*

62. **(A)** Because of the volatility of alcohol, it is not suitable in dosage forms from which it may slowly evaporate. If ingredients were dissolved in alcohol and incorporated into either ointments or suppositories, crystals of the ingredients would slowly appear on the surface of the dosage unit. However, one would expect alcohol to remain within the lotion formula until placed on the skin. *(1)*

63. **(E)** The solution also contains Polysorbate 80. This nonionic surfactant is included to disperse the water-insoluble components of coal tar, which will precipitate when the highly alcoholic solution is mixed with an aqueous preparation.

    (B—incorrect) The Latin name of coal tar solution is Liquor Carbonis Detergens (LCD). *(20; 24)*

64. **(A)** This prescription uses mineral oil as the solvent. It is not suited for administration into the eye. Ephedrine is used as a topical decongestant when administered by the intranasal route. The product would be ineffective if placed in the ear. *(1; 24)*

65. **(A)** Ephedrine sulfate is water soluble. It is best to request the prescriber's permission to use ephedrine base, which is soluble in nonpolar solvents such as mineral oil. Solid chemicals such as phenol, camphor, and menthol will liquefy when mixed together even at room temperature without heating. This phenomenon is known as forming a eutectic mixture. *(1)*

66. **(B)** Camphor is soluble in alcohol or organic solvents but is only slightly soluble in water (1 g in 800 mL). *(1)*

67. **(D)** Methyl salicylate can be used in small quantities as a flavoring or perfuming agent. It is also included in many topical products such as rubbing alcohol, gels, and liniments as a counterirritant. *(1; 2)*

68. **(A)** Tetracaine is a weak organic base with poor water solubility (1 g in 1 L of water). The hydrochloride salt, which is very soluble (1 g needs less than 1 mL of water), should be used. Boric acid, which is a very weak acid, is chemically compatible with both tetracaine free base and the HCl salt. Tetracaine, epinephrine (Adrenalin), and cocaine combinations are used as local anesthetics and are known as "TAC Topical Solutions." *(1; 20)*

69. **(D)** Boric acid is an effective buffer in ophthalmic solutions because it will maintain a slightly acidic pH, but when placed in the eye, it is quickly neutralized by the buffers in the lacrimal fluid. Boric acid has weak antimicrobial activity. *(1; 4)*

70. **(B)** This problem may be solved using the "E" values for the chemicals.

| Drug | Wt. of Drug | × | "E" values | Equiv. Amt. of NaCl |
|------|-------------|---|------------|---------------------|
| Tetracaine | 600 mg | | 0.18 | = 108 mg |
| Boric acid | 300 mg | | 0.50 | = 150 mg |
| Total | | | | = 258 mg |

60 mL of solution × 0.9% NaCl = 540 mg of NaCl
540 − 258 mg = 282 mg of NaCl to adjust for tonicity
*(1; 23)*

71. **(C)** Membrane filtration represents one of the most convenient sterilization methods available to the pharmacist performing extemporaneous compounding. It involves the passing of solutions through a 0.2 μm filter using one of the commercially available sterile filter units

such as Millipore's Millex or Swinnex units. The method does not involve heat, therefore there is no decomposition of heat labile drugs as might occur with autoclaving. Ethylene oxide gas is not practical for solutions because it would have to penetrate the solution and residues may be left behind. *(1; 13)*

72. **(C)** Because the exact density of the PEG 400/6000 mixture is not known, the pharmacist must prepare a trial batch in a mold to determine the weight of an individual suppository. In this prescription, the volume occupied by 20 mg of progesterone is insignificant, and it is not necessary to determine its bulk density. However, when a drug represents a large proportion of the total suppository weight, one must prepare a trial suppository that includes the active drug to calculate its bulk density. For example, boric acid has been prescribed at a dose of 600 mg per suppository. Progesterone has been extemporaneously incorporated into vaginal suppositories for the maintenance of pregnancy in luteal phase dysfunction. The usual dose has been 25 mg. *(1; 4; 24)*

73. **(C)** Vaginal suppositories or pessaries are traditionally larger in size and weight (5 g) than rectal suppositories (2 g). However, a regular rectal suppository mold could be used if the larger vaginal mold is not available. For many suppository formulas, a water-soluble base, such as the polyethylene glycols (PEGs) or glycerinated gelatin, are preferred over oil bases such as cocoa butter. *(1; 24)*

74. **(C)** Cocoa butter, a mixture of triglycerides, has been used for more than 100 years as a suppository base. A disadvantage of cocoa butter is its inability to absorb aqueous solutions. It melts at slightly below body temperature, and its melting point might be affected by drugs. Fattibase is a mixture of triglycerides from palm, palm kernel, and coconuts oils + glyceryl mononstearate SE and polyoxylstearate emulsifiers. Other suppository bases that melt include the Witepsols and the Wecobees. Although cocoa butter suppositories can be hand rolled or prepared by fusion in molds, the other bases are intended for mold use.

Different molecular weight PEGs can be blended and formed into suppositories by fusion using molds. However, the PEG suppositories do not melt in the body; instead, they slowly dissolve in the limited amount of water in the rectum. *(1; 4; 19)*

75. **(C)**

$$\frac{15,000 \text{ units}}{g} \times 30 \text{ g} = 450,000 \text{ units}$$

$$\frac{5000,000 \text{ U}}{10 \text{ mL}} = \frac{15,000 \text{ U}}{x \text{ mL}}$$

$$x = 9 \text{ mL of solution}$$

The 9 mL of solution should be incorporated into 21 g of an absorption base such as hydrophilic petrolatum or Aquaphor. Hydrophilic ointment is probably a poor choice since the 9 mL of liquid will thin the base too much. The pharmacist would not incorporate 9 mL of antibiotic solution directly into 30 g of ointment base because the final concentration of drug would be incorrect. *(4; 23)*

76. **(A)** Product inserts are the best sources of information concerning appropriate diluents for a given drug powder. However, BSWFI should not be used for reconstituting single-dose units because the preservative present would serve no useful purpose, and large amounts of the preservative could increase the incidence or severity of toxicity. The use of BSWFI may be appropriate if a powder in a multidose vial is being reconstituted. *(13; 24)*

77. **(C)** Currently there are two major reference sources in the United States that present detailed information concerning the compatibilities and incompatibilities of parenteral products. Trissel is the author of the *Handbook on Injectable Drugs*. The second book, King's *Guide to Parenteral Admixtures* presents similar material and is available in both print and on a regularly updated CD-ROM. Not only do the references describe mixing of drug solutions, but also compatibilities when mixing solutions in syringes and adding solutions into the Y-tubes on administration sets. *(1; 13; 21)*

78. **(A)** *Drug Facts and Comparisons* has a section which lists all commercial amino acid solutions by total concentration, individual amino acids present in each formula, and other pertinent information such as grams of nitrogen present, and other miscellaneous ingredients. *(3)*

79. **(A)** The pH of diazepam solution is slightly acidic (pH of 6.2–6.9). To solubilize diazepam, a mixed solvent system of 40% propylene glycol, 10% alcohol, and water is necessary. When diazepam solution is added to an aqueous solution, a portion of the diazepam may precipitate. *(21:333)*

80. **(E)** There is a large variety of parenteral amino acids formulas on the market. Some contain a mixture of both the essential and the nonessential amino acids while others contain almost exclusively the essential amino acids. Some formulas contain significantly higher levels of branched chained amino acids which are believed to be more readily assimilated in the body. When comparing similar formulas containing the same total amino acids concentration, the relative amounts of the individual amino acids present may vary slightly. These minor differences may be ignored when selecting one company's product versus another. *(4; 10)*

81. **(C)** Amphotericin B is available in vials containing 50 mg of drug as a powder. Because of the colloidal nature of the product, only sterile water for injection without preservatives is suitable as a reconstituting vehicle. Other vehicles such as normal saline may cause a precipitate. Amphotericin B is administered by slow intravenous infusion over a 2- to 6-h period. *(21)*

82. **(C)** Abelcet is a sterile suspension and Amphotec is a sterile lyophilized powder for reconstitution, both intended for intravenous administration. While both are liposome formulas, the particle sizes of each differ. Thus, they are used or are targeted for different organs and are not interchangeable. A second liposomal amphotericin product that needs reconstitution is AmBisome. Doxil is a liposome form of doxorubicin HCl which appears to have less toxicity than the parent compound. The product may have a slightly red color which does not affect its activity. *(24)*

83. **(C)** Liposomal powders are usually reconstituted using sterile water for injection. Other diluents such as sodium chloride injection may cause breakage of the liposomal system. Since many of the liposomal products are formulated as "targeted drug delivery systems," the drug present will concentrate in areas of the body in which they are most active. Thus, the drug dose required is often less. Consequently, if the larger conventional dose is given, toxic levels of the drug may occur. Conversely, if the conventional drug is required and the liposomal drug dose is given, the dose may be subtherapeutic. *(24)*

84. **(D)** Most total parenteral nutrition solutions are hypertonic because of the high concentrations of dextrose present. This is not a problem if they are slowly infused through major blood vessels. Essential fatty acid deficiencies are avoided by including certain vegetable oils in the formulas. BEE is the acronym for basal energy expenditure. This is the calculated minimum calories that must be provided to a patient for his/her daily needs. However, in the malnourished patient, larger amounts of calories should be provided. *(4; 14)*

85. **(D)** Multicomponent admixtures that contain dextrose, amino acids, and fat oil emulsions are referred to as total nutrition admixtures (TNAs), or 3 in 1s. Although these combinations simplify administration of calories and protein, the cloudy nature of the product precludes examination of the product for fine precipitants. The designation MCT has been used to represent medium chain triglycerides, which may be used in patients suffering from malabsorption. *(21; 24)*

86. **(A)** The concentration of dextrose in parenteral infusion solutions is based upon the official form of hydrous dextrose. Its caloric density (or count) is 3.4 kcal/g. *(4)*

87. **(B)** While the exact amount of nitrogen in an amino acid structure varies with the molecular weight of the amino acid, approximately 16% of any mixture of common amino acids will consist of nitrogen.

Therefore,

100 mL of 10% amino acids injection
= 10 g amino acids

10 g amino acids × 16% = 1.6 g of nitrogen *(4)*

88. **(C)** Because the pharmacist has only $D_{50}W$ and Aminosyn II packaged in 500-mL bottles, it is most convenient to transfer each solution aseptically to an evacuated sterile glass bottle or plastic bag. *(3)*

89. **(A)** Each 1 L of the TPN solution contains 500 mL each of the Aminosyn II solution and 50% dextrose injection.

500 mL × 50% = 250 g of dextrose

Since the caloric density of hydrated dextrose = 3.4 kcal/g,

250 g × 3.4 kcal/g = 850 kcal     *(4)*

90. **(A)** From the previous problem, the amount of dextrose requested was calculated to be 250 g. Using 360 mL of $D_{70}W$ will give 360 mL × 70% = 250 g (the correct amount).

Answer II is incorrect since the calories provided by the amino acids usually are not included as a supply of energy.

Answer III using 200 mL of $D_{70}W$ + 300 mL of $D_{20}W$ will give 200 mL × 70% = 140 g dextrose + 300 mL × 20% = 60 g dextrose which equals 200 g dextrose not the 250 g requested. *(23)*

91. **(C)** Many calcium salts, such as the phosphate and carbonate, have limited water solubility. When calcium salts and phosphate salts are included in the same admixture, it is possible that the very insoluble calcium phosphates may form. The pharmacist must recognize the potential danger of infusing such solutions into patients. Several reference sources list the limits of each salt that is compatible with the other. However, the precipitate may form slowly and would be invisible if a fat emulsion is included in the TPN. *(4; 21)*

92. **(A)** It is often possible to reduce the likelihood of a precipitation if the potassium phosphate is dissolved or mixed with the vehicle first followed by the calcium solution, which is added slowly while stirring. The pharmacist could also alternate the calcium and the phosphate solutions in the series of TPN containers. However, he or she should inform the prescriber, and double the amount of ion added each time. *(4)*

93. **(A)** Phosphorus is an essential mineral for the body and is readily available in the phosphate ion. When the potassium ion is required, the chloride or acetate salts are used. *(13)*

94. **(D)** Most electrolytes are ordered in terms of milliequivalents. The exception are the phosphates. Commercially available potassium phosphate injections consist of a mixture of monobasic (potassium) and dibasic (dipotassium) phosphates. Because body phosphate requirements are usually expressed in terms of millimoles (mM) per kg per day and the available solutions are mixtures of the two salts, it is more convenient to express the phosphate additive in terms of mM/L rather than mEq/L. The average adult needs 10–15 mmol of phosphorus per day. *(4; 13)*

95. **(C)** Low-dose insulin syringes are calibrated to contain 0.5 mL (50 units) of insulin. The 40 units of insulin (0.4 mL) could also be measured accurately using the tuberculin syringe, which has the capacity of 1 mL. The smallest calibrations on 10-mL syringes will not allow accurate enough measurements of 0.4 mL. *(13; 322)*

96. **(A)** When low concentrations of insulin are included in LVPs, the percentage of insulin adsorbed onto the walls of the containers and also onto the administration sets is significant. One can expect at least 50% insulin loss when only 40 units are added to the container. *(13; 24)*

The other answers are incorrect. Because the insulin dosage is expressed in units, the strength of the insulin is not needed. Most likely, the U-100 solution will be used. Only insulin solution is given intravenously; the suspension forms are intended for subcutaneous administration.

97. **(C)** Liposyn is a fatty acid emulsion with a physical appearance similar to that of milk. When included in TPN solutions, the resulting product will be somewhat cloudy. The intent of the Liposyn is to correct or prevent fatty acid deficiencies by providing linoleic and linolenic acids, which are present in either soybean or safflower oil. The fat emulsions also provide calories. For example, every mL of the 10% strength contributes 1.1 kcal, and a mL of the 20% provides 2.0 kcal. Because the fat emulsions have been adjusted for tonicity, they do not adversely affect the osmolarity of TPN solutions. *(4; 21)*

98. **(A)** Fatty oil emulsions are stabilized by the presence of egg phospholipids. As such they are usually contraindicated in those patients with serious allergies to eggs. *(4; 5)*

99. **(A)** Depending upon the reference source, the caloric density of the 10% fatty oil emulsions is reported as either 1 kcal/mL, or probably the more accurate 1.1 kcal/mL. The 20% fatty oil emulsions use a value of 2 kcal/mL.

> Using 1 kcal/mL, 500 mL × 1 = 500 kcal
> Using 1.1 kcal/mL 500 mL × 1.1 = 550 kcal

100. **(B)** The TPN formula calls for 500 mL of 8.5% amino acids solution per bottle. Since three bottles are administered per day, the total amount of amino acids is 500 mL × 3 bts × 8.5% = 127.5 g.

The average amount of nitrogen in amino acids is 16%, therefore,

$$127.5 \text{ g} \times 16\% = 20.4 \text{ g} \qquad (4)$$

101. **(C)** Selenium deficiencies may cause muscle pain, tenderness, and cardiomyopathy. *(3)*

102. **(C)** There are several sterile solutions that contain the most popular trace metals likely to be requested for TPNs. Iron is not included mainly because of compatibility problems. *(3)*

103. **(B)** Milliequivalent expressions allow direct comparisons of ions when different salt forms are being used. In other words, 40 mEq of sodium acetate will contain the same weight of sodium as will 40 mEq of sodium chloride. *(23)*

104. **(A)** While the exact cause of the cloudy solution is unknown, it is likely due to a calcium/phosphate interaction. This slight precipitate may worsen as time elapses, especially if infused into the patient since calcium phosphate's solubility decreases with higher temperatures. Use of an in-line filter will slow down the infusion with eventual clogging of the line. *(4)*

105. **(A)** PCA is the acronym for "Patient Controlled Analgesia," the name given to small devices worn outside the body that can provide constant, slow infusion of analgesics into patients. Pharmacists compound these units by aseptically placing the analgesic solution plus diluent into the flexible plastic cartridge which is then placed in an outer unit which controls the flow rate and pumping mechanism. The solution is slowly infused into the patient at a constant preset rate. The drug reservoir provides several days of therapy. Many of the units have a mechanism for bolus dosing if the patient is experiencing break-through pain. While the original units were used for strong analgesics such as morphine and Dilaudid, other drug solutions, such as 5-fluorouracil, may be infused through the PCA. Several companies manufacture these ambulatory infusion devices including Pharmacia's CADD. *(22)*

106. **(B)** Disposable infusion pumps such as the Block Medical's Homepumps and Baxter's Intermates are ideal for home infusion of parenterals at intermittent intervals. The elastomeric balloon present gives constant flow of solution without the need of pump device or gravity flow. The usual volume capacity of the units varies from 50 mL to 250 mL. Pharmacists fill the units by drawing up active drug solution plus diluent into plastic syringes then injecting through a filling port on the unit. The units have small diameter tubing already attached which allows the patient to attach the unit to a previously inserted infusion catheter. *(22)*

# CHAPTER 5

# Biopharmaceutics and Pharmacokinetics

Biopharmaceutics is a scientific discipline concerned with the relationship between the physicochemical properties of a drug in a dosage form and the biological response observed after its administration. It includes the study of the release of the drug from its dosage form. Pharmacokinetics is the study of the absorption, distribution, metabolism, and elimination (ADME) of drugs. As more quantitative and sophisticated assay techniques have been developed, a better understanding of the therapeutic pathways for drugs has emerged. This chapter tests the reader's knowledge of the principles of biopharmaceutics and pharmacokinetics, which is fundamental to the rational selection of quality drug products, the determination of appropriate dose and dosing schedules, and the monitoring of therapy.

# Questions

DIRECTIONS (Questions 1 through 92): Each of the numbered items or incomplete statements in this section is followed by answers or by completions of the statement. Select the ONE lettered answer or completion that is BEST in each case.

1. A prime consideration in biopharmaceutics is a drug's "bioavailability" which refers to the relative amount of drug that reaches the

   (A) small intestine
   (B) stomach
   (C) systemic circulation
   (D) liver
   (E) kidneys

2. The AUC can be described as

   I. a theoretic value
   II. a measure of drug concentration–time curve
   III. having units of weight and time/volume

   (A) I only
   (B) III only
   (C) I and II only
   (D) II and III only
   (E) I, II, and III

3. The relative bioavailability of a drug product can be determined by comparing which of the following values to similar control drug values?

   I. areas under the curve (AUC)
   II. total drug urinary excretion
   III. peak blood drug concentrations

   (A) I only
   (B) III only

   (C) I and II only
   (D) II and III only
   (E) I, II, and III

4. What is potentially the first rate-limiting process when a tablet dosage form is administered?

   (A) ionization of the drug
   (B) diffusion of the drug through the GI epithelium
   (C) dissolution of the drug in the GI fluids
   (D) dissolution of the drug in the blood
   (E) disintegration of the tablet

5. Which of the following could be the rate-limiting steps for drug absorption from an orally administered drug product?

   I. disintegration of the unit
   II. dissolution of the active drug
   III. diffusion of active drug through the intestinal wall

   (A) I only
   (B) III only
   (C) I and II only
   (D) II and III only
   (E) I, II, and III

6. Dissolution may be described by using which one of the following equations or laws?

   (A) Fick's second law
   (B) Fick's first law
   (C) Noyes-Whitney equation
   (D) Poiseuille's law
   (E) Stoke's law

7. The AUC of a drug can be determined from a graph by using which of the following methods?

    I.   law of diminishing returns
    II.   rule of nines
    III.  trapezoidal rule

    (A)  I only
    (B)  III only
    (C)  I and II only
    (D)  II and III only
    (E)  I, II, and III

8. Based upon graphic comparisons of AUCs, under which of the following criteria may a generic drug product be considered by the FDA to be bioequivalent with a trade name product?

    I.   The generic's AUC may be superimposed on that of the brand name product.
    II.   The generic's overall AUC is 15% lower than the brand name product.
    III.  The generic's overall AUC is 18% higher than the brand name product.

    (A)  I only
    (B)  III only
    (C)  I and II only
    (D)  II and III only
    (E)  I, II, and III

9. The peak of the serum concentration versus time graph approximates the

    (A)  point in time when the maximum pharmacological effect occurs
    (B)  point in time when absorption and elimination of the drug have equalized
    (C)  maximum concentration of free drug in the urine
    (D)  time required for essentially all of the drug to be absorbed from the GI tract
    (E)  point in time when the drug begins to be metabolized

10. In which of the following sites may drugs be metabolized?

    I.   skin
    II.   lungs
    III.  liver

    (A)  I only
    (B)  III only
    (C)  I and II only
    (D)  II and III only
    (E)  I, II, and III

11. When compared to their parent compound, metabolites usually have

    (A)  greater water solubility
    (B)  lower water solubility
    (C)  greater therapeutic activity
    (D)  no therapeutic activity
    (E)  greater diffusion through the blood/brain barrier

12. Differences in bioavailability are most frequently observed with drug products administered by which one of the following routes?

    (A)  subcutaneous
    (B)  intravenous
    (C)  oral
    (D)  sublingual
    (E)  intramuscular

13. When graphed, nonlinear pharmacokinetics are characterized by data that

    (A)  does not yield a straight line at any time
    (B)  exhibits a straight line only when plotted as log-log functions
    (C)  is dose dependent
    (D)  follows first-order kinetics
    (E)  will have a negative slope

14. The "F" value for a drug product is ideally compared to its

    (A)  absolute bioavailability
    (B)  dosing rate
    (C)  clearance rate
    (D)  relative bioavailability
    (E)  route of administration

15. Determine the F value for a drug available as a 100-mg capsule with a calculated AUC of 20 mg/dL/h when a 100-mg IV bolus of the same drug exhibits an AUC of 25 mg/dL/h.

    (A)  0.2
    (B)  0.4
    (C)  0.8
    (D)  1.25
    (E)  20

16. What is the F value for an experimental drug tablet based on the following data?

| Drug Dosage Form | Dose | AUC ($\mu$g/mL/h) |
|---|---|---|
| Tablet | 100 mg po | 20 |
| Solution (control) | 100 mg po | 30 |
| Injection (control) | 50 mg IV push | 40 |

    (A)  0.25
    (B)  0.38
    (C)  0.50
    (D)  0.66
    (E)  0.90

17. If an oral capsule formulation of a drug produces a serum concentration–time curve having the same area under the curve as that produced by an equivalent dose of the drug given IV, it can generally be concluded that

    (A)  the IV route is preferred to the oral route
    (B)  the capsule formulation is essentially completely absorbed
    (C)  the drug is very rapidly absorbed
    (D)  all oral dosage forms of drug A will be bioequivalent
    (E)  there is no advantage to the IV route

18. The term therapeutic window refers to the

    (A)  time interval between administration and the beginning of activity
    (B)  concentration differential between drug's MTC and MEC
    (C)  concentration which must be reached before activity begins

    (D)  concentration versus time curve
    (E)  time period before administration of the next dose

19. For two drug products to be considered "pharmaceutical equivalents," the products must

    I.  have the same active drug (therapeutic moiety)
    II.  consist of the same salt
    III.  contain the same excipients

    (A)  I only
    (B)  III only
    (C)  I and II only
    (D)  II and III only
    (E)  I, II, and III

20. Requirements for drug products to be considered "pharmaceutical alternatives" include having the same

    I.  active drug or precursor
    II.  dosage form
    III.  salt or ester

    (A)  I only
    (B)  III only
    (C)  I and II only
    (D)  II and III only
    (E)  I, II, and III

21. Based upon the pH partition theory, weakly acidic drugs are most likely to be absorbed from the stomach because

    (A)  the drugs will exist primarily in the unionized, more lipid-soluble form
    (B)  the drugs will exist primarily in the ionized, more water-soluble form
    (C)  weak acids are more soluble in acid media
    (D)  the ionic form of the drug facilitates dissolution
    (E)  weak acids will further depress pH

22. Gastric emptying is slowed by all of the following EXCEPT

(A) vigorous exercise

(B) fatty foods

(C) hot meals

(D) hunger

(E) emotional stress

23. Reducing drug particle size to enhance drug absorption is limited to those situations in which the

(A) absorption process occurs by active transport

(B) absorption process is rate-limited by the dissolution of drug in GI fluids

(C) drug is very water soluble

(D) drug is very potent

(E) drug is irritating to the GI tract

24. Which of the following statements concerning the blood protein albumin is (are) true?

I. It is a very site-specific binding agent.

II. It will generally bind acidic drugs.

III. Blood levels are approximately 3.5–5.0 g/dL.

(A) I only

(B) III only

(C) I and II only

(D) II and III only

(E) I, II, and III

25. Drugs that are absorbed from the GI tract are generally

(A) absorbed into the portal circulation and pass through the liver before entering the general circulation

(B) filtered from the blood by the kidney, then reabsorbed into the general circulation

(C) absorbed into the portal circulation and are distributed by an enterohepatic cycle

(D) not affected by liver enzymes

(E) stored in the liver

26. Which of the following routes of administration is (are) unlikely to be influenced by the First-Pass effect?

I. IM or subcutaneous injection

II. inhalation

III. transdermal

(A) I only

(B) III only

(C) I and II only

(D) II and III only

(E) I, II, and III

27. The biological half-life of a drug

(A) is a constant physical property of the drug

(B) is a constant chemical property of the drug

(C) is the time for one-half of the therapeutic activity to be lost

(D) may be decreased by giving the drug by rapid IV injection

(E) depends entirely on the route of administration

28. The biological half-life of a drug that is eliminated by first-order kinetics is represented mathematically by _____, where $k$ is the first-order rate constant for elimination.

(A) $1/k$

(B) $\log k$

(C) $0.693/k$

(D) $2.303/k$

(E) peak serum concentration/$2k$

29. A specific drug has a first-order biological half-life of 4 h. This half-life value will

(A) be independent of the initial drug concentration

(B) increase when the concentration of the drug increases

(C) decrease when the concentration of the drug increases

(D) decrease if the patient has renal impairment

(E) be the same whether the drug level is determined in the blood or by observing the pharmacological action

**30.** A drug that follows linear pharmacokinetics has a half-life of 4 h. How many mg of the drug will remain in the body 12 h after the administration of a 400-mg dose?

(A) 10
(B) 25
(C) 50
(D) 100
(E) 200

**31.** Determine the half-life of furosemide if it appears to be eliminated from the body at a rate constant of 46% per hour. Assume that first-order kinetics occurs.

(A) <1 h
(B) 1.5 h
(C) 3.0 h
(D) 4.0 h
(E) >5 h

**32.** The volume of distribution of a drug is

I. a mathematical relationship between the total amount of drug in the body and the concentration of drug in the blood
II. a measure of an individual's blood volume
III. a measure of an individual's total body volume

(A) I only
(B) III only
(C) I and II only
(D) II and III only
(E) I, II, and III

**33.** The volume of distribution ($V_d$) of a particular drug will be

(A) greater for drugs that concentrate in tissues rather than in plasma
(B) greater for drugs that concentrate in plasma rather than in tissues
(C) independent of tissue concentration
(D) independent of plasma concentration
(E) approximately the same for all drugs in a given individual

**34.** A knowledge of $V_d$ for a given drug is useful because it allows us to

(A) estimate the elimination rate constant
(B) determine the biological half-life
(C) calculate a reasonable loading dose
(D) determine the best dosing interval
(E) determine the peak plasma concentration

**35.** Estimate the plasma concentration of a drug when 50 mg is given by IV bolus to a 140-lb patient if her volume of distribution is 1.6 L/kg.

(A) 0.1 mg/L
(B) 0.5 mg/L
(C) 1 mg/L
(D) 5 mg/L
(E) 31 mg/L

**36.** The time needed to achieve a steady-state plasma level for a drug administered by infusion will depend upon

I. amount of drug being infused
II. volume of distribution of the drug
III. half-life of the drug

(A) I only
(B) III only
(C) I and II only
(D) II and III only
(E) I, II, and III

**Questions 37 through 41: The following graph represents drug blood level curves. Answer the next five questions based upon this graph.**

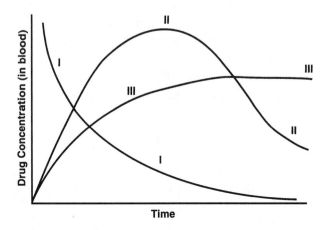

37. Curve I represents the blood level concentration of a drug administered by

 I. the oral route
 II. intramuscular injection
 III. intravenous injection

 (A) I only
 (B) III only
 (C) I and II only
 (D) II and III only
 (E) I, II, and III

38. The upward slope of curve II could represent

 I. increased absorption of drug from a capsule dosage form
 II. absorption of drug from an intramuscular injection
 III. absorption of drug from a sustained-release tablet

 (A) I only
 (B) III only
 (C) I and II only
 (D) II and III only
 (E) I, II, and III

39. Which one of the following statements concerning the graph is completely true?

 (A) Once the peak in curve II has been reached, no further drug absorption is likely to occur.
 (B) Doubling the administered dose will double the height of curve II.
 (C) The *Y*-axis (concentration of drug in the blood) is being expressed as a log function.
 (D) The *X*-axis (time) is being expressed as a log function.
 (E) The curves in lines II and III indicate that the absorption rate ($k_a$) is greater than the elimination rate ($k_e$).

40. Curve III would best illustrate a drug administered by

 (A) intravenous push
 (B) intravenous infusion

 (C) intramuscular injection
 (D) intrathecal injection
 (E) either intravenous push or infusion

41. The time needed to reach optimum drug blood levels (the plateau portion of curve III) during constant-rate intravenous infusion is

 (A) directly proportional to the rate of infusion
 (B) inversely proportional to the rate of infusion
 (C) independent of the rate of infusion
 (D) independent of the biological half-life
 (E) not related to either the infusion rate or the biological half-life

42. What factor besides the desired steady-state concentration ($C_{ss}$) is most important for determining an infusion rate of a parenteral solution?

 (A) half-life of the drug
 (B) metabolism rate
 (C) renal elimination
 (D) total clearance
 (E) volume of distribution

43. Compartmental models are often used to illustrate the various principles of pharmacokinetics. A compartment is best defined as

 (A) any anatomic entity that is capable of absorbing drug
 (B) a kinetically distinguishable pool of drug
 (C) specific body organs or tissues that can be assayed for drug
 (D) any body fluid—such as blood or urine—that may contain drug
 (E) any component of the blood, including blood proteins that would have a tendency to absorb drug

**44.** Which of the following is/are true of nonlinear pharmacokinetics

  I. follows zero-order kinetics
  II. elimination half-life will change as the dose is increased
  III. half-life is expressed in terms of fraction per unit of time

  (A) I only
  (B) III only
  (C) I and II only
  (D) II and III only
  (E) I, II, and III

**45.** The difference between peak and trough concentrations is greatest when a drug is given at dosing intervals

  (A) much longer than the half-life
  (B) about equal to the half-life
  (C) much shorter than the half-life
  (D) equal to the half-life times serum creatinine
  (E) equal to the time it takes to reach peak concentration following a single oral dose

**46.** Which of the following pharmacokinetic parameters is (are) likely to decrease in the geriatric population when compared to the average population?

  I. renal elimination
  II. drug metabolism
  III. volume of distribution

  (A) I only
  (B) III only
  (C) I and II only
  (D) II and III only
  (E) I, II, and III

**47.** The pharmacokinetic parameter known as clearance is essentially the

  (A) rate at which the plasma is cleared of all waste materials and foreign substances (e.g., drugs)
  (B) volume of blood that passes through the kidneys per unit of time

  (C) volume of blood that passes through the liver per unit of time
  (D) rate at which a drug is removed (cleared) from its site of absorption
  (E) volume of blood that is completely cleared of drug per unit of time

**48.** A knowledge of the clearance (CL) of a given drug is useful because it allows the

  (A) calculation of the maintenance dose required to sustain a desired average steady-state plasma concentration
  (B) determination of a loading dose but not the maintenance dose
  (C) determination of the ideal dosing interval
  (D) decision whether a loading dose is necessary
  (E) determination if the drug is metabolized or excreted unchanged

**49.** In dosing drugs that are primarily excreted by the kidneys, one must have some idea of the patient's renal function. A calculated pharmacokinetic parameter that gives us a reasonable estimate of renal function is the

  (A) blood urea nitrogen (BUN)
  (B) serum creatinine ($Sr_{cr}$)
  (C) creatinine clearance ($CL_{cr}$)
  (D) urine creatinine ($U_{cr}$)
  (E) free water clearance ($CL_{fw}$)

**50.** If the rate of elimination of a drug is reduced because of impaired renal function, the effect on the drug half-life and the time required to reach steady-state plasma levels (steady-state concentrations—$C_{ss}$) will

  (A) both increase
  (B) both decrease
  (C) be an increase in half-life and a decrease in the time to reach $C_{ss}$
  (D) be a decrease in half-life but an increase in the time to reach $C_{ss}$
  (E) be negligible

51. For many drugs, bioavailability can be evaluated using urinary excretion data. This is based on the assumption that

    (A) bioavailability studies can be done only on drugs that are completely excreted unchanged by the kidneys
    (B) drug levels can be measured more accurately in urine than in blood
    (C) a drug must first be absorbed into the systemic circulation before it can appear in the urine
    (D) all of the administered dose can be recovered from the urine
    (E) only drug metabolites are excreted in the urine

52. Estimating bioavailability from urinary excretion data is less satisfactory than estimates based on blood level data because accurate urinary excretion studies require

    I.   complete urine collection
    II.  normal or near-normal renal function
    III. that the drug be completely excreted unchanged by the kidney

    (A) I only
    (B) III only
    (C) I and II only
    (D) II and III only
    (E) I, II, and III

**Questions 53 through 55 are to be answered using the following data collected by testing various dosage forms of the same drug manufactured by two companies.**

| Product by Company | Dosage Form | Dose Administered | Cumulative Urinary Amount (mg) |
|---|---|---|---|
| A | Parenteral injection | 10 mg IV | 9.4 |
| A | Tablet | 20 mg po | 12.0 |
| B | Tablet | 20 mg po | 8.2 |
| B | Capsule | 15 mg po | 6.8 |

53. The absolute bioavailability of Company B tablets is best estimated to be

    (A) 25%
    (B) 40%
    (C) 44%
    (D) 68%
    (E) 87%

54. What is the relative bioavailability of Company B tablets?

    (A) 25%
    (B) 40%
    (C) 44%
    (D) 68%
    (E) 76%

55. What is the relative bioavailability of Company B tablets when compared to the capsule formula?

    (A) 44%
    (B) 68%
    (C) 76%
    (D) 90%
    (E) 120%

56. Company A conducts a study comparing the AUCs for its generic version of a drug with Company B's tradename product. The respective AUCs for each company's 10 mg oral tablets were 80 µg h/mL and 76 µg h/mL. Which of the following statements is (are) true?

    I.   The absolute bioavailability of Company A's product cannot be determined from this data.
    II.  The relative bioavailability of Company A's product is 0.95.
    III. The study is flawed since Company A's drug has a higher AUC than Company B's.

    (A) I only
    (B) III only
    (C) I and II only
    (D) II and III only
    (E) I, II, and III

57. The above drug follows linear pharmacokinetics and has a half-life of 8 h with complete renal clearance. What is the elimination rate for this drug when a 10 mg dose is given?

    (A)  0.087/h
    (B)  0.33/h
    (C)  1.25 mg/h
    (D)  4 mg/h
    (E)  5.5 L/h

58. The half-life of an antibacterial drug has been reported as ranging between 4 and 10 h. What is the estimated clearance of this drug in a patient receiving a 50-mg bolus dose of a drug at 1000? A blood sample drawn at 1400 assays at 10 mg/L.

    (A)  0.8 L/h
    (B)  1.25 L/h
    (C)  1.6 L/h
    (D)  2.5 L/h
    (E)  5 L/h

59. Which of the following factors is (are) included in the Cockcroft and Gault equation for estimating creatinine clearance?

    I.   patient's age
    II.  patient's height and weight
    III. patient's calculated BEE

    (A)  I only
    (B)  III only
    (C)  I and II only
    (D)  II and III only
    (E)  I, II, and III

60. What is the approximate creatinine clearance in a 140 lb, 50-year-old patient if the lab reports a serum creatinine value of 1.5 mg/dL?

    (A)  50–55 mL/min
    (B)  100–105 mL/min
    (C)  110–118 mL/min
    (D)  120–125 mL/min
    (E)  130–140 mL/min

61. The patient in the previous problem is a female. What correction, if any, should be made in calculating her creatinine clearance value?

    (A)  The value will be 50% of the male value.
    (B)  The value will be 75% of the male value.
    (C)  The value will be 80% of the male value.
    (D)  The value will be 85% of the male value.
    (E)  No correction is needed.

62. When converting a patient from theophylline to aminophylline, a dose adjustment

    (A)  is not needed
    (B)  with an increase of 20% is suggested
    (C)  with an increase of 50% is suggested
    (D)  with a decrease of 20% is suggested
    (E)  with a decrease of 50% is suggested

63. Determine the loading dose of aminophylline needed in a 55-year-old male patient weighing 70 kg if the targeted theophylline plasma level is 10 mg/L. The patient's estimated volume of distribution is 0.5 L/kg.

    (A)  150 mg
    (B)  350 mg
    (C)  400 mg
    (D)  500 mg
    (E)  800 mg

64. What maintenance dose is appropriate in the above patient if the clearance is estimated to be 0.35 mL/min/kg?

    (A)  10 mg/h
    (B)  14 mg/h
    (C)  17 mg/h
    (D)  20 mg/h
    (E)  25 mg/h

65. A drug with a half-life of 6 h has a targeted steady-state concentration of 1 mg/dL. What infusion rate (mg/min) should be established on a patient if the total clearance is approximately 0.04 L/h?

    (A)  0.007
    (B)  0.07

(C) 0.04

(D) 0.4

(E) 4

66. The metabolism of drugs generally results in

(A) less acidic compounds

(B) more acidic compounds

(C) compounds having a higher oil/water partition coefficient

(D) more polar compounds

(E) compounds with lower aqueous solubility

67. The pharmacist may suspect that a drug undergoes a significant First-Pass effect when

I. the average oral dose is significantly higher than the parenteral bolus dose

II. the drug is marketed in a sustained-release dosage form

III. the drug is contraindicated when renal impairment is present

(A) I only

(B) III only

(C) I and II only

(D) II and III only

(E) I, II, and III

68. All of the following drugs are believed to undergo significant First-Pass hepatic biotransformation EXCEPT

(A) lidocaine

(B) morphine

(C) nitroglycerin

(D) phenytoin

(E) propranolol

69. Dosage forms of nitroglycerin that are minimally affected by the First-Pass effect include

I. intravenous

II. transdermal patches

III. sublingual tablets

(A) I only

(B) III only

(C) I and II only

(D) II and III only

(E) I, II, and III

70. All of the following drugs have shown an increase in their bioavailability with the coadministration of concentrated grapefruit juice EXCEPT

(A) coumadin

(B) cyclosporine

(C) felodipine

(D) phenytoin

(E) saquinavir

71. The equation that describes the process of "passive transport" is

(A) Fick's law

(B) Henderson-Hasselbalch

(C) Noyes-Whitney

(D) Stoke's law

(E) Michaelis-Menten

72. The rate of diffusion of drugs across biological membranes is most commonly

(A) independent of the concentration gradient

(B) directly proportional to the concentration gradient

(C) dependent on the availability of carrier substrate

(D) dependent on the route of administration

(E) directly proportional to membrane thickness

73. Which one of the following statements concerning active transport is NOT correct? Active transport systems

(A) are also known as carrier-mediated transport

(B) may be adversely affected by certain chemicals

(C) are structure specific

(D) reach equilibrium faster than passive transport systems

(E) consume energy

74. When the active transport system described in Question 73 becomes saturated, the rate process will be

    (A) zero order
    (B) pseudo-zero order
    (C) first order
    (D) pseudo-first order
    (E) second order

75. When comparing a highly protein-bound drug to its less- or nonprotein-bound analog, the highly bound drug will probably have

    I.   faster metabolism rate
    II.  a longer biological half-life
    III. slower diffusion into tissue

    (A) I only
    (B) III only
    (C) I and II only
    (D) II and III only
    (E) I, II, and III

76. Which one of the following drugs does NOT bind to plasma protein to any significant extent?

    (A) allopurinol (Zyloprim)
    (B) furosemide (Lasix)
    (C) phenytoin (Dilantin)
    (D) propranolol (Inderal)
    (E) warfarin (Coumadin)

77. Which of the following is (are) likely to occur with highly protein-bound cephalosporin drugs?

    I.   The drug's half-life will be longer.
    II.  The renal clearance value will be greater.
    III. Transfer into tissue will be easier.

    (A) I only
    (B) III only
    (C) I and II only
    (D) II and III only
    (E) I, II, and III

78. Dialysis is most successful with drugs that

    I.   have relatively low molecular weights
    II.  are protein bound
    III. have high volumes of distribution

    (A) I only
    (B) III only
    (C) I and II only
    (D) II and III only
    (E) I, II, and III

79. Which of the following drugs are poor candidates for removal from the body by hemodialysis?

    I.   digoxin
    II.  amphotericin B
    III. doxycycline

    (A) I only
    (B) III only
    (C) I and II only
    (D) II and III only
    (E) I, II, and III

80. The excretion of a weakly acidic drug (e.g., p$K_a$ of 3.5) will be more rapid in alkaline urine than in acidic urine because

    (A) all drugs are excreted more rapidly in alkaline urine
    (B) the drug will exist primarily in the un-ionized form, which cannot be reabsorbed easily
    (C) the drug will exist primarily in the ionized form, which cannot be reabsorbed easily
    (D) weak acids cannot be reabsorbed from the kidney tubules
    (E) active transport mechanisms function better in alkaline urine

81. Which one of the following characteristics is most accurately reflected in a drug's apparent volume of distribution value?

    (A) rate of metabolism
    (B) rate of renal clearance
    (C) extent of distribution in the body

(D) areas in body where the drug is concentrating

(E) degree of protein binding

82. A drug has an elimination half-life of 3 h and its apparent volume of distribution is 100 mL/kg. What is the total body renal clearance of this drug in a 70 kg male in terms of liters per hour?

(A) 0.5 L/h

(B) 1.6 L/h

(C) 8 L/h

(D) 14.6 L/h

(E) 16.3 L/h

83. The rectal route of administration may be preferred over the oral route for some systemic-acting drugs because

(A) the drug does not have to be absorbed

(B) absorption is predictable and complete

(C) a portion of the absorbed drug does not pass through the liver before entering the systemic circulation

(D) inert binders, diluents, and excipients cannot interfere with absorption

(E) the dissolution process is avoided

84. If a drug appears in the feces after oral administration,

(A) the drug cannot have been completely absorbed from the GI tract

(B) the drug must not have completely dissolved in the GI fluids

(C) the drug must have complexed with materials in the GI tract

(D) parenteral administration of the drug may determine the contribution of the biliary system to the amount of drug in the feces

(E) parenteral administration of the drug will be useful to determine the bioavailability of the oral formulation

85. Drugs that are poorly lipid soluble, polar, or extensively ionized at the pH of blood generally

(A) penetrate the CNS very slowly and may be eliminated from the body before a significant concentration in the CNS is reached

(B) penetrate the CNS very slowly but are centrally active in much lower concentration

(C) achieve adequate CNS concentrations only if given IV

(D) must be metabolized to a more polar form before they can gain access to the CNS

(E) can gain access to the CNS if other drugs are used to modify blood pH

86. The term "prodrug" refers to a

(A) chemical substance that is part of the synthesis procedure in preparing a drug

(B) compound that liberates an active drug in the body

(C) compound that may be therapeutically active but is still under clinical trials

(D) drug that has only prophylactic activity in the body

(E) drug that is classified as being "probably effective"

87. Which of the following drugs is/are classified as prodrugs?

I. clorazepate (Tranxene)

II. enalapril (Vasotec)

III. lisinopril (Zestril)

(A) I only

(B) III only

(C) I and II only

(D) II and III only

(E) I, II, and III

88. For which one of the following purposes is haloperidol formulated as the decanoate?

(A) better water solubility

(B) longer duration of therapeutic activity

(C) greater stability

(D) immediate activity

(E) sustained release from a capsule

89. Which of the following agents may be utilized as targeted drug delivery systems?

    I.   lyophilized powders
    II.  liposomes
    III. MABs

    (A) I only
    (B) III only
    (C) I and II only
    (D) II and III only
    (E) I, II, and III

90. Which of the following properties of a drug may preclude its formulation into a sustained-release dosage form?

    I.   half-life less than 2 h
    II.  erratic absorption from the GI tract
    III. low therapeutic index

    (A) I only
    (B) III only
    (C) I and II only

    (D) II and III only
    (E) I, II, and III

91. Which one of the following oral dosage forms is likely to exhibit the longest lag time?

    (A) delayed-release tablet
    (B) elixir (20% alcohol)
    (C) enteric-coated tablet
    (D) osmotic tablet
    (E) sustained-release capsule

92. The biological half-life of many drugs is often prolonged in newborn infants because of

    (A) a higher degree of protein binding
    (B) microsomal enzyme induction
    (C) more complete absorption of drugs
    (D) incompletely developed enzyme systems
    (E) incompletely developed barriers to the distribution of drugs in the body

# Answers and Explanations

1. **(C)** For most drugs, a dose-response relationship can be correlated with the amount of drug that gains access to the general circulation. In many cases, the amount of drug that is present in the blood (blood level) directly relates to the intensity and duration of the pharmacological effect. The relative amount of drug that is biologically available compared to the total amount of drug in the dosage form administered is a measure of bioavailability. Usually, bioavailability is expressed as the fraction or percentage of the administered drug that is absorbed. The term "absolute bioavailability" compares the amount of drug absorbed with the "gold standard" of the amount present in the blood after administration by an IV bolus. *(15)*

2. **(D)** The AUC can be calculated mathematically by the use of equations or evaluation of a graph when concentration (drug w/v) is plotted on the Y axis and time is plotted on the X axis. Units for AUC are weight and time/volume. *(17)*

3. **(C)** The availability of a drug from a specific formulation is compared to a reference standard that is administered at the same dose level. The standard for oral drugs is usually a solution of the pure drug. The relative bioavailability is then calculated by dividing either the AUC of the drug or the total amount of the drug excreted in the urine by respective values for the reference standard. The absolute bioavailability can be calculated by comparing similar data for the drug product to an IV bolus dose. *(17)*

4. **(E)** The surface area of a drug is so limited in the intact tablet that dissolution of drug from the intact tablet is negligible except for very water-soluble drugs. Therefore, although a drug must dissolve before it can be absorbed, a tablet must generally disintegrate before the drug can dissolve. *(17)*

5. **(E)** The rate-limiting step is considered the slowest step in the kinetics of drug absorption. For some drugs, especially tablet dosage forms, the slow release of the drug from the dosage form may be due to slow tablet disintegration due to excessive tablet hardness or excessive amounts of water-insoluble lubricant. Once disintegration has occurred, a poorly water-soluble drug may only slowly dissolve, thus limiting absorption. If a drug has high water solubility and the tablet has disintegrated rapidly, the rate-limiting step may be the ability of the drug to diffuse through the GI tract wall. *(17)*

6. **(C)** Terms in the Noyes-Whitney equation reflect the rate at which a drug dissolves from the surface of a solid mass followed by diffusion through the stagnant layer that surrounds the solid particle. The Noyes-Whitney equation is a modified form of Fick's first law used to describe diffusion. *(17)*

7. **(B)** By employing the mathematical technique known as the trapezoidal rule, one may calculate an AUC. The AUC is subdivided into individual segments and the area of each is determined. By totaling these areas, an accurate estimate of the total AUC is obtained. *(17)*

8. **(E)** The area under the plasma level time curve (AUC) is a measurement that allows

comparisons of similar drug products. For two products of the same drug to be considered bioequivalent, their AUCs must be similar in size and shape. However, the FDA does allow some leeway for overall AUCs. Differences of less than 20% in either the AUC or the maximum concentration ($C_{max}$) are unlikely to be clinically significant in patients. Thus, a generic house may present data illustrating that their product has an AUC of 2000 µg h/mL while the trade named product has an AUC of only 1600 µg h/mL.

9. **(B)** Prior to the peak time, the rate of absorption is greater than the rate of elimination, and the curve ascends. After the peak, the rate of elimination is greater than the rate of absorption, and the curve descends. If these rates are equal for some time interval, the curve will show a plateau rather than a distinct peak. *(1; 17)*

10. **(E)** Drug metabolism or biotransformation is usually associated with the liver and its numerous enzymes. However, enzymes present in other body organs and tissues may metabolize some drugs. These sites include the lungs, skin, kidney and small intestine. *(7; 15)*

11. **(A)** Drug metabolites such as the glucuronides, sulfates, or glycine conjugates are more polar, i.e., water soluble than their parent compound. There are exceptions such as the acetylated compounds which are less polar. The greater water solubility results in more rapid excretion through the kidneys. Some metabolites are less therapeutic than the original compound but others are more active. In fact, some drugs must first metabolize in the body before biological activity occurs. These are known as prodrugs. *(17; 24)*

12. **(C)** Differences in bioavailability of various drug products might be anticipated with any route of administration that requires the drug to be absorbed into the blood compartment. The oral route is most often involved because it is the most common route of administration and the drug must pass through the GI lumen,

gut wall, and the hepatic circulation system before reaching the general circulation. *(15; 17)*

13. **(C)** Linear pharmacokinetics is characterized by straight-line (linear) relationships when plotted as a log function ($Y$ axis) versus time ($X$ axis). Some drugs deviate from this straight line, especially when their doses are increased or multidoses are given. Such drugs are described as following dose-dependent or non-linear pharmacokinetics. The classic example is a drug that demonstrates a saturable elimination process. *(17)*

14. **(A)** F values are calculated for drugs in their dosage forms by comparing AUCs, or total amount of drug excreted, to the control reference of an IV bolus dose, as outlined in Question 3. An ideal F value would be 1.0, which indicates complete absorption of the drug and no losses from other mechanisms such as hepatic First-Pass effect. The F value is also known as the bioavailability factor. *(17; 23)*

15. **(C)** As outlined in Question 14, the F value can be estimated by using the equation

$$F = \frac{AUC_{cap}}{AUC_{IV}} = \frac{20}{25} = 0.8$$

Because in this example the comparison of AUCs relates to the absolute standard of an IV bolus dose, the drug's absolute bioavailability was calculated. If the comparison had been to another standard, such as to an oral solution or another product of the same drug, the F value would be the relative bioavailability. *(17)*

16. **(A)** This problem is similar to Question 15, except that a correction factor is necessary since different amounts of drug were given by tablet versus IV. If 50 mg IV had an AUC of 40, 100 mg IV would theoretically have an AUC of 80. The F ratio would be

$$F = \frac{AUC_{tab}}{AUC_{IV}} = \frac{20}{80} = 0.25 \qquad (17)$$

17. **(B)** If the areas under the respective curves are equal, it can be concluded that the total amount

of drug delivered to the body by each dosage form was equal. Because the intravenous administration did not involve an absorption process, the fact that the same amount of drug administered in a capsule formulation delivered the same total amount of drug indicates that the absorption of the drug from the oral capsule was essentially complete. *(1)*

18. **(B)** The therapeutic window is calculated by determining the minimum toxic concentration (MTC) and the minimum effective concentration (MEC). The difference between these two concentrations is usually referred to as the "therapeutic window" of the drug. *(15; 17)*

19. **(C)** Pharmaceutical equivalents are considered to be drug products that are almost identical in all aspects and are expected to exhibit almost identical therapeutic activity. Bioavailablity data submitted to the FDA must show that similar values for onset of action, duration, peak concentrations, and time to peak concentration are obtained. One of the few variables allowed is the choice of excipients. These excipients, or "inactive ingredients," include binders, diluents, lubricants, and so on. Naturally the manufacturers must include data proving that these excipients do not adversely affect the performance of their product. *(17; 24)*

20. **(A)** Drug products considered to be pharmaceutical alternatives are allowed greater variation from each other. Although they must contain the same active drug or its precursor, they may consist of different dosage forms, strengths, or contain a different salt of the drug. *(17; 24)*

21. **(A)** The ionic equilibrium that is established in the acid contents of the stomach will favor a relatively higher concentration of un-ionized drug in solution. The unionized molecule, because of the absence of a charge, is more lipid soluble than the ionic species and will be able to cross biological membranes more easily. If the drug reaches the more alkaline contents of the intestines before absorption is complete, the higher pH will then favor the ionic form of the drug, which has considerably less lipid solubility and

is much less readily absorbed. It should be pointed out, however, that because of the extremely large surface area of the intestine, weakly acidic drugs can be absorbed from the intestine in spite of the unfavorable ion/molecule ratio. *(15)*

22. **(D)** Gastric emptying appears to be a process with a normal half-life of between 20 and 60 min. However, many factors can influence the rate of this process. It is slowed by the A, B, C, and E choices and is speeded by hunger, mild exercise, cold meals, dilute solutions, and lying on the right side. Because some drugs and some dosage forms (e.g., enteric-coated tablets) are absorbed at rather specific sites along the GI tract, alterations in the rate of gastric emptying may lead to erratic and unpredictable absorption. For example, if an acid-labile drug that is preferentially absorbed from a portion of the small intestine is consumed as an enteric-coated tablet, a greatly reduced gastric emptying rate may permit the tablet to dissolve in the stomach and be degraded by the acid fluids of the stomach. Similarly, if the gastric emptying rate is greatly increased, the tablet may not dissolve before it reaches its primary site of absorption. *(17)*

23. **(B)** Drugs must be in solution for significant absorption from the GI tract to occur. Thus, drugs with poor water solubility may have their dissolution rate as the rate-limiting factor. However, making a drug dissolve faster (e.g., by particle size reduction) will not increase the rate of its absorption if the absorption process itself is the rate-limiting step in the overall transport of the drug from its intact dosage form to the blood. The classical example of a drug formulated as a micronized powder is griseofulvin (Fulvicin U/F). This poorly water-soluble drug will dissolve faster in the GI tract due to an increase in surface area. Thus, larger quantities are available for absorption. *(1; 17)*

24. **(D)** Albumin will bind numerous drugs that have an acid functional group. Because of its nonspecificity and high blood levels (3.5–5%), the loading doses of some drugs must be high to at least partially saturate the protein binding sites. *(1; 15)*

25. **(A)** Drugs are generally absorbed from the GI tract through capillaries that empty into the portal vein. This vessel carries the absorbed drugs to the liver, where they are subjected to varying degrees of metabolism before they are carried into the general circulation. This initial passage through the liver is therapeutically significant, primarily for drugs that are metabolized to a less active or inactive form by the liver. *(17)*

26. **(D)** Routes of administration that avoid the First-Pass effect include intravenous injections, inhalation, and transdermal. By these routes the drug is distributed within the body before metabolism by the liver. The "F" value, may be approximated by dividing the AUC of a non-IV dose by the AUC of an IV bolus dose which represents absolute bioavailability. The F value is a fraction and the higher the fraction, the greater the bioavailability of the non-IV drug. A second, more accurate method to evaluate the First-Pass effect is determining the liver extraction ratio (ER). *(17)*

27. **(C)** Generally, when a particular drug has a half-life of 6 h, there is reasonable certainty that in spite of as much as a one- to twofold intersubject variation, the mean biological half-life in any group of subjects will be approximately 6 h. Alterations in biological half-life can be expected when a particular drug is primarily excreted unchanged by the kidneys. The presence of renal impairment slows the process of excretion and thereby increases the biological half-life of the drug in the blood. *(1; 24)*

28. **(C)** *(1; 24)*

29. **(A)** Most drugs have biological half-lives that follow first-order kinetics. A basic characteristic of first-order kinetics is that the rate constants for metabolism or excretion are independent of the initial drug concentration. That is, a specific fraction of drug will be lost in a given time period. Doubling the drug concentration will not change the rate constant, even though the amount of drug lost in a given time period would increase.

(D—incorrect) Renal impairment may affect the biological half-life of drugs eliminated by the kidneys. However, the half-life would be expected to increase (not decrease), because the drug remains in the circulation for longer periods of time.

(E—incorrect) Two methods for determining half-life are (1) to determine drug blood levels with respect to time, and (2) to quantify with respect to time actual biological responses to the drug. Ideally, the half-life values determined by each method should be identical. However, they will be identical only when there is a direct and measurable relationship between drug blood concentrations and the biological response. *(17)*

30. **(C)** One-half (200 mg) of the administered dose will be eliminated in 4 h. Of the remaining 200 mg, one-half (100 mg) will be eliminated in the second 4-h period. In the next 4-h span, an additional 50 mg of drug will be lost. Therefore, after 12 h (or three half-lives), only 50 mg of drug remains. If graphed as log drug remaining (*Y* axis) versus time (*X* axis), the data will appear as a straight line (first-order kinetics). *(1; 23)*

31. **(B)** A rate constant of 46% per hour refers to a fractional loss of 0.46 per hour. The equation for determining half-lives for first-order reactions is

$$t_{0.5} = \frac{0.693}{k}, \quad \text{or} \quad \frac{0.693}{0.46} = 1.5 \text{ h} \quad (23)$$

32. **(A)** Volume of distribution ($V_d$) is an "apparent volume" measured in terms of a reference compartment, usually the blood, because of the accessibility of this compartment to sampling. Because the drug dose is known and the blood concentration can be determined, the $V_d$ may be calculated by

$$V_d = A_b/C_b$$

where $A_b$ is the total amount of unchanged drug in the body and $C_b$ is the concentration of drug in the blood.

Knowledge of the $V_d$ for a particular drug permits calculation of the total amount of drug in the body ($A_b$) at any time by measuring the drug concentration in the blood (because $A_b = V_d$) accumulation in specific body areas. Also, because only the unbound fraction of drug is available for biotransformation and excretion, protein-bound drugs have a tendency to remain in the body longer (i.e., delayed elimination and longer half-lives). *(1; 17)*

33. **(A)** Following a given dose of a drug, the greater its concentration in various tissue compartments, the smaller its concentration in plasma. Therefore, according to the relationship Dose = $C_{ss} \times V_d$, the volume of distribution of a particular drug will be greater for those drugs that tend to concentrate in tissues than remain in the plasma. *(1; 15)*

34. **(C)** Because the $V_d$ is a parameter that allows accountability for all of the drug in the body, it can be used to calculate the loading dose that would rapidly result in a desired plasma concentration ($C_p$).

$$\text{Loading dose} = \frac{V_d C_p}{SF}$$

where $S$ is the portion of the salt form that is active drug and $F$ is the fraction of dose absorbed. *(15; 17)*

35. **(B)** One can easily picture that the plasma concentration of the drug ($C_p$) will be equal to the amount of drug ($D$) administered or absorbed divided by the body volume ($V_d$) in which it is distributed.

$$C_p = D \quad \text{or} \quad \text{Dose} = C_p \times V_d$$

In this problem:

Step 1: 140 lb $\times$ 1 kg/2.2 lb = 64 kg (body wt)
Step 2: $V_d$ = 64 kg $\times$ 1.6 L/kg = 102 L
Step 3: 50 mg = ($C_p$) (102 L)
Step 4: $C_p$ = 0.5 mg/L       *(6; 23)*

36. **(B)** For any drug that is eliminated by first-order kinetics, the time required to achieve

steady-state plasma levels is dependent only on the biological half-life of that drug in a given individual. As a drug is repeatedly administered in constant dosage and at constant time intervals (that are short enough to preclude complete elimination of the drug), the elimination rate of the drug increases as the concentration of drug in plasma increases. The tendency of a drug to accumulate on repeated dosing is, therefore, balanced by increased amounts of drug being eliminated. Eventually, a steady state will be reached in which the amount of drug absorbed will equal the amount of drug being eliminated. The time to reach steady state corresponds to about four to five half-lives and is more completely described in the following table:

| Time Plasma (Half-Lives) | Concentration (% of Steady-State Level) |
|---|---|
| 1 | 50 |
| 2 | 75 |
| 3 | 88 |
| 4 | 94 |
| 5 | 97 |
| 6 | 98 |
| 7 | 99 |

37. **(B)** Curve I shows an initial high concentration of drug in the blood with a steadily decreasing concentration. This curve is characteristic of drugs administered by rapid intravenous injection. *(17)*

38. **(E)** Any of the listed dosage forms could exhibit blood level curves similar to curve II. The first portion of the curve shows an increasing concentration of drug in the blood. This pattern would be expected whenever there is steady drug absorption (i.e., when absorption is greater than elimination), either from the GI tract or from a tissue injection site. Curve III is also a good representation for a sustained-release product as it illustrates a plateau effect. *(17)*

39. **(E)** For any drug to exhibit high blood levels it must be absorbed at a rate significantly greater than the rate by which it is eliminated. That is, $K_a$ must be greater than $K_e$, at least in the early period of its therapeutic curve. Obviously the

manufacturer bases dosing amounts on the relative speed and extent of absorption versus how quickly the drug is being eliminated. *(15)*

(A—incorrect) Blood levels of drug increase until a peak occurs where the rate of absorption equals the rate of elimination. Drug absorption will usually continue to occur even after the peak blood concentration has been reached. However, the blood level curve is then declining, because the rate of elimination is greater than the rate of absorption.

(B—incorrect) Because most of the factors affecting pharmacokinetics are first order, doubling a drug dose will seldom double the height of a blood level curve. However, the total area under the drug curve can be expected to double, because the AUC is directly proportional to the dose.

(C—incorrect) The pharmacokinetics of most drugs follow a first-order pattern. Therefore, if the concentration of drug in the blood is plotted as a log function on the $Y$ axis, a straight line will be obtained rather than a curve, as shown on the graph.

(D—incorrect) The time factor is a constant variable plotted at regular intervals (hours, days, etc.). It is very seldom expressed as a log function.

40. **(B)** Administration of drugs by intravenous infusion, which implies slow flow into a vein, will result in a plateau effect in respect to drug blood levels. The resulting steady-state levels are directly proportional to the infusion rate.

(A—incorrect) An intravenous push (bolus dose) will give a curve similar to curve I on the graph.

(D—incorrect) The blood level curve for an intrathecal (spinal) injection will probably resemble curve II as the drug slowly diffuses into the blood. *(15)*

41. **(C)** The time in which the optimum drug blood level is obtained is independent of the infusion rate. It is dependent only on the biological half-life of the particular drug. The time required to reach the plateau (steady state) is approximately four to five half-lives. At the blood concentration plateau, the $K_e$ equals the infusion rate. *(15)*

42. **(D)** Determination of the rate of infusion of a parenteral solution may be accomplished using the equation:

$$R \text{ (infusion rate)} = C_{ss} \times CL$$

It is obvious that the higher the total clearance rate, the faster the infusion rate to maintain a specific steady-state concentration. Although renal clearance predominates for many drugs, hepatic metabolism, or other elimination processes may be present. *(15; 17)*

43. **(B)** Although various organs, tissues, and fluids in the body can be considered to be compartments for a specific drug, a compartment does not necessarily have to be an anatomic entity. Any body site or fluid that appears to contain the drug may be described as a compartment or "pool" in the model. *(17; 24)*

44. **(C)** Nonlinear pharmacokinetics follows zero-order kinetics in which the half-life changes as the drug dose is changed. It usually reflects the effect of enzymes or the presence of carrier-mediated systems. In these situations, the elimination half-life of the drug will increase when the dose is increased. *(15; 17)*

45. **(A)** Drugs (e.g., aminoglycosides) given at intervals that are much longer than one half-life are almost completely eliminated from the body before the next dose is given. This results in a large difference between peak and trough drug concentrations, thus timing of blood sample(s) becomes crucial to interpretation of results. At the other extreme, drugs given at intervals that are much shorter than one half-life (e.g., phenobarbital) are slowly cleared from the body; consequently, their peak-to-trough concentration differences are relatively small. *(17)*

46. **(E)** Decreased efficiency in renal function occurs in approximately 70% of the geriatric population. Also, both blood circulation and hepatic function decrease in many of the elderly. Because both extracellular and other body fluids may decrease in volume, reported

volume of distributions in some geriatric patients may be lower than expected. *(15; 17)*

47. **(E)** This is the definition of total systemic (whole body) clearance, which is the sum of all the separate clearances (i.e., renal, hepatic, etc.). *(17)*

48. **(A)** When the clearance (CL) of a drug is known, the maintenance dose required to sustain a desired average steady-state plasma concentration can be calculated by

$$\text{Maintenance dose} = \frac{CL \times C_p \times \tau}{S \times F}$$

where $C_p$ = average steady-state plasma concentration
$\tau$ = dosing interval (tau)
$S$ = portion of salt that is active drug
$F$ = fraction of dose absorbed *(17)*

49. **(C)** Drug elimination by the kidneys can often be correlated with blood urea nitrogen (BUN), serum creatinine ($Sr_{cr}$), and creatinine clearance ($CL_{cr}$). The BUN and $Sr_{cr}$, however, are less useful indices of renal function than the $CL_{cr}$ because they are influenced by other factors (e.g., state of hydration, age, etc.). For example, as patients age, both the production and clearance of creatinine decrease. Therefore, an elderly patient with a normal serum creatinine of 1 mg/dL may have a $CL_{cr}$ of much less than 100 mL/min (normal $CL_{cr}$ is 100–120 mL/min for a 70-kg adult). There are a number of methods used to calculate $CL_{cr}$. One equation, the Cockcroft and Gault equation reads:

$$CL_{cr}\text{(for a male)} = \frac{(40 - \text{age})(\text{weight})}{72\,(Sr_{cr})}$$

Units include age in years, weight in kilograms, and serum creatinine measurements in mg/dL. For females, the calculated CL value is reduced by multiplying by 0.85. *(17; 23)*

50. **(A)** If the biological half-life of a drug increases in patients with impaired renal function, the time required to reach steady-state plasma

levels will also be increased. This time factor is only dependent on the biological half-life of a given drug in a given individual. *(17)*

51. **(C)** Once a drug gains access to the systemic circulation, it may be metabolized to varying degrees and/or be excreted unchanged. For most drugs and their metabolites, the kidneys are the primary organ of excretion. The presence of a drug and/or its metabolites in the urine must be preceded by the presence of drug in the blood. When an appreciable amount of drug is excreted in the urine, it is often possible to use urinary excretion data—such as cumulative amount of drug in the urine and maximum urinary excretion rate—to evaluate the systemic availability of various drug formulations. *(17)*

52. **(C)** Urinary excretion studies require complete urine collection so that the total quantity of drug that is excreted in the urine can be determined. Normal or near-normal renal function is also a prerequisite for accurate urinary excretion studies because sufficiently impaired renal function can alter the composition of various body fluids that, in turn, can alter the pharmacokinetic properties of many drugs. Although urinary excretion studies are usually conducted on drugs that are primarily excreted unchanged by the kidney, it is not necessary that a drug be completely excreted unchanged by the kidney. *(17)*

53. **(C)** The best measure of absolute bioavailability is considered to be AUC data obtained after a bolus IV injection of a drug. Because AUC data are not available for these drug products, the next best comparison will be the use of cumulative drug amounts found in the urine. Because the IV injection dose was 10 mg whereas the oral tablet dose was 20 mg, a correction factor of $2x$ is needed. Cumulative amount if 20 mg had been injected will be $9.4 \times 2 = 18.8$. Dividing 8.2 mg by 18.8 mg = 0.44, or 44%. *(17)*

54. **(D)** Relative bioavailability of Company B's tablet when compared to Company A's tablet

will be 8.2 mg divided by 12 mg = 0.68, or 68%. *(17)*

55. **(D)** To determine the relative bioavailability of Company B's tablet when compared to the capsule formula , one must correct for the fact that the capsule dose was 15 mg. That is, determine the mg of drug that would accumulate in the urine if a 20 mg capsule dose had been administered.

$$\frac{15 \text{ mg cap}}{6.8 \text{ mg (in urine)}} = \frac{20 \text{ mg}}{x \text{ mg (in urine)}}$$

$$x = 9.1 \text{ mg}$$

Relative bioavailability of the tablet will equal 8.2 divided by 9.1 mg or 0.90 (90%). One may expect higher amounts of drug from a capsule to reach the urine since most capsules disintegrate in the GI tract faster. Neither of Company B's dosage forms, tablet, or capsule, can be considered bioequivalent to Company A's tablet because neither is within 80% of the cumulative amount of drug in the urine. This 80% guideline has been accepted by the FDA for determining bioequivalency of similar drug products. *(17)*

56. **(A)** Since there are no data based upon calculated AUCs after intravenous bolus dosing the absolute bioavailability of Company A's drug cannot be determined. The relative bioavailability can be determined by

$$\text{Relative bioavailability} = \frac{\text{AUC(Company A)}}{\text{AUC(Company B)}}$$

$$= \frac{80 \ \mu g \, h/mL}{76 \ \mu g \, h/mL} = 1.05$$

As shown above, it is possible for the experimental drug to have greater bioavailability than the standard or control drug. *(17)*

57. **(A)** Linear pharmacokinetics indicate first-order rates, thus half-life = 0.693/$k$.

$$8h = \frac{0.693}{k} = 0.087/h \qquad (17)$$

58. **(B)** The fastest estimation of clearance may be obtained using the equation:

$$\text{Dose} = C_{ss} \times \text{CL}$$

$$\frac{50 \text{ mg}}{4 \text{ h}} = \frac{10 \text{ mg}}{L} \times \text{CL}$$

$$\text{CL} = 1.25 \text{ L/h} \qquad (17)$$

59. **(A)** The Cockcroft and Gault equation allows estimations of a patient's creatinine clearance. It reads:

$$\text{CL}_{cr} = \frac{[140 - \text{age}] \, [\text{body wt}]}{72[\text{serum creatinine conc.}]}$$

The age is expressed in years and the body weight in kilograms.
While the patient's weight is needed, his/her height is not. A patient's BEE refers to basal energy expenditure, a useful measurement in determining caloric needs of a patient. *(17; 23)*

60. **(A)**

$$\text{CL}_{cr} = \frac{[140 - \text{age}] \, [\text{body wt}]}{72[\text{serum creatinine conc.}]}$$

Body weight of 140 lb × 1 kg/2.2 lb = 63.6 kg

$$\text{CL}_{cr} = \frac{[140 - 50] \, [63.6 \text{ kg}]}{72 \, [1.5 \text{ mg/dL}]}$$

$$\text{CL}_{cr} = 52.9 \text{ mL/min}$$

61. **(D)** Female creatinine clearance values are approximately 85% of the values calculated for a male. Other factors that affect creatinine clearance values include relative obesity. For these patients the lean body mass should be used in the equation rather than the total body weight. *(15; 17; 23)*

62. **(B)** The water solubility of theophylline is enhanced by combining it with ethylenediamine, forming the drug aminophylline. Because the active moiety, theophylline, contributes 80% of the molecular weight of aminophylline, a correction factor is needed to convert between the two drugs when predicting

therapeutic activity. This conversion factor is often referred to as the "S" factor, and is expressed as a fraction. In some books, a correction of 85% is used instead of 80. This minor discrepancy is based on whether the hydrous or anhydrous form of aminophylline is present. *(1; 5; 17)*

63. **(C)** (F) (Loading dose) = (plasma conc.) × (volume of distribution)

1. Patient's total $V_d$ will be 0.5 L/kg × 70 kg = 35 L
2. Since aminophylline consists of 85% theophylline, its F value will be 0.85.

$$(0.85)(LD) = (10 \text{ mg/L})(35 \text{ L})$$

$$LD = 412 \text{ mg} \qquad (5; 17)$$

64. **(C)** Convert the clearance to L/h and eliminate the kg weight,

$$0.35 \text{ mL/min/kg} \times 60 \text{ min/h} \times 70 \text{ k}$$
$$= 1470 \text{ mL/h or } 1.47 \text{ L/h}$$

(F) (Maintenance dose)
= (Plasma conc.)(Clearance)

$$(0.85)x = (10 \text{ mg/L})(1.47 \text{ L/h})$$

$$x = 17.3 \text{ mg/h} \qquad (5)$$

65. **(A)** Using the equation R (infusion rate) = $[C_{ss}][CL]$

$$R = \frac{1 \text{ mg}}{dL} \times \frac{0.4 dL}{h}$$

$$R = 0.4 \text{ mg/h} \quad \text{and} \quad \frac{0.4 \text{ mg}}{60 \text{ min}} = \frac{x \text{ mg}}{1 \text{ min}}$$

$$x = 0.0067 \text{ mg/min} \qquad (15; 17)$$

66. **(D)** Drug metabolites are usually more polar and less lipid soluble than the parent compound. Because of these changes, metabolites are usually not as tightly nor as extensively protein bound. They are ionized to a greater degree and are less likely to cross biological membranes than the parent compound. Drug metabolism, therefore, is generally a process that inactivates a drug and changes it to a form that can be excreted more easily and rapidly. For some drugs, however, metabolism may

result in activation of an inactive substance, or an active substance may be transformed into (an) active metabolite(s). In these cases, either further biotransformation takes place to inactivate the metabolite(s), or it (they) is (are) excreted unchanged. *(1)*

67. **(A)** The term "First-Pass" refers to the first passage of drug molecules through a designated organ such as the lungs or the liver. Biotransformation will often occur at this site, thereby altering the absolute bioavailability of a drug. Commercial preparations of such drugs are formulated to contain sufficient quantities of drug to compensate for loss due to First-Pass biotransformation. Although acetylsalicylic acid does not appear to undergo a significant First-Pass hepatic biotransformation, some drug loss does occur in the intestinal lumen or during absorption through the GI mucosa. *(17)*

68. **(D)** Only 5% of phenytoin is metabolized in the liver; most of the drug is excreted unchanged. When significant amounts of a drug are metabolized by the liver immediately after absorption through the GI tract wall (First-Pass effect), manufacturers may compensate by increasing the dose present in oral dosage forms. For example, propranolol is available as 40- and 80-mg tablets, whereas the parenteral form is 2-mL ampules containing 2 mg/mL. *(17; 24)*

69. **(E)** All three routes of administration are used for delivering nitroglycerin. In each case, the drug enters systemic blood before significant loss occurs due to the First-Pass effect. *(17)*

70. **(D)** All of the listed drugs have shown improvement in their bioavailability when administered with grapefruit juice. Most notable is saquinavir, which normally has only a 4% bioavailability, but demonstrated a 150 to 220% increase with the juice. It is believed that the bioflavonoid naringin, found in grapefruit juice inhibits the liver cytochrome P450 enzyme. *(17)*

71. **(A)** Fick's first law states that the rate of diffusion is directly related to the diffusion coefficient and the surface area of the membrane and

inversely proportional to the thickness of the membrane. The driving force in the equation is the concentration gradient, because the greater the difference in concentrations on each side of the membrane, the greater the amount of drug diffusing (first-order kinetics). One form of the equation used for the passage of drug through the intestinal wall reads:

$$J_W = P_W \; C_W$$

in which $J_w$ is the drug flux, $P_w$ is the permeability of the intestinal membrane, and $C_w$ is the drug concentration at the membrane surface. *(17; 24)*.

72. **(B)** The greater the difference between the drug concentrations on each side of a biological membrane, the greater the rate of transfer from the side having the higher concentration to the side having the lower concentration. *(24)*

73. **(D)** As the name implies, carrier-mediated or active transport involves active participation of a membrane in transferring molecules from one side to the other. The "carrier," such as an enzyme in the membrane, aids in transporting the molecules of drug across the membrane. Because this transfer process is continuous, it can work against a concentration gradient and continue until all of the drug has been transported. Therefore, equilibrium does not occur.

(A—incorrect) Active transport requires energy. Facilitated diffusion is a carrier-mediated transport process that does not require energy.

(B—incorrect) Certain chemicals, known as poisons, can reduce active transport, probably by destroying, or inactivating the drug carriers.

(C—incorrect) Carriers are often very specific in respect to the drug they will transport. Only a certain chemical structure, or similar chemical structures may be actively transported by a given carrier. Because of the chemical specificity and limited capacity of carriers, active transport systems may become saturated. When this occurs, the active transport rate becomes a constant value until the drug concentration is reduced. *(6; 23; 17)*

74. **(A)** A characteristic of a zero-order process or reaction is a constant rate of change. When the active transport system is saturated, there are not enough carriers to handle the large number of transferable molecules. Therefore, the carriers work at maximum capacity, transferring molecules at a constant rate until the drug concentration is reduced to less than the capacity of the carrier system. At this time, the number of molecules transferred will be a fraction of those present for transfer (i.e., a first-order rate will exist). *(1)*

75. **(D)** Only the unbound fraction of a drug is available for biotransformation and excretion. Protein-bound drugs have a tendency to remain in the body longer because they do not readily enter hepatocytes for metabolism by the liver. Protein-bound drugs are larger molecules and cannot as readily diffuse through the renal glomeruli for eventual excretion, thus their half-lives will be longer. *(17; 24)*

76. **(A)** When administered in therapeutic doses, allopurinol does not appear to bind to plasma proteins. All of the other choices are drugs known to undergo significant protein binding. The pharmacist should carefully monitor drug therapy when two or more drugs that exhibit significant protein-binding properties are prescribed. Relatively small changes in the degree of protein binding caused by competition for binding sites can result in significant changes in plasma concentration of free drug and in the intensity of the clinical response. *(1; 17)*

77. **(A)** Cephalosporins are mainly eliminated from the body by renal excretion. The greater the degree of protein binding, the slower the excretion clearance thus increasing both the body half-life and the elimination half-life. For example, ceftriaxone is 96% protein bound with a half-life of 8 h and a clearance of 10 mL/min/1.73 m$^2$. Cefazolin which is 70% protein bound has values of 2.7 h half-life and 56 mL/min/1.73 m$^2$ clearance. Since a protein bound drug is less able to diffuse through membranes, the elimination through the kidneys will be less resulting in a longer half-life. *(17)*

78.  **(A)** Drugs that can be dialyzed include those that are water soluble and have relatively low molecular weights. Protein bound drugs do not readily diffuse through membranes. A high volume of distribution indicates that the drug is distributed throughout the body or concentrated in certain organs or tissue, therefore not readily available for fast dialysis. *(17)*

79.  **(E)** It is unlikely if any of the drugs in this question will be removed by hemodialysis to any significant extent. Digoxin has a very high volume of distribution meaning that it is distributed throughout the body. Amphotericin B and doxycycline are large molecules and will not diffuse readily through membranes. *(1: 17)*

80.  **(C)** Just as shifting the ionic equilibrium in favor of the ionic species reduces the probability that a weakly acidic drug will be absorbed from the alkaline fluids of the intestines, it also reduces the probability that the drug will be reabsorbed from the renal tubules into the blood. Consequently, a greater fraction of drug in the tubules cannot be reabsorbed and will be excreted in the urine. *(15; 17)*

81.  **(C)** The calculated apparent volume of distribution of a drug gives some indication of how widely distributed a drug may be in the body. Two useful, simple equations are

$$t_{0.5} = \frac{0.693 \times V_d}{CL} \quad \text{and} \quad \text{dose} = C_{ss} \times V_d$$

The apparent volume of distribution may be calculated after determination of the blood level of a drug soon after a loading dose has been administered. A low value such as 6 L usually indicates a drug that remains in the blood while very high values such as 240 L implies wide distribution or concentration in specific organs or tissues. While a drug that is highly bound to proteins will demonstrate a low volume of distribution, a low volume of distribution does not necessarily mean protein bonding is occurring. In other words, other reasons for a low value are possible. *(15; 17)*

82.  **(B)** Since the volume of distribution is given as 100 mL/kg body weight, convert this to liters.

$$100 \text{ mL/kg} \times 70 \text{ kg} = 7000 \text{ mL or } 7 \text{ L}$$
$$t_{0.5} = \frac{0.693 \times V_d}{CL}$$
$$3 \text{ h} = \frac{0.693 \times 7 \text{ L}}{CL}$$
$$CL = 1.6 \text{ L/h}$$

*(17)*

83.  **(C)** Although it is desirable for drugs that are rapidly metabolized by the liver to bypass absorption into the portal circulation, the value of using the rectal route for this purpose is limited. This is due to the fact that while three principal veins drain the blood supply to the rectum, only the middle and inferior hemorrhoidal veins actually bypass the liver. The superior hemorrhoidal vein enters the portal circulation via the inferior mesenteric vein. *(17; 24)*

84.  **(D)** If an orally administered drug appears in the feces, it might be desirable to determine whether this is the result of incomplete absorption or secretion of the drug into the GI tract via biliary excretion. The clinical significance of biliary excretion or enterohepatic cycling of the drug depends on the fraction of the dose excreted in the bile. By administering the drug parenterally, this fraction can be determined. *(15; 17)*

85.  **(A)** The "blood–brain barrier" appears to behave as a lipid membrane toward foreign compounds. This barrier may be due to a sheath of glial cells surrounding the capillaries of the brain. The rate of entry of a drug can often be correlated with its oil/water partition coefficient and degree of ionization at plasma pH. *(17)*

86.  **(B)** In order to take advantage of certain desirable characteristics, some drugs are marketed as prodrugs. These are chemical modifications of biologically active drugs and are not active themselves. However, the active form of the drug, the metabolite, is liberated in the body by biotransformation. Prodrugs may be better absorbed, possess better water solubility, be more stable, have a less objectionable taste, or give higher blood levels than the parent compound. *(17; 24)*

87. **(C)** Clorazepate (Tranxene) is rapidly decarboxylated in the acidic stomach to an active metabolite that possesses antiepileptic properties. Enalapril (Vasotec) is hydrolyzed to enalaprilat, which is the active angiotensin-converting enzyme (ACE) inhibitor for hypertension. However, lisinopril (Zestril) does not undergo metabolism, and instead is excreted unchanged in the urine. Other drugs, such as verapamil (Calan) form a large number of metabolites. *(10; 24)*

88. **(B)** The antipsychotic drug, haloperidol (Haldol) is available in several dosage forms including tablets, oral liquid, and parenteral. The injectable forms are designed for IV use with immediate activity and an elimination half-life of about 14 h. The IM form has peak concentrations after 0.3 h with an elimination half-life of 21 h. Haloperidol decanoate in sesame oil is intended for sustained activity. It reaches peak concentrations in about 6 days with an elimination half-life of 3 weeks. Other drugs formulated as esters for slow (depot) release include fluphenazine decanoate (Prolixin). *(5; 17)*

89. **(D)** Targeted drug delivery or site-specific systems are intended to place a drug near or at its receptor site. This concept is especially useful when concentrating a drug in the cells of a tumor since lower concentrations of the drug are needed with less toxic effects throughout the body. One mechanism for drug targeting is the use of drugs enveloped in liposomes, which when injected, will concentrate at the tumor site. A second method is the administration of monoclonal antibodies (MAB) which are very receptor site specific, thus effective drug delivery carriers. Lyophilized powders are not classified as targeted drug delivery systems; instead they are powders which have been dried to increase their stability. *(17; 24)*

90. **(E)** All of these drug characteristics are probably undesirable for a sustained-release dosage form. For a successful sustained-release product, the rate-limiting step must be drug release from the dosage form. If the drug has poor solubility, the dissolution rate may become the rate-limiting step. In this case, the patient may not absorb the quantity of drug needed for desired blood levels and therapeutic activity. Drugs with very long half-lives do not need to be formulated for sustained release because they will be biologically present for a long period of time. Intelligent dosing, such as every 12 or 24 h (depending on the actual half-life), ensures sufficient blood levels. The release of drug from most sustained-release dosage forms is subject to individual biological variations. This patient-to-patient variability may result in the release of two or three times the normal dose in a particular patient. Therefore, a dangerous situation may develop if very large amounts of very potent drugs are formulated as sustained-release products. Thus, drugs that possess high therapeutic indexes are desired. Conversely, a drug with a very short half-life is also a poor candidate for sustained release. A very large amount of drug would have to be included in the dosage form, and rapid release of the drug would be necessary. *(17; 24)*

91. **(C)** The lag time is the time delay between drug administration and the beginning of absorption, usually reflected in the appearance of drug in the plasma. Enteric-coated tablets are intended for disintegration in the small intestine, which could slow absorption for several hours. Both delayed-release and sustained-release tablets are usually designed to begin some drug release shortly after administration. *(15)*

92. **(D)** The metabolic pathways of newborn infants are incompletely developed at birth; most notably, the oxidative and conjugative mechanisms that are known to metabolize many drugs. The reduced capacity to metabolize certain drugs will therefore result in prolonged biological half-lives of these drugs in newborn infants. Because of inadequate metabolic inactivation, the plasma concentration of chloramphenicol is higher in infants younger than 2 weeks of age than in older infants. Kidney function also varies. Many drugs such as penicillin and gentamicin have longer half-lives in neonates than in adults (3.2 h versus 0.5 h for penicillin and 5 h versus 2–3 h for gentamicin. *(17)*

# CHAPTER 6

# Pharmaceutical Care

Pharmaceutical care is a term many have found difficult to define. A U.S. Supreme Court Justice, when challenged to define pornography, is said to have replied that although he could not define it, he was sure he could recognize it if he saw it. One definition of pharmaceutical care states that it is "the responsible provision of drug therapy for the purpose of achieving definite outcomes that improve a patient's quality of life."[1] With this example in mind, we have assembled a series of questions for this chapter that we believe fall under the category of pharmaceutical care—that is, they relate to patients, diseases, drugs, information, and pharmacists.

---

[1] C. D. Hepler and L. M. Strand. *Opportunities and responsibilities in pharmaceutical care.* Am J Hosp Pharm 47:533–543, 1990.

# Questions

DIRECTIONS (Questions 1 through 210): Each of the numbered items or incomplete statements in this section is followed by answers or by completions of the statement. Select the ONE lettered answer or completion that is BEST in each case.

1. The antiemetic effect of which of the following drugs is the result of increased rate of gastric emptying?

   (A) promethazine (Phenergan)
   (A) hyoscyamine (Nulev)
   (C) olsalazine (Dipentum)
   (D) baclofen (Lioresal)
   (E) metoclopramide (Reglan)

2. Which of the following agents is (are) indicated for the treatment of Parkinson's disease?

   I. amantadine (Symmetrel)
   II. bromocriptine (Parlodel)
   III. entacapone (Comtan)

   (A) I only
   (B) III only
   (C) I and II only
   (D) II and III only
   (E) I, II, and III

3. Patients diagnosed with Alzheimer's disease may be treated with which of the following agents?

   I. gabapentin (Neurontin)
   II. donepezil (Aricept)
   III. tacrine (Cognex)

   (A) I only
   (B) III only
   (C) I and II only
   (D) II and III only
   (E) I, II, and III

4. Patients receiving metformin (Glucophage) for the treatment of diabetes mellitus should be monitored for the development of

   (A) lactic acidosis
   (B) hearing loss
   (C) gastroparesis
   (D) respiratory alkalosis
   (E) agranulocytosis

5. A pharmacist tells a young mother about clinical (fever) thermometers and advises her to report to the pediatrician both the degrees of temperature and whether the temperature was taken rectally or orally. This is good advice because

   (A) oral temperature is about 1° Fahrenheit (1°F) higher than rectal temperature
   (B) oral thermometers have degree calibrations that differ from rectal thermometers
   (C) the normal temperature (marked with an arrow) is 99.6°F on the rectal thermometer and 98.6°F on the oral one
   (D) rectal temperature is about 1°F higher than oral temperature
   (E) the bulb on the rectal thermometer is round and contains more mercury than in the thin cylindrical bulb of the oral thermometer

6. The best emergency advice that a pharmacist could give an individual who has just suffered a minor burn is to

   (A) apply bacitracin cream onto the burn site
   (B) immerse the burned area in warm water followed by cold water
   (C) contact a physician immediately
   (D) immerse the burned area in cold water
   (E) apply Vaseline to the burn

7. A patient who is to use montelukast sodium (Singulair) should be advised to

   I. use one inhalation at the onset of an asthma attack
   II. stop using bronchodilator drugs
   III. take the drug daily as prescribed even when they are asymptomatic

   (A) I only
   (B) III only
   (C) I and II only
   (D) II and III only
   (E) I, II, and III

8. Which of the following is an effect associated with the use of pilocarpine ophthalmic products?

   I. mydriasis
   II. cholinergic agonism
   III. pupillary constriction

   (A) I only
   (B) III only
   (C) I and II only
   (D) II and III only
   (E) I, II, and III

9. Patients using amiodarone (Cordarone) should be monitored for

   I. pulmonary toxicity
   II. visual changes
   III. intestinal polyp formation

   (A) I only
   (B) III only
   (C) I and II only
   (D) II and III only
   (E) I, II, and III

10. Which of the following should NOT be administered to a patient being treated for narrow-angle glaucoma?

   (A) latanoprost
   (B) dorzolamide
   (C) homatropine
   (D) phospholine iodide
   (E) carbachol

11. Advantage(s) of levobetaxolol (Betaxon) over pilocarpine for the reduction of elevated intraocular pressure include(s)

   I. longer duration of activity
   II. little or no effect on visual acuity or accommodation
   III. little or no effect on pupil size

   (A) I only
   (B) III only
   (C) I and II only
   (D) II and III only
   (E) I, II, and III

12. Which of the following is true of GoLYTELY?

   I. contains bisacodyl
   II. ingredients are enzymatically converted to active form in colon
   III. must be reconstituted before use

   (A) I only
   (B) III only
   (C) I and II only
   (D) II and III only
   (E) I, II, and III

13. Which of the following is true of orlistat (Xenical)?

    I.   inhibits absorption of dietary fats
    II.  patient should consume diet that contains about 30% of calories from fat
    III. not more than one dose should be taken in any 24-h period

    (A) I only
    (B) III only
    (C) I and II only
    (D) II and III only
    (E) I, II, and III

14. Scabies is a contagious skin disease caused by a

    (A) herpes virus
    (B) fungus
    (C) flea
    (D) mite
    (E) tick

15. Psoriasis is characterized by

    (A) granulomatous lesions
    (B) silvery gray scales
    (C) small, water-filled blisters
    (D) small red vesicles
    (E) pustules

16. A patient with a documented allergy to morphine should NOT receive which one of the following analgesics?

    I.   pentazocine
    II.  fentanyl
    III. codeine

    (A) I only
    (B) III only
    (C) I and II only
    (D) II and III only
    (E) I, II, and III

17. Which of the following agents are classified as immunosuppressive agents?

    I.   fluconazole
    II.  tacrolimus
    III. cyclosporine

    (A) I only
    (B) III only
    (C) I and II only
    (D) II and III only
    (E) I, II, and III

18. Patients using alendronate should be advised to

    I.   lie down for 30 min after taking each dose
    II.  take each dose with food
    III. take each dose first thing in the morning

    (A) I only
    (B) III only
    (C) I and II only
    (D) II and III only
    (E) I, II, and III

19. Which of the following antihypertensive agents is available in a transdermal patch dosage form?

    (A) penbutolol
    (B) benazepril
    (C) clonidine
    (D) telmisartan
    (E) terazosin

20. Ideally, an antacid should raise the pH of the stomach contents to a value of approximately

    (A) 5.5
    (B) 3.5
    (C) 6.5
    (D) 7.5
    (E) 9.5

21. Which of the following is an indication for the use of epoetin alfa (Epogen, Procrit)?

    I.   treatment of anemia associated with chronic renal failure
    II.  treatment of anemia associated with cancer chemotherapy
    III. treatment of severe chronic neutropenia

    (A) I only
    (B) III only
    (C) I and II only
    (D) II and III only
    (E) I, II, and III

22. A patient with Parkinson's disease has been receiving levodopa (1 g four times daily) with fairly good response but excessive side effects. The patient's physician wishes to switch from levodopa to Sinemet. An approximate dose of Sinemet would be

    (A) one 10/100 tablet daily
    (B) one 10/100 tablet four times daily
    (C) one 25/250 tablet daily
    (D) four 25/250 tablets four times daily
    (E) one 25/250 tablet four times daily

23. A patient is being treated effectively for Parkinson's disease with levodopa. Suddenly, all therapeutic benefits of the levodopa are lost and the adverse effects also disappear. Which one of the following facts obtained from a medication history would most likely explain this phenomenon?

    (A) The patient has forgotten to take two doses of the medication.
    (B) The patient began using an OTC multivitamin product.
    (C) Selegiline was added to the drug regimen for 1 week.
    (D) Antacids were taken occasionally.
    (E) The patient regularly consumed alcoholic beverages.

24. Patients receiving miglitol should be advised to

    I.   expect some flatulence and diarrhea to occur
    II.  take each dose on an empty stomach
    III. expect to use a higher insulin dose while on the medication

    (A) I only
    (B) III only
    (C) I and II only
    (D) II and III only
    (E) I, II, and III

25. Which of the following drugs is associated with the "gray baby syndrome" in infants?

    (A) demeclocycline
    (B) ciprofloxacin
    (C) chloramphenicol
    (D) amphotericin B
    (E) kanamycin

26. Stomatitis refers to an inflammation of the

    (A) eyelid
    (B) oral mucosa
    (C) stoma formed by intestinal surgery
    (D) stomach wall
    (E) tongue

27. An obese individual would most likely be suffering from

    (A) polymorphism
    (B) hypotonia
    (C) nystagmus
    (D) polyhydrosis
    (E) polyphagia

28. The mechanism of action of ezetimibe can best be described as a (an)

    (A) bile acid binding agent
    (B) central nervous system agonist
    (C) selective norepinephrine reuptake inhibitor
    (D) inhibitor of cholesterol absorption
    (E) antipsoriatic agent

29. Which of the following is true of misoprostol?

    I.   It is in pregnancy category X.
    II.  It is a prostaglandin analog.
    III. It is available in inhalation form.

    (A)  I only
    (B)  III only
    (C)  I and II only
    (D)  II and III only
    (E)  I, II, and III

30. All of the following terms relate directly to body muscles EXCEPT

    (A)  myalgia
    (B)  myopia
    (C)  myoclonus
    (D)  myocardia
    (E)  myositis

31. Patients taking lithium products should be advised to

    I.   reduce their salt intake
    II.  drink 8–12 glasses of water each day
    III. stop taking the medication if tremors or diarrhea occur

    (A)  I only
    (B)  III only
    (C)  I and II only
    (D)  II and III only
    (E)  I, II, and III

32. Which of the following drug products would be most useful in treating a patient with a diagnosis of irritable bowel syndrome (IBS) whose primary bowel symptom is constipation?

    (A)  tegaserod
    (B)  alosetron
    (C)  granisetron
    (D)  hyoscyamine
    (E)  dicyclomine

33. When dispensing Adderal, the patient should be told

    I.   to take the medication at bedtime
    II.  that it may cause weight gain
    III. that it may cause palpitations

    (A)  I only
    (B)  III only
    (C)  I and II only
    (D)  II and III only
    (E)  I, II, and III

34. A 60-year-old patient with congestive heart failure who has been stabilized for three months on digoxin, furosemide, and potassium chloride is gradually placed on the following additional medicines. Which of these drugs is most likely to cause a problem?

    (A)  quinidine
    (B)  temazepam (Restoril)
    (C)  meperidine HCl (Demerol)
    (D)  aspirin
    (E)  nitroglycerin

35. Which of the following diuretics would be LEAST likely to produce a hypokalemic effect in a patient?

    (A)  ethacrynic acid (Edecrin)
    (B)  torsemide (Demadex)
    (C)  chlorthalidone (Hygroton)
    (D)  furosemide (Lasix)
    (E)  eplerenone (Inspra)

36. Mannitol is used therapeutically primarily as a (an)

    (A)  osmotic diuretic
    (B)  sucrose substitute
    (C)  antianginal agent
    (D)  cardiac stimulant
    (E)  plasma expander

37. Which of the following drugs are indicated for the treatment of enuresis?

    I.   imipramine (Tofranil)
    II.  desmopressin (DDAVP)
    III. isosorbide (Ismotic)

(A) I only

(B) III only

(C) I and II only

(D) II and III only

(E) I, II, and III

38. In monitoring acute MI patients who are using warfarin sodium (Coumadin), their INR should ideally be between

(A) 0.1–0.2

(B) 2–3

(C) 4–5.5

(D) 9–14

(E) 80–120

39. Patients using phenytoin should be monitored for the development of

I. pseudomembranous enterocolitis

II. nystagmus

III. gingival hyperplasia

(A) I only

(B) III only

(C) I and II only

(D) II and III only

(E) I, II, and III

40. A potential problem of using nalbuphine (Nubain) in a patient who is dependent on codeine is

(A) additive respiratory depression

(B) increased tolerance to codeine

(C) precipitation of narcotic withdrawal symptoms

(D) impaired renal excretion of codeine

(E) excessive CNS stimulation

41. The advantage of nalmefene (Revex) over naloxone (Narcan) is

(A) its longer duration of action

(B) that it is not addictive

(C) its availability as sublingual tablets

(D) that it does not have to be reconstituted immediately before use

(E) its more rapid onset of action

42. Which of the following would be appropriate for the treatment of candidal vulvovaginitis?

I. miconazole

II. nystatin

III. clotrimazole

(A) I only

(B) III only

(C) I and II only

(D) II and III only

(E) I, II, and III

43. Polycythemia refers to an elevated number of

(A) reticulocytes

(B) leukocytes

(C) thrombocytes

(D) erythrocytes

(E) granulocytes

44. In treating excessive heparin therapy with protamine sulfate, caution must be exercised to avoid using more protamine than is necessary because

(A) protamine sulfate is toxic in small amounts

(B) protamine sulfate is a cardiotoxic agent

(C) the production of endogenous heparin will be stimulated

(D) the strongly basic protamine will produce alkalosis

(E) protamine sulfate is also an anticoagulant

45. Which of the following agents has the longest duration of effect as a bronchodilator?

(A) isoetharine

(B) albuterol

(C) salmeterol

(D) terbutaline

(E) bitolterol

46. Which of the following would be the best choice for use in providing anticoagulant therapy for a pregnant patient near the anticipated time of delivery?

    (A) ticlopidine (Ticlid)
    (B) heparin
    (C) aspirin
    (D) warfarin (Coumadin, Panwarfin)
    (E) dipyridamole (Persantine)

47. The use of zolmitriptan is contraindicated in patients

    I.   with angina pectoris
    II.  using MAO inhibitors
    III. who have received an ergotamine derivative within the past 24 h

    (A) I only
    (B) III only
    (C) I and II only
    (D) II and III only
    (E) I, II, and III

48. The most likely organism to cause an acute uncomplicated urinary tract infection is

    (A) *E. coli*
    (B) *S. aureus*
    (C) *Candida albicans*
    (D) *S. epidermidis*
    (E) *H. influenza*

49. The Schilling test is useful for the detection of pernicious anemia. This test utilizes orally administered, radiolabeled

    (A) folic acid
    (B) intrinsic factor
    (C) iron
    (D) cyanocobalamin
    (E) pyridoxine

50. Lipodystrophy experienced by patients using insulin can be avoided by recommending the

    (A) rotation of injection sites
    (B) use of shorter-acting insulin
    (C) use of longer-acting insulin

    (D) use of protamine-containing insulins
    (E) avoidance of protamine-containing insulins

51. Insulin lispro (Humalog) is generally administered

    (A) 1 h after the morning meal
    (B) 1 h after dinner
    (C) at bedtime
    (D) 15 min before a meal
    (E) in a commercial mixture with NPH insulin

52. Which of the following insulins would be expected to exert the longest duration of action?

    (A) semilente
    (B) NPH
    (C) protamine zinc
    (D) lente
    (E) lantus

53. A patient has been told by his physician to consume foods that are high in lycopene because it may decrease his chance of developing prostate cancer. Which of the following foods would be the BEST dietary source of lycopene?

    (A) tomato sauce
    (B) walnuts
    (C) cabbage
    (D) aged cheeses
    (E) cold-water fish

54. Patients receiving analgesic doses of morphine should be monitored for the development of

    I.   diarrhea
    II.  respiratory depression
    III. nausea

    (A) I only
    (B) III only
    (C) I and II only
    (D) II and III only
    (E) I, II, and III

55. Which of the following is true of combination oral contraceptive products?

    I.   They suppress FSH and LH.
    II.  They decrease viscosity of cervical mucus.
    III. Most contain medroxyprogesterone and ethinyl estradiol.

    (A) I only
    (B) III only
    (C) I and II only
    (D) II and III only
    (E) I, II, and III

56. A 28-year-old female visits a neighborhood clinic complaining of flu-like symptoms that began about 24 h ago. She is diagnosed as having uncomplicated influenza A. Which of the following would be appropriate to prescribe for this patient?

    I.   oseltamivir
    II.  zanamivir
    III. penciclovir

    (A) I only
    (B) III only
    (C) I and II only
    (D) II and III only
    (E) I, II, and III

57. Which of the following drugs is particularly useful for the treatment of acute hypoglycemic reactions when oral or IV administration of glucose is not possible?

    (A) insulin lispro
    (B) glucocorticoids
    (C) glucagon
    (D) pancreatin
    (E) glimepiride (Amaryl)

58. Which of the following would be the best drug to use in treating a pregnant patient who is HIV positive in order to reduce the likelihood of transmission of HIV to the newborn child?

    (A) ritonavir (Norvir)
    (B) nevirapine (Viramune)

    (C) didanosine (Videx)
    (D) zidovudine (Retrovir)
    (E) enfurvitide (Fuzeon)

59. A patient is admitted to the emergency room (ER) with marked hypotension and appears to be in shock. The drug of choice to treat the condition is probably

    (A) dobutamine (Dobutrex)
    (B) dopamine HCl (Intropin)
    (C) epinephrine HCl (Adrenalin)
    (D) milrinone (Primacor)
    (E) nitroprusside (Nitropres)

60. Which of the following oral contraceptive products could be prescribed for a woman who does not wish to use an estrogen-containing contraceptive product?

    I.   Modicon
    II.  Ovrette
    III. Micronor

    (A) I only
    (B) III only
    (C) I and II only
    (D) II and III only
    (E) I, II, and III

61. The erythrocytes of an iron-deficient patient would be described as

    (A) macrocytic and hypochromic
    (B) microcytic and hyperchromic
    (C) normocytic and hyperchromic
    (D) macrocytic and hyperchromic
    (E) microcytic and hypochromic

62. Which of the following drug products is indicated for the treatment of trigeminal neuralgia?

    (A) procainamide (Pronestyl)
    (B) moexipril (Univasc)
    (C) epoprostenol sodium (Flolan)
    (D) carbamazepine (Tegretol)
    (E) sumatriptan (Imitrex)

63. Which of the following is NOT an ingredient of a product used to induce an abortion?

    I.   propafenone
    II.  misoprostol
    III. mifepristone

    (A) I only
    (B) III only
    (C) I and II only
    (D) II and III only
    (E) I, II, and III

64. Lomotil should NOT be given to patients taking oral clindamycin because

    (A) the antimicrobial action of clindamycin will be impaired
    (B) aplastic anemia may be more likely to occur
    (C) an insoluble complex will be formed
    (D) the rate of hydrolytic destruction of clindamycin in the GI tract will increase
    (E) toxic effects of clindamycin may be enhanced

65. An advantage of loperamide (Imodium) over diphenoxylate (Lomotil) as an antidiarrheal is the fact that loperamide

    (A) does not cause drowsiness or dizziness
    (B) has a direct effect on the CNS and therefore works more rapidly than does diphenoxylate
    (C) is available in a parenteral form
    (D) does not appear to have opiate-like effects
    (E) has significant adsorbent action

66. A woman has had two unplanned pregnancies. Each pregnancy was associated with failure to correctly use the oral contraceptive prescribed for the patient. Which of the following would be a reasonable alternative for this patient to reduce the likelihood of future pregnancies?

    I.   Norplant
    II.  Preven
    III. Clomid

    (A) I only
    (B) III only
    (C) I and II only
    (D) II and III only
    (E) I, II, and III

67. A patient using felodipine (Plendil) should be advised to

    (A) take the product on an empty stomach
    (B) avoid aspirin while taking the product
    (C) take the product at bedtime
    (D) take each dose with a fatty food
    (E) avoid the use of grapefruit juice while using the product

68. A patient under the influence of crack cocaine is brought to an acute-care facility. The symptoms of cocaine intoxication are most similar to

    (A) dextroamphetamine
    (B) heroin
    (C) ethanol
    (D) tetrahydrocannabinol (THC)
    (E) morphine

69. The initiation of therapy with which one of the following agents would be LEAST likely to cause therapeutic problems in a patient already taking warfarin (Coumadin)?

    (A) metronidazole
    (B) acetaminophen
    (C) phenytoin
    (D) aspirin
    (E) cimetidine

70. Which of the following is (are) true of valsartan (Diovan)?

    I.   It is angiotensin II receptor blocker.
    II.  It must be taken on an empty stomach.
    III. It is useful for the treatment of herpes zoster (shingles).

    (A) I only
    (B) III only
    (C) I and II only

(D) II and III only

(E) I, II, and III

71. A nutritional product is said to contain 11 g of protein, 22 g of carbohydrate, and 5 g of fat in each 100-mL serving. The caloric content of a serving would be

(A) 238 kcal

(B) 198 kcal

(C) 218 kcal

(D) 177 kcal

(E) 378 kcal

72. Patients experiencing toxicity as a result of methotrexate administration should be given

(A) EDTA

(B) sodium bicarbonate

(C) bioflavinoids

(D) leucovorin calcium

(E) *para*-aminobenzoic acid

73. A 19-year-old college student visited Mexico during her spring break and acquired an acute GI disorder characterized by severe diarrhea. Over the past week, she has lost 5 lb and feels weak and run down. Which of the following would be most appropriate to administer to this patient?

(A) Lyphocin

(B) K-Lyte

(C) Isomil

(D) Pedialyte

(E) Lypressin

74. Parenteral administration of 1 L of 5% dextrose in water provides the patient with approximately how many kilocalories of energy?

(A) 150–200 kcal

(B) 350–400 kcal

(C) 450–500 kcal

(D) 800–850 kcal

(E) 1000 kcal

75. Which of the following is true of Hepatitis B vaccine?

I. administered intradermally

II. will also protect against hepatitis A

III. must be stored in a refrigerator

(A) I only

(B) III only

(C) I and II only

(D) II and III only

(E) I, II, and III

76. A patient is said to have a significantly elevated PSA level. This could be indicative of

(A) thyroid carcinoma

(B) lymphocytic leukemia

(C) BPH

(D) chronic renal failure

(E) cholestatic hepatitis

77. Which of the following would be (a) good alternative(s) to penicillin V in a pregnant patient allergic to penicillins?

I. erythromycin (Ilotycin)

II. trimethoprim (Trimpex)

III. demeclocycline (Declomycin)

(A) I only

(B) III only

(C) I and II only

(D) II and III only

(E) I, II, and III

78. Which one of the following sulfonamides is best suited for the topical prophylactic treatment of burns?

(A) sulfacetamide (Sulamyd)

(B) sulfamethoxazole (Gantanol)

(C) sulfisoxazole (Gantrisin)

(D) silver sulfadiazine (Silvadene)

(E) sulfasalazine (Azulfidine)

79. Which of the following drugs would be most appropriate to use for the treatment of an uncomplicated gonorrhea infection in a poorly compliant patient?

    (A) ceftriaxone (Rocephin)
    (B) pipericillin (Pipracil)
    (C) tetracycline (Achromycin V)
    (D) clindamycin (Cleocin)
    (E) itraconazole (Sporanox)

80. Which of the following drugs used in the treatment of acute gouty arthritis does (do) NOT affect urate metabolism or excretion?

    I.   allopurinol (Zyloprim)
    II.  probenecid (Benemid)
    III. indomethacin (Indocin)

    (A) I only
    (B) III only
    (C) I and II only
    (D) II and III only
    (E) I, II, and III

81. A pharmacist wishes to dispense cromolyn sodium 4% ophthalmic solution for use by a patient. This product is usually used to treat

    (A) cytomegalovirus (CMV)
    (B) herpes simplex keratitis
    (C) open-angle glaucoma
    (D) bacterial infections
    (E) vernal keratoconjunctivitis

82. Which of the following is (are) true of adalimumab (Humira)?

    I.   tumor necrosis factor antagonist
    II.  used to treat rheumatoid arthritis
    III. liposome

    (A) I only
    (B) III only
    (C) I and II only
    (D) II and III only
    (E) I, II, and III

83. An important advantage of using dopamine (Intropin) in cardiogenic shock is that dopamine

    (A) will not cross the blood-brain barrier and cause CNS effects
    (B) has no effects on alpha and beta receptors
    (C) can be given orally
    (D) will not increase blood pressure
    (E) produces dose-dependent increases in cardiac output and renal perfusion

84. A patient is experiencing signs of acute chlordiazepoxide (Librium) toxicity after having consumed approximately 15 doses in a suicide attempt. An appropriate agent to administer is

    (A) naloxone (Narcan)
    (B) flumazenil (Romazicon)
    (C) lorazepam (Ativan)
    (D) naltrexone (ReVia)
    (E) physostigmine (Antilirium)

85. A male patient who has been stabilized on 300 mg of Dilantin Kapseals once daily is having difficulty swallowing capsules. His physician writes a new prescription for Dilantin suspension 300 mg once daily. This change is likely to

    (A) reduce the phenytoin level because of decreased bioavailability from the suspension
    (B) increase the phenytoin level because of increased bioavailability from the suspension
    (C) have no impact on the phenytoin level
    (D) decrease the phenytoin level because the 300 mg dose of suspension contains less of the active form of the drug
    (E) increase the phenytoin level because the 300 mg dose of suspension contains more of the active form of the drug

86. A terminally ill hospice patient is experiencing severe pain associated with metastatic colon cancer. Which of the following would be an appropriate regimen to treat his pain?

(A)  morphine sulfate PO, 15 mg p.r.n. pain

(B)  codeine sulfate 30 mg PO q.i.d.

(C)  Duragesic-50 applied q72h

(D)  meperidine 50 mg PO q.i.d.

(E)  acetaminophen 500 mg PO q4h

87.  A patient has been complaining of easy bruising. Hematological studies reveal that the patient has thrombocytopenia. An appropriate choice for treating this condition is

(A)  Epogen

(B)  Neumega

(C)  Neupogen

(D)  Leukine

(E)  ReoPro

88.  Patients who are about to use metronidazole (Flagyl) should be advised that

   I.  the drug should be taken on an empty stomach

  II.  they should avoid alcohol while using the medication

 III.  their urine will be discolored by the drug

(A)  I only

(B)  III only

(C)  I and II only

(D)  II and III only

(E)  I, II, and III

89.  A male diabetic patient reports that he is planning a four-week trip to Europe and will not have continued access to a refrigerator to store insulin. What information would you give him?

(A)  Store the insulin in a small styrofoam box that can be kept cold with several ice cubes.

(B)  Be sure that insulin is available wherever you travel and purchase a fresh vial at least every third day

(C)  Increase your insulin dose by 10% to compensate for any deterioration.

(D)  The insulin will remain stable at room temperature during the time period in which a single vial will be used.

(E)  See your doctor to prescribe a mixture of insulins that will be more stable.

90.  Which of the following are true of isotretinoin (Accutane)?

   I.  vitamin D derivative

  II.  likely to cause cheilitis

 III.  pregnancy category X

(A)  I only

(B)  III only

(C)  I and II only

(D)  II and III only

(E)  I, II, and III

91.  Peripheral veins are seldom used for the administration of total parenteral nutrition (TPN) fluids because

(A)  TPN fluids tend to infiltrate surrounding tissue

(B)  the blood flow in peripheral vessels is not great enough to protect the peripheral vessels from irritation

(C)  large-bore needles must be used

(D)  the hypotonic solution causes local hemolysis

(E)  the vessels are easily occluded

92.  A patient is diagnosed with a beta-lactamase–producing streptococcal infection. Which of the following would be suitable for treating this patient?

   I.  gentamicin

  II.  ticarcillin

 III.  dicloxacillin

(A)  I only

(B)  III only

(C)  I and II only

(D)  II and III only

(E)  I, II, and III

93. A patient who began using Procardia XL a week ago calls to complain of the appearance of the tablet in his stool. You should tell the patient that

(A) he should crush or chew the tablet before swallowing

(B) if he takes the medication with an alkaline food such as milk, the problem will not occur

(C) he should return the remaining tablets to the pharmacy for replacement

(D) if he takes the medication with an acidic food such as orange juice, the problem will not occur

(E) he should not be concerned because this is a normal occurrence

94. Which of the following complications associated with the administration of TPN solutions is most likely to occur after the infusions have been discontinued?

(A) hypoglycemia
(B) hyperchloremic metabolic acidosis
(C) hyperosmotic nonketotic hyperglycemia
(D) alkalosis
(E) pulmonary edema

95. Which one of the following provides the greatest number of calories per gram?

(A) ethanol
(B) proteins
(C) anhydrous dextrose
(D) fats
(E) hydrous dextrose

96. A patient requires several administrations of high-dose cisplatin (Platinol) therapy for the treatment of advanced bladder cancer. During the first cisplatin administration, the patient develops severe nausea and vomiting. Which of the following drugs would be appropriate to administer to control these symptoms for future administrations?

(A) ritodrine (Yutopar)
(B) buspirone (BuSpar)
(C) danazol (Danocrine)

(D) amantadine (Symmetrel)
(E) tropisetron (Navoban)

97. The mechanism of action of amiloride (Midamor) is most similar to that of

(A) spironolactone (Aldactone)
(B) hydrochlorothiazide (HydroDIURIL)
(C) metolazone (Zaroxolyn)
(D) triamterene (Dyrenium)
(E) chlorthalidone (Hygroton)

98. A 50-year-old hypertensive patient has been maintained on spironolactone with hydrochlorothiazide (Aldactazide), methyldopa (Aldomet), and potassium (K-Tabs). The patient is admitted to the hospital for elective surgery and is found to be hyperkalemic (serum K of 6.4 mEq/L; normal range is 3.5–5.5 mEq/L) with no symptoms and a normal electrocardiogram. This patient should be treated with

(A) rectal sodium polystyrene sulfonate
(B) IV sodium nitrite
(C) IV normal saline
(D) flumazenil (Romazicon)
(E) oral EDTA

99. A 55-year-old patient is to receive dalteparin sodium (Fragmin) for the prevention of deep vein thrombosis. Which of the following is true of dalteparin sodium?

I. It is administered by IV infusion.
II. It should not be used if the patient is allergic to pork products.
III. It is a low molecular weight heparin.

(A) I only
(B) III only
(C) I and II only
(D) II and III only
(E) I, II, and III

100. Which of the following drug products are indicated for use in type 2 diabetes mellitus patients?

I. miglitol (Glyset)
II. repaglinide (Prandin)
III. rosiglitazone (Avandia)

(A) I only

(B) III only

(C) I and II only

(D) II and III only

(E) I, II, and III

101. Which of the following drugs is generally considered a drug of choice in treating status epilepticus?

(A) carbamazepine (Tegretol)

(B) ethosuximide (Zarontin)

(C) buspirone (Buspar)

(D) lorazepam (Ativan)

(E) phenytoin (Dilantin)

102. The use of which of the following drugs has resulted in the development of a syndrome strongly resembling systemic lupus erythematosus (SLE)?

(A) pirbuterol (Maxair)

(B) lamotrigine (Lamictal)

(C) hydralazine (Apresoline)

(D) methyldopa (Aldomet)

(E) diazoxide (Hyperstat IV)

103. The antiparkinson effect of levodopa may be inhibited by

(A) nicotinic acid

(B) D-alpha tocopherol

(C) riboflavin

(D) dihydrotachysterol

(E) pyridoxine HCl

104. In terms of its major pharmacological effect, atenolol (Tenormin) is most similar to

(A) pindolol (Visken)

(B) metaproterenol (Alupent)

(C) fenoldopam (Corlopam)

(D) albuterol (Ventolin)

(E) isoproterenol (Isuprel)

105. The pharmacist should advise a patient that he or she may experience dizziness and syncope after taking the first dose of

(A) trandolapril (Mavik)

(B) fosinopril (Monopril)

(C) clonidine (Catapres)

(D) terazosin (Hytrin)

(E) labetalol (Trandate)

106. A common measure in assessing the degree of immunodeficiency in acquired immunodeficiency syndrome (AIDS) patients is the determination of levels of

(A) CD4 cells

(B) *Pneumocystis carinii* organisms

(C) leukocytes

(D) serotonin

(E) erythrocyte sedimentation rate (ESR)

107. In the treatment of acute hypertensive crisis, nitroprusside (Nitropress) is administered

(A) sublingually

(B) subcutaneously

(C) as an IV bolus

(D) transdermally

(E) as an IV infusion

108. Which of the following drugs should NOT be used to treat bacteremias?

(A) azithromycin

(B) erythromycin lactobionate

(C) clarithromycin

(D) dirithromycin

(E) amoxicillin

109. An IV admixture should not be prepared with tobramycin sulfate and

I. phenytoin sodium

II. ticarcillin sodium

III. acetazolamide

(A) I only

(B) III only

(C) I and II only

(D) II and III only

(E) I, II, and III

110. Which of the following agents has NOT been suggested as an agent to use to eradicate *Helicobacter pylori* from the gastrointestinal (GI) tract?

    (A) clarithromycin
    (B) bismuth subsalicylate
    (C) metronidazole
    (D) terbinafine
    (E) tetracycline

111. Cholestyramine (Questran) will probably interfere with the GI absorption of

    I.   warfarin sodium
    II.  levothyroxine sodium
    III. pyridoxine HCl

    (A) I only
    (B) III only
    (C) I and II only
    (D) II and III only
    (E) I, II, and III

112. A clinically noticeable drug interaction resulting from the displacement of drug A by drug B from common plasma protein–binding sites is most often seen when

    (A) drug A has a high association constant (K) for binding the protein
    (B) drug B has a low association constant (K) for binding the protein and is given in large doses
    (C) drug B has a high association constant (K) for binding the protein and is given in large doses
    (D) drug B is more toxic than drug A
    (E) drug B is rapidly absorbed

113. Tinsaparin (Innohep) should be administered

    (A) transdermally
    (B) subcutaneously
    (C) rectally
    (D) intramuscularly
    (E) by IV infusion

114. Which of the following agents would likely affect the platelet aggregation of an adult?

    I.   dipyridamole
    II.  clopidogrel
    III. acetylsalicylic acid

    (A) I only
    (B) III only
    (C) I and II only
    (D) II and III only
    (E) I, II, and III

115. A microorganism that is particularly dangerous to the eye is

    (A) *Streptococcus thermophilus*
    (B) *Bacillus subtilis*
    (C) *Pseudomonas aeruginosa*
    (D) *Aspergillus niger*
    (E) *Escherichia coli*

116. Purulent boils in the ear are usually caused by species of

    (A) *Streptococcus*
    (B) *Candida*
    (C) *Pseudomonas*
    (D) *Aspergillus*
    (E) *Staphylococcus*

117. The treatment of choice for herpes simplex infection of the eyelids and conjunctiva is

    (A) metronidazole (Flagyl)
    (B) bacitracin (Baciguent)
    (C) amphotericin B (Fungizone)
    (D) idoxuridine (Stoxil)
    (E) mupirocin (Bactroban)

118. Which of the following antifungal agents is ineffective against *Candida* organisms?

    (A) miconazole (Micatin)
    (B) clotrimazole (Lotrimin)
    (C) amphotericin (Fungizone)
    (D) tolnaftate (Tinactin)
    (E) nystatin (Mycostatin)

119. Tolterodine has been shown to be of clinical use in the management of

    (A) overactive bladder
    (B) scabies
    (C) venereal warts
    (D) ringworm infections of the skin
    (E) psoriasis

120. Important potential complications of corticosteroid therapy include(s)

    I.   dissemination of local infection
    II.  masking symptoms of an infection
    III. increased susceptibility to infection

    (A) I only
    (B) III only
    (C) I and II only
    (D) II and III only
    (E) I, II, and III

121. The primary advantage of oxaprozin over most other nonsteroidal anti-inflammatory drugs (NSAIDs) is that it

    (A) does not interact with warfarin
    (B) may be used concomitantly with aspirin
    (C) may be given on a once-a-day schedule
    (D) has a cytoprotective effect
    (E) has essentially no adverse GI effects

122. Which of the following is (are) true of adalimumab (Humira)?

    I.   It is a leukotriene inhibitor.
    II.  It is indicated for the treatment of type II diabetes mellitus.
    III. It is a monoclonal antibody.

    (A) I only
    (B) III only
    (C) I and II only
    (D) II and III only
    (E) I, II, and III

123. A patient who is having difficulty with GI tolerance of ibuprofen may be more tolerant to which of the following NSAIDS?

    (A) aspirin
    (B) piroxicam
    (C) indomethacin
    (D) rofecoxib
    (E) naproxyn

124. When dispensing isotretinoin (Accutane) capsules to a 19-year-old female college student with acne, the pharmacist should advise the patient to

    I.   avoid pregnancy while using the drug
    II.  discontinue the drug if the acne gets worse
    III. increase her exposure to sunlight to help eliminate lesions

    (A) I only
    (B) III only
    (C) I and II only
    (D) II and III only
    (E) I, II, and III

125. Which of the following best describes the condition known as hypoprothrombinemia?

    (A) the development of transient ischemic attacks (TIAs)
    (B) the development of deep vein thromboses (DVTs)
    (C) a low level of iron in the blood
    (D) a decrease in the production of red blood cells by the bone marrow
    (E) a reduced capability for blood to clot

126. The rapid reversal of warfarin-induced hemorrhage can be accomplished by the administration of

    I.   dihydrotachysterol (Hytakerol)
    II.  ergocalciferol (Drisdol)
    III. phytonadione (AquaMEPHYTON)

    (A) I only
    (B) III only
    (C) I and II only
    (D) II and III only
    (E) I, II, and III

127. A patient complains of a reddish discoloration of his or her urine. Which of the following drugs would most likely produce such an effect?

    (A) naratriptan
    (B) clindamycin HCl
    (C) sulfamethoxazole
    (D) cilostazol (Pletal)
    (E) phenazopyridine

128. Which of the following is true of menotropins?

    I. It is a gonadotropin.
    II. It is only administered parenterally.
    III. It may be administered to pregnant women to reduce spontaneous abortion.

    (A) I only
    (B) III only
    (C) I and II only
    (D) II and III only
    (E) I, II, and III

129. Patients using amiloride tablets should be advised to

    I. avoid large quantities of potassium rich foods
    II. take the medication on an empty stomach
    III. avoid the use of acetaminophen while using the drug

    (A) I only
    (B) III only
    (C) I and II only
    (D) II and III only
    (E) I, II, and III

130. The clinical investigation of a new drug consists of four phases. Phase I of the clinical testing involves administering the drug

    (A) to animals for toxicity studies
    (B) by select clinicians to healthy volunteers
    (C) to animals to determine the effectiveness of the drug
    (D) by select clinicians to patients suffering from the disease
    (E) by general practitioners to patients suffering from the disease

131. Which of the following best describes the common clinical manifestations of hypoparathyroidism?

    (A) hypercalcemia and hypochlorhydria
    (B) hypocalcemia and hypophosphatemia
    (C) hypercalcemia and hypophosphatemia
    (D) hypocalcemia and hyperphosphatemia
    (E) hypercalcemia and hyperphosphatemia

132. Which of the following is true of atomoxetine HCl?

    I. It is indicated for the treatment of ADHD.
    II. It is a CNS stimulant.
    III. It may be used concomitantly with MAOIs.

    (A) I only
    (B) III only
    (C) I and II only
    (D) II and III only
    (E) I, II, and III

133. An adult patient who is hypothyroid may have

    I. a goiter
    II. Hashimoto's disease
    III. elevated levels of TSH

    (A) I only
    (B) III only
    (C) I and II only
    (D) II and III only
    (E) I, II, and III

134. Enuresis refers to

    (A) gout
    (B) urinary retention
    (C) bedwetting
    (D) diminished stature
    (E) urinary tract infection

135. Which of the following should NOT be used in patients who are allergic to aspirin?

   (A) Fiorinal
   (B) Panadol
   (C) Excedrin PM
   (D) Stadol
   (E) BuSpar

136. Which of the following phrases best defines the clinical disorder known as hemochromatosis?

   (A) excessive storage of iron by the body
   (B) spontaneous hemolysis of red blood cells
   (C) a lack of circulating antibodies
   (D) abnormally shaped red blood cells
   (E) absence of pigmentation in circulating red blood cells

137. A reversible cholestatic hepatitis with fever and jaundice has been observed as an adverse drug reaction in patients taking erythromycin

   (A) ethylsuccinate (EES granules)
   (B) estolate (Ilosone)
   (C) base (E-Mycin tablets)
   (D) stearate (Erythrocin Filmtab)
   (E) gluceptate (Ilotycin)

138. A patient who has been diagnosed with cystic fibrosis is likely to benefit from the use of which of the following?

   I. isotretinoin
   II. dornase alfa
   III. pancrelipase

   (A) I only
   (B) III only
   (C) I and II only
   (D) II and III only
   (E) I, II, and III

139. Lansoprazole (Prevacid) inhibits gastric acid secretion as a result of what kind of activity?

   (A) $H_2$-receptor antagonism
   (B) Proton pump inhibition
   (C) Prokinetic action

   (D) Inhibition of the amine pump
   (E) *Helicobacter pylori* inhibition

140. Patients with chronic inflammatory bowel disease who are allergic to sulfa drugs may safely use

   I. Azulfidine
   II. Dipentum
   III. Pentasa

   (A) I only
   (B) III only
   (C) I and II only
   (D) II and III only
   (E) I, II, and III

141. Which of the following is true of ezetimibe?

   I. It may be used in combination with a "statin" drug.
   II. It inhibits the intestinal absorption of cholesterol.
   III. It should not be administered to diabetic patients.

   (A) I only
   (B) III only
   (C) I and II only
   (D) II and III only
   (E) I, II, and III

142. Which of the following agents are indicated for the treatment of the human immunodeficiency virus (HIV) infection?

   I. ifosfamide
   II. enfuvirtide
   III. didanosine

   (A) I only
   (B) III only
   (C) I and II only
   (D) II and III only
   (E) I, II, and III

143. A patient complains about a headache that is localized in the periorbital area and seems to be worse in the morning than the afternoon. Which of the following would be the best way to characterize the headache?

   (A) tumorigenic
   (B) vascular-migraine
   (C) muscle contraction
   (D) eye strain
   (E) sinus

144. The purpose of combination drug treatment in tuberculosis is to

   I.  increase the tuberculostatic effects of the drugs
   II. delay the emergence of drug resistance
   III. reduce the duration of therapy

   (A) I only
   (B) III only
   (C) I and II only
   (D) II and III only
   (E) I, II, and III

145. Patients taking the antitubercular drug rifampin (Rifadin) should be told that the drug

   (A) may cause diarrhea
   (B) may cause them to sunburn more easily
   (C) may impart an orange color to their urine and sweat
   (D) may produce nausea and vomiting if used with alcoholic beverages
   (E) should be swallowed whole (i.e., not chewed) to prevent staining of the teeth

146. A patient using ticlopidine (Ticlid) should be monitored for the development of

   (A) pseudomembranous enterocolitis
   (B) renal toxicity
   (C) respiratory impairment
   (D) abnormal bleeding
   (E) hyperpyrexia

147. A penicillin derivative that has significantly greater activity against *Pseudomonas* than amoxicillin is

   (A) bacampicillin (Spectrobid)
   (B) dicloxacillin (Dynapen)
   (C) nafcillin (Unipen)
   (D) mezlocillin (Mezlin)
   (E) oxacillin (Bactocill)

148. Antimicrobial-induced pseudomembranous colitis is most commonly treated with

   (A) attapulgite (Kaopectate)
   (B) loperamide (Imodium)
   (C) metronidazole (Flagyl)
   (D) tobramycin (Nebcin)
   (E) sulfasalazine (Azulfidine)

149. Cushing syndrome is a condition associated with

   (A) hyperthyroidism
   (B) excessive accumulation of copper in the body
   (C) hypothyroidism
   (D) adrenal hyperplasia
   (E) polyuria

150. The aminoglycoside antibiotics are

   I.  metabolized by the liver
   II. may be used orally for serious systemic pseudomonas infections
   III. bactericidal for a wide range of gram-positive and gram-negative micro-organisms

   (A) I only
   (B) III only
   (C) I and II only
   (D) II and III only
   (E) I, II, and III

151. Which of the following is an infectious complication associated with HIV?

   I.   MAC
   II.  PCP
   III. SARS

(A) I only

(B) III only

(C) I and II only

(D) II and III only

(E) I, II, and III

152. A disadvantage of using cromolyn sodium in asthma treatment is

(A) that it is ineffective in treating acute attacks

(B) its nephrotoxicity

(C) that it may cause tachyphylaxis

(D) its brief duration of action

(E) that it causes cardiac stimulation

153. An asthmatic patient who is currently taking terbutaline (Brethine) 5-mg tablets (t.i.d.), prednisone 5 mg (q.i.d.), and Proventil Inhaler (p.r.n.) presents you with a prescription for Vanceril Inhaler. The directions on the prescription are "one inhalation PRN breathing difficulty." The most appropriate action for you to take is to

(A) fill the prescription

(B) advise the prescriber to discontinue the terbutaline tablets

(C) inform the prescriber that the prednisone should be discontinued before Vanceril therapy is initiated

(D) advise the patient to stop using the Proventil Inhaler

(E) inform the prescriber that Vanceril (beclomethasone) is a prophylactic drug that should be taken regularly

154. A common name for the antidiuretic hormone elaborated by the posterior pituitary gland is

(A) ACTH

(B) renin

(C) luteotropic hormone

(D) vasopressin

(E) secretin

155. Which of the following is true of lithium carbonate (Eskalith, Lithane)?

I. It is used to treat manic depressive illness.

II. Baseline liver function tests must be performed prior to initiating therapy.

III. It should not be used within 1 h of pyridoxine ($B_6$).

(A) I only

(B) III only

(C) I and II only

(D) II and III only

(E) I, II, and III

156. Patients on lithium carbonate therapy should be advised

(A) not to restrict their normal dietary salt intake

(B) to stop taking the drug if they experience drowsiness

(C) to limit water intake

(D) to take the medication as a single dose in the morning

(E) not to take the drug with food

157. Hemolytic anemia due to erythrocyte deficiency of glucose-6-phosphate dehydrogenase (G6PD) would most likely be precipitated by

(A) phenytoin (Dilantin)

(B) primaquine

(C) isoniazid (INH)

(D) pyridoxine HCl

(E) gentamicin (Garamycin)

158. The anticoagulant action of heparin is monitored by the

(A) complete blood count

(B) antiplatelet clotting time

(C) prothrombin time (PT)

(D) international normalization ratio (INR)

(E) activated partial thromboplastin time (APTT)

159. Two hours after receiving the last dose of heparin (9000 units IV), a male patient begins bleeding from the gums after brushing his teeth. What is the most appropriate clinical action?

    (A) inject 30 mg of protamine sulfate IM

    (B) inject 10 mg of phytonadione (Aqua-MEPHYTON) IM

    (C) inject 10 mg of phytonadione (Aqua-MEPHYTON) IV

    (D) swab a small amount of epinephrine 1:100 onto the gum tissue to produce local vasoconstriction

    (E) discontinue heparin administration and wait for the anticoagulant effect to subside

160. A 40-year-old woman with a history of deep-vein thrombosis (DVT) is stabilized on 5 mg of warfarin daily. The administration of which of the following medications to this patient would increase the risk of hemorrhage?

    (A) acetaminophen (Tylenol) 650 mg q4h

    (B) captopril (Capoten) 25 mg b.i.d.

    (C) milk of magnesia 30 mL hs

    (D) cimetidine (Tagamet) 300 mg q.i.d.

    (E) diazepam (Valium) 5 mg q.i.d.

161. A blood sugar concentration within normal limits for a fasting adult is

    (A) 100 mg/dL

    (B) 200 mg/dL

    (C) 300 mg/dL

    (D) 400 mg/dL

    (E) 500 mg/dL

162. Which of the following drugs can interfere with the diagnosis of pernicious anemia?

    (A) ascorbic acid

    (B) pyridoxine

    (C) thiamine

    (D) folic acid

    (E) phytonadione

163. Which of the following is (are) true of clomiphene citrate (Clomid)

    I.   It is used to treat polycystic ovary disease.

    II.  It has antiestrogenic effects.

    III. It promotes the secretion of gonadotropin-releasing hormone.

    (A) I only

    (B) III only

    (C) I and II only

    (D) II and III only

    (E) I, II, and III

164. Which of the following are appropriate agents to administer in treating severe hyperkalemia?

    I.   calcium gluconate

    II.  insulin

    III. sodium polystyrene sulfonate

    (A) I only

    (B) III only

    (C) I and II only

    (D) II and III only

    (E) I, II, and III

165. Which of the following drugs is MOST likely to result in elevations of serum creatinine levels?

    (A) metoprolol

    (B) benazepril

    (C) valsartan

    (D) nifedipine

    (E) clonidine

166. The hematocrit (HCT) measures the

    (A) total number of blood cells per volume of blood

    (B) weight of red blood cells per volume of blood

    (C) number of red blood cells per volume of blood

    (D) weight of hemoglobin per volume of blood

    (E) percentage of red blood cells per volume of blood

**167.** Which of the following is NOT a white blood cell (or leukocyte)?

(A) basophil

(B) lymphocyte

(C) monocyte

(D) eosinophil

(E) reticulocyte

**168.** The best product to use in a 7-year-old child with otitis media (and no history of drug allergies) is

(A) tetracycline HCl

(B) mupirocin

(C) trimethoprim-sulfamethoxazole

(D) ciprofloxacin

(E) bacitracin

**169.** Which of the following agents is (are) capable of producing an antipyretic action in humans?

  I. acetaminophen

 II. acetylsalicylic acid

III. ibuprofen

(A) I only

(B) III only

(C) I and II only

(D) II and III only

(E) I, II, and III

**170.** Patients receiving clozapine (Clozaril) must be monitored for the development of

(A) pseudomembranous enterocolitis

(B) heptatocellular necrosis

(C) hyperlipidemia

(D) congestive heart failure

(E) agranulocytosis

**171.** Zollinger-Ellison syndrome can be best treated with which of the following agents?

(A) lithium carbonate

(B) pantoprazole

(C) zolmitriptan

(D) atorvastatin

(E) betaserone

**172.** Intermittent IV therapy is used to

  I. avoid anticipated or potential stability or compatibility problems

 II. reduce the potential of thrombophlebitis

III. promote better diffusion of some drugs into the tissues because of a greater concentration gradient

(A) I only

(B) III only

(C) I and II only

(D) II and III only

(E) I, II, and III

**173.** Which of the following drugs are classified as mitotic inhibitors?

  I. methotrexate

 II. vinorelbine

III. vinblastine

(A) I only

(B) III only

(C) I and II only

(D) II and III only

(E) I, II, and III

**174.** Which of the following statements is (are) true of aspirin?

  I. High doses of aspirin may decrease plasma uric acid levels.

 II. Low doses of aspirin may increase plasma uric acid levels.

III. Aspirin should not be used during the last trimester of pregnancy.

(A) I only

(B) III only

(C) I and II only

(D) II and III only

(E) I, II, and III

175. Which of the following reference sources would be appropriate to use to find an American equivalent of a British drug?

   (A) *Martindale's Extra Pharmacopoeia*
   (B) *The Royal Compendium*
   (C) *USPDI*
   (D) *AHFS Drug Information*
   (E) *Facts and Comparisons*

176. Which of the following is (are) classified as a debriding agent?

   I. collagenase
   II. fibrinolysin
   III. lipase

   (A) I only
   (B) III only
   (C) I and II only
   (D) II and III only
   (E) I, II, and III

177. Which of the following cephalosporins would be appropriate to use in treating a CNS infection?

   I. cefotetan (Cefotan)
   II. ceftriaxone (Rocephin)
   III. cefotaxime (Claforan)

   (A) I only
   (B) III only
   (C) I and II only
   (D) II and III only
   (E) I, II, and III

178. A patient has been diagnosed with herpes labialis. Which of the following agents would be most appropriate to recommend for treatment of this condition?

   (A) ritonavir
   (B) saquinavir
   (C) penciclovir
   (D) zalcitabine
   (E) amphotericin B

179. A patient with fungal blepharitis should be treated with

   (A) idoxuridine (Herplex)
   (B) natamycin (Natacyn)
   (C) gentamicin (Garamycin)
   (D) cyclopentolate (Cyclogyl)
   (E) sulfacetamide sodium (Bleph-10)

180. Patients receiving doses of plantago (psyllium) should be advised to

   (A) take the product with lots of water
   (B) take the medication with food
   (C) mix the product with water and let stand for 30 min before administering
   (D) avoid driving or operating heavy machinery within 1 h of taking the medication
   (E) avoid dairy products

181. The cation most prevalent in the extracellular fluid of the human body is

   (A) potassium
   (B) chloride
   (C) phosphate
   (D) sodium
   (E) magnesium

182. Systemic toxic effects of atropine sulfate should be treated by administering which of the following antidotes?

   (A) EDTA
   (B) physostigmine
   (C) naloxone
   (D) Romazicon
   (E) calcium hydroxide

183. The blood concentration of which of the following cations would normally rise if a patient became hypophosphatemic?

   (A) phosphorus
   (B) magnesium
   (C) calcium
   (D) iron
   (E) potassium

184. Products containing nicotine polacrilex should be avoided in

I. smokers

II. patients with severe angina

III. pregnant women

(A) I only

(B) III only

(C) I and II only

(D) II and III only

(E) I, II, and III

185. Large overdoses of acetaminophen are likely to cause

(A) tinnitis

(B) seizures

(C) hepatic necrosis

(D) renal tubular necrosis

(E) pseudomembranous enterocolitis

186. An adult patient who ingested 30 acetaminophen tablets (325 mg/tab) 6 hours ago should be treated with/by

(A) EDTA infusion

(B) ipecac syrup

(C) activated charcoal

(D) *N*-acetylcysteine

(E) probenecid

187. Which of the following statements is (are) correct descriptions of sulfasalazine (Azulfidine)?

I. used in treating ulcerative colitis and regional enteritis

II. poorly absorbed from the GI tract

III. available as oral tablets and IM injection

(A) I only

(B) III only

(C) I and II only

(D) II and III only

(E) I, II, and III

188. Asthmatic patients with a documented allergy to aspirin should NOT receive

(A) meloxicam (Mobic)

(B) acetaminophen (Tylenol)

(C) salmeterol (Serevent)

(D) pentazocine (Talwin)

(E) albuterol (Proventil)

189. Nonselective beta-adrenergic blocking agents should be used with caution in patients with

I. asthma

II. type I diabetes mellitus

III. sinus bradycardia

(A) I only

(B) III only

(C) I and II only

(D) II and III only

(E) I, II, and III

190. Which of the following agents would be most dangerous to use in a patient already receiving high doses of gentamicin?

(A) tetracycline HCl

(B) torsemide (Demadex)

(C) fosinopril (Monopril)

(D) hydroDIURIL

(E) temazepam (Restoril)

191. A patient arriving in a hospital emergency room suffering from severe hypertensive crisis would most likely be treated initially with

(A) guanethidine (Ismelin)

(B) methyldopa (Aldomet)

(C) nitroprusside sodium (Nitropress)

(D) minoxidil (Loniten)

(E) benazepril (Lotensin)

192. A patient with left ventricular failure is likely to exhibit which of the following signs or symptoms?

I. peripheral edema

II. dyspnea

III. orthopnea

(A) I only

(B) III only

(C) I and II only

(D) II and III only

(E) I, II, and III

**193.** Which of the following would be considered a level within normal range for a healthy adult?

    I.   total cholesterol  175 mg/dL
    II.  triglycerides  245 mg/dL
    III. LDL cholesterol 180 mg/dL

(A) I only
(B) III only
(C) I and II only
(D) II and III only
(E) I, II, and III

**194.** Food containing tyramine should NOT be part of the diet of patients taking which of the following agents?

(A) selegeline (Eldepryl)
(B) hydralazine (Apresoline)
(C) cefixime (Suprax)
(D) methyldopa (Aldomet)
(E) clonidine (Catapres)

**195.** Which of the following symptoms would be LEAST likely to be exhibited by a patient suffering from diabetes mellitus?

(A) weight loss
(B) excessive thirst
(C) urinary retention
(D) glycosuria
(E) weakness

**196.** Hyperphosphatemia assocated with hypoparathyroidism can be effectively treated by administering

    I.   calcium carbonate
    II.  aluminum hydroxide
    III. magnesium hydroxide

(A) I only
(B) III only
(C) I and II only
(D) II and III only
(E) I, II, and III

**197.** Which of the following therapeutic agents is specifically contraindicated for use in patients who have bronchial asthma?

(A) sotalol (Betapace)
(B) quinapril (Accupril)
(C) nifedipine SR
(D) digoxin
(E) entacapone (Comtan)

**198.** Which of the following are uses for bupropion HCl?

    I.   antidepressant
    II.  smoking deterrent
    III. treatment of narcotic dependence

(A) I only
(B) III only
(C) I and II only
(D) II and III only
(E) I, II, and III

**199.** Which of the following potential adverse effects of the phenothiazines is thought to be irreversible?

(A) akathisia
(B) muscular rigidity
(C) tardive dyskinesia
(D) orthostatic hypotension
(E) tremor

**200.** Which of the following agents can be classified as an antagonist of angiotensin II receptors?

    I.   labetalol (Trandate)
    II.  trandolapril (Mavik)
    III. valsartan (Diovan)

(A) I only
(B) III only
(C) I and II only
(D) II and III only
(E) I, II, and III

**201.** Which of the following agents is NOT employed in the treatment of depression?

(A) zolpidem (Ambien)
(B) nefazodone (Serzone)
(C) paroxetine (Paxil)

(D) sertraline (Zoloft)

(E) venlafaxine (Effexor)

202. The use of olsalazine (Dipentum) is contraindicated in patients with a history of hypersensitivity to

(A) sulfonamides

(B) imidazolines

(C) phenothiazines

(D) salicylates

(E) beta-adrenergic–blocking agents

203. A patient has been receiving 50 mg of hydrocortisone (Solu-Cortef) by IV every 6 h for an acute exacerbation of ulcerative colitis. After several days of IV therapy, the physician wishes to switch the patient to an equivalent dose of oral prednisone. The equivalent total daily dose of prednisone would be

(A) 50 mg

(B) 100 mg

(C) 200 mg

(D) 400 mg

(E) 600 mg

204. A 50-year-old patient with congestive heart failure is stabilized on digoxin 0.25 mg daily, hydrochlorothiazide 50 mg daily, and a low-sodium, potassium-rich diet. The patient then develops polyarteritis, which requires corticosteroid therapy. Which of the following glucocorticoids would be most appropriate for this patient?

(A) hydrocortisone

(B) cortisone

(C) prednisolone

(D) dexamethasone

(E) prednisone

205. An asthmatic patient is stabilized to a therapeutic theophylline level on an IV aminophylline (dihydrate) infusion of 50 mg/h. The physician wishes to put the patient on an equivalent amount of sustained-release anhydrous theophylline (e.g., Theo-Dur). An appropriate total daily dose of Theo-Dur would be

(A) 1500 mg

(B) 1200 mg

(C) 900 mg

(D) 600 mg

(E) 300 mg

206. A 20-year-old asthmatic patient has been treated with zileuton (Zyflo) 600 mg q.i.d. While the patient seems to tolerate the drug well, she has brief episodes of bronchospasm several times a week. Which of the following drugs would NOT be appropriate to recommend for the treatment of acute bronchospasm in this patient?

I. zafirlukast (Accolate)

II. triamcinolone acetonide (Azmacort)

III. salmeterol (Serevent)

(A) I only

(B) III only

(C) I and II only

(D) II and III only

(E) I, II, and III

207. A patient with rheumatoid arthritis cannot swallow tablets or capsules. Which of the following salicylates is available in an oral liquid dosage form?

(A) choline salicylate

(B) magnesium salicylate

(C) salsalate

(D) sodium salicylate

(E) salicylic acid

208. A prescriber wishes to prescribe Lanoxicaps for a patient who has been receiving Lanoxin 0.25 mg tablets. The pharmacist should recommend which strength of Lanoxicaps?

(A) 0.05 mg

(B) 0.1 mg

(C) 0.2 mg

(D) 0.3 mg

(E) 0.5 mg

**209.** A secondary means of contraception should be recommended to patients using oral contraceptives when which of the following drugs is (are) also to be taken?

    I.  rifampin
   II.  cetirizine (Zyrtec)
  III.  acetaminophen

  (A)  I only
  (B)  III only
  (C)  I and II only
  (D)  II and III only
  (E)  I, II, and III

**210.** Which of the following agents are used as an aid to smoking cessation?

    I.  bupropion
   II.  nicotine
  III.  disulfiram

  (A)  I only
  (B)  III only
  (C)  I and II only
  (D)  II and III only
  (E)  I, II, and III

# Answers and Explanations

1. **(E)** Metoclopramide exerts a potent antiemetic effect by inhibiting dopamine receptors in the chemoreceptor trigger zone of the brain. It also stimulates GI motility and increases the rate of gastric emptying. This enhances the antiemetic activity by eliminating stasis that precedes vomiting. All of the other drugs listed, decrease the rate of gastric emptying. *(3)*

2. **(E)** Most antiparkinson agents act by increasing dopaminergic activity. *(3)*

3. **(D)** Tacrine (Cognex) and donepezil (Aricept) are centrally-acting cholinesterase inhibitors that increase acetylcholine levels in cortical neurons and may, therefore, slow progression of Alzheimer's disease symptoms. *(3)*

4. **(A)** Metformin is a biguanide that, in rare cases, may cause lactic acidosis. This is a condition that may be fatal in 50% of cases. *(3)*

5. **(D)** A satisfactory approximation of the temperature of the internal organs can be made by inserting a clinical thermometer into either the mouth or rectum. Both of these are closed cavities with good blood supply. The accepted average oral temperature is 98.6°F, with the recognition that both individual and diurnal variations occur regularly. The rectum is about 1°F warmer. Rectal and oral thermometers have the same temperature scales and markings, differing only in the shape of the bulb. To avoid the potential confusion and errors in subtracting or adding degrees from readings, physicians prefer that the actual temperature and the method be reported; for instance, 102.5°F taken rectally.

6. **(D)** Immediate treatment of the burn is recommended. Application of cold water will often reduce the severity of the burn. The burn area should be kept in cold water until no further pain is experienced whether in or out of the water. If necessary, a physician may then be contacted. *(3)*

7. **(B)** Montelukast sodium (Singulair) is an orally active leukotriene receptor antagonist used to provide prophylaxis and chronic treatment of asthma. It should be taken daily to prevent asthma attacks, even when the patient is asymptomatic. If required, bronchodilator drugs may be used to control acute attacks. *(3)*

8. **(D)** Pilocarpine is a cholinergic drug that produces a miotic effect (pupillary constriction). *(3)*

9. **(C)** Amiodarone (Cordarone) is a Class III antiarrhythmic agent that can produce a number of serious adverse effects including visual impairment, pulmonary toxicity and proarrhythmic effects. *(3)*

10. **(C)** Homatropine will produce mydriasis, which will further aggravate the patient's condition and possibly lead to blindness. The other agents are all useful in glaucoma treatment. *(3)*

11. **(E)** Pilocarpine is a relatively short-acting drug that causes accommodative spasm and miosis. Levobetaxolol (Betaxon), a beta-receptor antagonist, is believed to reduce elevated intraocular pressure by decreasing the production of aqueous humor. Levobetaxolol exerts its maximal effect within 1–2 h and maintains a significant effect for as long as 24 h following a

single topical dose. There seems to be little or no effect on pupil size, visual acuity, or accommodation. *(3)*

12. **(B)** GoLYTELY is a bowel evacuant product that is used to cleanse the bowel prior to GI examination. It contains polyethylene glycol and a mixture of electrolytes that must be reconstituted with water before it is administered. The usual dose is 4 L of reconstituted solution consumed in doses of 240 mL every 10 min., until the contents of the container have been consumed or the rectal effluent is clear. *(3)*

13. **(C)** Xenical (Orlistat) is a lipase inhibitor that inhibits the absorption of dietary fats. It is used in the management of obesity by having patients to take one 120 mg capsule of the drug three times daily with each main meal containing fat. A dose may be skipped if a meal is low in fat or if a meal is skipped. *(3)*

14. **(D)** Scabies is a disorder caused by the mite *Sarcoptes scabeii*. The mite burrows into the skin. Its droppings cause a hypersensitivity reaction characterized by intense itching. *(3)*

15. **(B)** The distinctive lesion is a vivid red macule, papule, or plaque covered by silvery lamellated scales. Usually the scalp, elbows, knees, and shins are affected first. *(3)*

16. **(B)** If morphine allergy is present, codeine should also be avoided because both codeine and morphine are structurally similar phenanthrene derivatives. Also, codeine is partially (10%) demethylated to morphine. *(3)*

17. **(D)** Tacrolimus (Prograf) and cyclosporine (Sandimmune, Neoral) are immunosuppressive drugs that are used to reduce organ rejection in patients who receive an organ transplant. *(3)*

18. **(B)** Alendronate (Fosamax) is a biphosphonate compound that inhibits normal and abnormal bone resorption. It is used for the treatment and prevention of osteoporosis in postmenopausal women. Patients should be advised to take their daily dose first thing in the morning, at least 30 min. before the first food, beverage or medication of the day is consumed. The drug should be taken with a full glass of plain water. The patient should be advised not to lie down for at least 30 min. following the administration of the drug, to reduce the possibility of esophageal irritation. *(3)*

19. **(C)** Clonidine is a central alpha-adrenergic stimulant that reduces peripheral vascular resistance and heart rate. Patients who use oral clonidine are susceptible to rebound hypertension if they discontinue their use of the tablets. The transdermal dosage form (Catapres TTS) releases clonidine at a constant rate for about 7 days, thereby improving compliance and reducing the likelihood of rebound hypertension. *(3)*

20. **(B)** Raising the intragastric pH from 1.5 to 3.5 neutralizes 99% of the acid and greatly reduces the proteolytic activity of pepsin. Buffering to a higher pH serves no useful purpose. *(3)*

21. **(C)** Epoetin alfa (Epogen, Procrit) is a glycoprotein that stimulates red blood cell production. It is not effective in treating patients with neutropenia (inadequate white blood cells). *(3)*

22. **(E)** Sinemet is a combination product containing carbidopa and levodopa in a ratio of 1:4 or 1:10. Because carbidopa inhibits the peripheral decarboxylation of levodopa, much smaller doses of levodopa can be used. This in turn generally reduces the peripheral side effects associated with high doses of levodopa. Dosage levels of levodopa can be decreased by approximately 75%. *(3)*

23. **(B)** The administraton of pyridoxine, even in small doses (5 mg or more) contained in ordinary vitamin preparations, is equivalent to a reduction in dosage of levodopa. Pyridoxine is believed to be a cofactor for the enzyme dopa decarboxylase, which is responsible for the peripheral metabolism of levodopa. The decarboxylated metabolic product cannot enter the brain, which is the desired site of action. *(3)*

**24. (A)** Miglitol (Glyset) is an alpha-glucosidase inhibitor that delays the digestion of ingested carbohydrates. This results in a smaller increase in blood glucose concentration after meals and permits better control of Type 2 diabetic patients who cannot control their hyperglycemia with diet alone. *(5)*

**25. (C)** The gray-baby syndrome occurs in premature and term newborn infants when chloramphenicol is administered during the first few days of life. The syndrome results from the inability of the infant to metabolize the drug because of a deficient enzyme, glucuronyl transferase, which is required to detoxify the drug by changing it to the glucuronide. Symptoms consist of cyanosis, vascular collapse, and elevated chloramphenicol levels in the blood. *(3)*

**26. (B)**
(A—incorrect) Inflammation of the eyelid is blepharitis.
(D—incorrect) Gastritis is an inflammation of the stomach wall.
(E—incorrect) Inflammation of the tongue would be known as glossitis. *(5)*

**27. (E)** Polyphagia is defined as an excessive craving for food. *(27)*

**28. (D)** Ezetimibe (Zetia) inhibits the absorption of cholesterol at the brush border of the small intestine, leading to decreased delivery of cholesterol to the liver. *(10)*

**29. (C)** Misoprostol is a synthetic prostaglandin E1 analog that inhibits gastric acid secretion. It is used orally to prevent NSAID-induced gastric ulcers. The drug is in pregnancy category X. *(3)*

**30. (B)** Myopia is the condition of nearsightedness.
(A—incorrect) Myalgia is pain in a muscle.
(D—incorrect) Myocardia pertains to the heart muscle.
(C—incorrect) Myoclonus is muscular twitching or contraction.
(E—incorrect) Myositis is inflammation of a voluntary muscle.

**31. (D)** Lithium products are used for the maintenance treatment of manic episodes of manic-depressive illness. Since lithium decreases renal sodium reabsorption, patients should be advised to maintain a normal salt and fluid intake. Anything that depletes the patient of sodium (e.g., sweating, diarrhea, use of diuretics, etc.) may increase lithium toxicity. Signs of lithium toxicity include the development of diarrhea and/or tremors. *(3)*

**32. (A)** Tegaserod (Zelnorm), a partial 5-HT4 agonist, is indicated for irritable bowel syndrome (IBS) that is constipation predominant. Alosetron (Lotronex) is a selective 5-HT3 receptor antagonist that is indicated for diarrhea predominant IBS. *(10)*

**33. (B)** Amphetamines (Adderal) are CNS stimulants. Patients should be advised to take the medication early in the day to avoid insomnia and warned that the drug may cause palpitations. With prolonged use, amphetamine products are likely to cause weight loss. *(3)*

**34. (A)** Although digoxin and quinidine are frequently used together, it is well documented that administering quinidine to a patient previously stabilized on digoxin will cause serum digoxin levels to rise to an average of 2- to 2.5-fold. The mechanism of this interaction may involve both a displacement of digoxin from tissue-binding sites and a reduction in renal clearance of digoxin. Even though the significance of this interaction remains controversial, many clinicians suggest reducing the dose of digoxin by 50% when adding quinidine. In any case, the patient should be monitored carefully for signs of digoxin toxicity. *(3)*

**35. (E)** Eplerenone (Inspra) is an aldosterone blocking agent that, like spironolactone (Aldactone), triamterene (Dyrenium), and amiloride (Midamor) may exert a potassium sparing action. Potassium supplements should not be used with these drugs because of the possibility of causing hyperkalemia. *(3)*

**36. (A)** Mannitol is usually administered by IV as a hypertonic 10% to 25% solution (an isotonic solution is about 5.5%). The introduction of a hypertonic solution promotes urine flow. Mannitol solutions are used in prophylaxis of acute renal failure, in the evaluation of acute oliguria, and for the reduction of the pressure and volume of the intraocular and cerebrospinal fluids. *(3)*

37. **(C)** Imipramine (Tofranil) is a tricyclic antidepressant that is used routinely to treat nocturnal enuresis. It is not recommended for children younger than 6 years of age. Doses of imipramine range from 25 to 75 mg, lower than those used for treatment of depression. Desmopressin (DDAVP) is a posterior pituitary hormone that has an antidiuretic effect. It is administered once daily as a nasal spray. *(3)*

38. **(B)** The international normalization ratio (INR) is used to monitor anticoagulant efficacy for patients using warfarin sodium (Coumadin). For patients who have had an acute MI, the INR should ideally be between 2 and 3. *(3)*

39. **(D)** Use of phenytoin (Dilantin) is associated with a number of adverse effects, including nystagmus (oscillation of the eyeball) and gingival hyperplasia (excessive gum growth). *(6)*

40. **(C)** Nalbuphine (Nubain) is a mixed narcotic agonist-antagonist capable of relieving moderate to severe pain. In subjects dependent on such narcotics as morphine and codeine, nalbuphine precipitates a withdrawal syndrome. Although it is capable of producing euphoria similar to morphine, its effect on respiration seems to exhibit a ceiling effect, such that doses higher than 30 mg produce no further respiratory depression. *(3)*

41. **(A)** Nalmefene (Revex) is a pure opioid antagonist that is used to reverse opioid effects. It has a longer duration of effect than naloxone (Narcan) and is, therefore, more effective in reversing the effects of long-acting opioid compounds. *(3)*

42. **(E)** Each of these agents exerts an antifungal action against candida (yeast) organisms. *(3)*

43. **(D)** Mild polycythemia is normal in persons who exercise excessively and in persons who live at high altitudes. Polycythemia vera is a state in which the rate of red cell production is far greater than normal, even though there is no apparent physiologic need for the increased production. It is believed that this disease may result from a malignancy of the bone marrow stem cells. Phlebotomy whenever the hematocrit rises higher than 55% may suffice as the only treatment for patients who do not have severe thrombocytosis. Drugs used to treat polycythemia include busulfan (Myleran) and radioactive phosphorus $^{32}$P. *(5)*

44. **(E)** Protamine is a strongly basic substance that combines with the strongly acidic heparin to produce a stable salt and a loss of anticoagulant activity. Because protamine itself possesses anticoagulant properties, it is unwise to administer more than 50 mg of protamine over a short period of time unless it is known that there is a definite need for a larger amount. *(3)*

45. **(C)** Salmeterol (Serevent) is the longest acting of these beta$_2$-adrenergic agonists. It has a duration of action of greater than 12 h. Isoetharine has the shortest duration (0.5–2.0 h), while the others have an intermediate duration of approximately 4–8 h. *(5)*

46. **(B)** Although the risk of hemorrhage in the fetus can be minimized by monitoring the prothrombin time of the mother closely, it is probably best to use heparin, if anticoagulant therapy is necessary, under these circumstances. Because heparin is a high molecular weight mucopolysaccharide, it does not cross the placenta. *(5)*

47. **(E)** Zolmitriptan (Zomig) is contraindicated in patients with angina pectoris, previous myocardial infarction and/or uncontrolled hypertension. It should also not be used if a patient has used an ergotamine derivative within the past 24 h, or within two weeks after discontinuing use of the MAO inhibitor *(5)*

48. **(A)** Acute uncomplicated urinary infections are most commonly caused by *E. coli*. Such

infections are most common in women and are characterized by the presence of dysuria, urinary urgency, and suprapubic discomfort. (5)

49. **(D)** In normal individuals, more than 50% of an oral dose of cyanocobalamin (vitamin $B_{12}$) is absorbed from the GI tract. This absorption occurs only in the presence of the intrinsic factor of Castle, with which the vitamin must presumably combine in order to pass through the intestinal walls. By means of radioactive cobalt–labeled cyanocobalamin, it has been shown that more than one-half of an oral dose soon appears in the blood. Normally, only a small amount of radioactivity appears in the urine. However, if a large flushing dose (1000 mg) of cyanocobalamin is given parenterally within an hour of the tagged oral dose, the renal threshold for cyanocobalamin is exceeded and radioactivity is observed in the urine. In patients with pernicious anemia, there is a deficiency in intrinsic factor that results in poor absorption of the radioactive cyanocobalamin. Most of the radioactivity in these patients will be detected in the feces. (5)

50. **(A)** Lipodystrophy is either the breakdown or accumulation of subcutaneous fat at the insulin injection site. It can best be avoided by having the patient rotate the site of insulin injection so that the same site is not used more frequently than once every 30 days. (3)

51. **(D)** Insulin lispro (Humalog) is the most rapidly acting insulin available. The onset of action takes about 15 min and its peak action occurs within 30–90 min. This form of insulin is generally given 15 min before a meal to permit effective utilization of the glucose that is absorbed. (3)

52. **(E)** Lantus insulin is a long-acting insulin that needs to be injected only once daily. Unlike other insulins that are formulated to have a pH of 7.4, Lantus insulin is formulated to have a pH of 8. For this reason Lantus insulin should never be mixed with other insulins. Lantus insulin is generally administered subcutaneously at bedtime and releases insulin from the injection site for approximately 24 h. The

shortest duration of the insulins listed is exhibited by regular insulin, which may act for only 6–8 h. (3)

53. **(A)** Lycopene is a carotenoid that contains 13 double bonds. This makes it a useful compound that is capable of neutralizing free radicals, substances that have been associated with the development of aging, cancers and other degenerative diseases. Foods that have a deep red color, such as tomatoes, watermelon, guava and pink grapefruit tend to have high levels of lycopene in the trans form. Processing these foods, particularly with heat, tends to convert the trans form of the lycopene into the cis form which is more biologically active. (28; Oct 2002)

54. **(D)** Morphine and its chemical derivatives commonly cause respiratory depression, nausea and constipation. (5)

55. **(A)** Combination oral contraceptive products usually contain norethindrone (a progestin) and ethinyl estradiol (an estrogen). The estrogen component suppresses the production of follicle-stimulating hormone (FSH) and luteinizing hormone (LH) and thereby prevents ovulation. The progestin component increases the viscosity of cervical mucus and makes the endometrial lining of the uterus less receptive to the implantation of a fertilized ovum. (3)

56. **(C)** Oseltamivir (Tamiflu) and zanamivir (Relenza) are antiviral drugs used for the treatment of uncomplicated influenza A or B. In order to be effective, therapy with these agents must begin within two days of symptom onset. Zanamivir is administered as a powder for inhalation while oseltamivir is administered orally. For treatment of influenza A or B, each medication should be administered twice daily for five days. Penciclovir (Denavir) is an antiviral drug used topically for the treatment of cold sores. (3)

57. **(C)** The usual method of treating an acute hypoglycemic reaction is to give glucose orally or, in unconscious patients, by IV in concentrated solutions. However, if these routes cannot be used, 0.5–1 mg of glucagon may be

given SC or IM as well as by IV. Glucagon is an endogenous hormone produced by the alpha cells of the pancreatic Islet of Langerhans. Glucagon increases blood glucose by stimulating hepatic gluconeogenesis and glycogenolysis. *(3)*

58. **(D)** Zidovudine (AZT, Retrovir) is a nucleoside reverse transcriptase inhibitor that is employed in treating pregnant women who are HIV positive in order to reduce the likelihood of transmission of the virus to their offspring. When used in this manner, zidovudine is administered orally to the pregnant women during the second and third trimesters of pregnancy. During labor, an IV dose of zidovudine is administered. After delivery zidovudine is administered orally to the newborn for approximately six weeks. *(3)*

59. **(B)** Dopamine exerts a positive inotropic effect by direct action on beta-adrenergic receptors and causes a release of norepinephrine from storage sites. A major advantage of the drug is that controlling the infusion rate can vary its hemodynamic effects. *(3)*

60. **(D)** Ovrette and Micronor are oral contraceptive products that contain only progestin. *(3)*

61. **(E)** In the iron-deficient state, the iron storage compartment becomes depleted. This is followed by a reduction in plasma transferrin saturation. Subsequently, the number and size of the erythrocytes as well as their hemoglobin content will be decreased. The lack of hemoglobin causes the erythrocytes to become paler (hypochromic) in color. *(5)*

62. **(D)** Trigeminal neuralgia is a disorder characterized by sudden attacks of severe pain along the distribution of the fifth cranial nerve. Attacks are often precipitated by stimulation of a trigger zone in the area of the pain. Carbamazepine (Tegretol) is remarkably effective in both relieving and preventing the pain of trigeminal neuralgia. Anticonvulsants such as phenytoin (Dilantin) may also be beneficial in some cases. Other drugs that have been effective are vitamin $B_{12}$ in massive

doses (1 mg) and injection of alcohol into the ganglion or the branches of the trigeminal nerve. *(3)*

63. **(A)** Mifepristone (Mifeprex) and misoprostol (Cytotec) are employed as ingredients in a product used to induce abortion in women in whom less than 49 days have elapsed since the beginning of their last menstrual period. To induce abortion several doses of mifepristone (an antiprogestin) are administered. After two days a dose of misoprostol (Cytotec) (a pregnancy category X drug) is administered. The use of these two agents in the manner described results in an abortion in over 95% of women (in the category described above). *(10)*

64. **(E)** The development of inflammatory conditions of the colon (e.g., nonspecific colitis or a more severe pseudomembranous colitis) has been associated with antibiotic therapy. Although many antibiotics have been implicated, there have been a disproportionate number of reports specifically involving clindamycin and lincomycin. Colitis has been associated with both oral and parenteral administration of these drugs, and no clear predisposing conditions have been identified. Because antiperistaltic drugs (e.g., diphenoxalate) used to treat the resulting diarrhea seem to prolong the disease (probably by retaining the toxins produced by the *Clostridium* causative organism), they should not be used. *(3)*

65. **(D)** Loperamide (Imodium) inhibits peristaltic activity by a direct effect on the musculature of the intestinal wall. Loperamide appears to be devoid of opiate-like effects. *(3)*

66. **(A)** The Norplant system consists of a number of silastic tubes containing levonorgestrel, a progestin. These tubes are generally surgically implanted under the skin of the forearm, where they will release the progestin over a period of 5 years. The advantage of this system is its long duration of action, its effectiveness, and its usefulness in patients who have a history of noncompliance in using oral contraceptive products. This product has recently been withdrawn from the market but many patients are

still utilizing this system. Preven is an emergency contraceptive used within 72 h of unprotected sex. Clomid is an ovulation stimulant. *(3)*

67. **(E)** Felodipine (Plendil) is a calcium channel blocking agent used in treating angina and hypertension. When taken with grapefruit juice, there is evidence that the AUC of felodipine will be increased. Therefore, grapefruit juice should be avoided when using this product. *(3)*

68. **(A)** Cocaine, like the amphetamines, is a potent CNS stimulant. The other agents listed are CNS depressants. *(3)*

69. **(B)** Acetaminophen will not displace warfarin from its protein-binding sites or interfere with warfarin metabolism. It is less likely, therefore to cause a therapeutic problem in this patient. All of the other choices either have a high affinity for plasma proteins or may alter warfarin metabolism. *(3)*

70. **(A)** Valsartan (Diovan) is an angiotensin II-receptor blocker (ARB) that is used to treat hypertension. *(10)*

71. **(D)** Each gram of protein supplies about 4 kcal, each gram of carbohydrate supplies about 4 kcal, and each gram of fat supplies about 9 kcal. It is obvious, therefore, that strictly on a weight basis, fats are better caloric sources than are other nutrients. *(26)*

72. **(D)** Leucovorin calcium (Wellcovorin) is a derivative of folic acid used as an antidote for drugs used as folic acid antagonists such as methotrexate. *(6)*

73. **(D)** Pedialyte is an orally administered electrolyte solution containing dextrose; potassium chloride; and sodium, calcium, and magnesium salts. It is used to supply water and electrolytes in a balanced proportion in order to prevent serious deficits from occurring in patients suffering from mild to moderate fluid loss. The product does not contain protein or fat. *(3)*

74. **(A)** Each gram of dextrose supplies approximately 3.4 kcal of energy to a patient. Because a liter of dextrose 5% solution contains 50 g of dextrose, the administration of the liter will supply the patient with approximately 170 kcal. *(26)*

75. **(B)** Hepatitis B vaccine is used to immunize people of all ages against all known subtypes of hepatitis B virus. It must be stored in a refrigerator and is usually administered intramuscularly (IM). *(3)*

76. **(C)** Prostate-specific antigen (PSA) is a glycoprotein produced only by prostate cells. Levels of PSA are determined for prostate cancer screening. PSA levels may also be elevated in men with acute prostatitis or benign prostatic hyperplasia (BPH). *(5)*

77. **(A)** Of the drugs listed, erythromycin has the lowest degree of toxicity and the spectrum of action most similar to penicillin. Demeclocycline may inhibit skeletal growth in the fetus. Deposition of tetracyclines in the teeth of the fetus has been associated with enamel defects and staining of the teeth. Trimethoprim is a teratogenic drug. *(3)*

78. **(D)** Silver sulfadiazine (Silvadene) cream applied topically to burns has been found to be quite effective in inhibiting the invasion of the affected site by both gram-positive and gram-negative bacteria. The cream is usually applied to a thickness of about 1/16 inch twice daily over the entire burned surface. Mafenide (Sulfamylon) cream is also used topically for the same purpose. *(3)*

79. **(A)** The drug of choice in treating most forms of gonorrhea is ceftriaxone (Rocephin). The drug is generally given in a single 125 mg IM dose. In patients who cannot tolerate a beta-lactam antimicrobial agent, ciprofloxacin (Cipro) 500 mg PO once or Ofloxacin (Floxin) 400 mg PO once may be given instead. *(5)*

80. **(B)** Indomethacin (Indocin) and other NSAIDs are effective agents in the treatment of acute

gouty arthritis. They act by reducing the joint inflammation responsible for the excruciating pain associated with the disease. While colchicine may also be used for this purpose, colchicine is much more likely to produce serious adverse effects. *(5:1463)*

81. **(E)** Cromolyn sodium 4% ophthalmic solution (Crolom) is used to treat ocular allergic disorders such as vernal keratoconjunctivitis. It is effective only if it is used at regular intervals. Cromolyn acts to inhibit degranulation of sensitized mast cells that occurs after exposure to specific antigens. *(3)*

82. **(C)** Adalimumab (Humira) is a monoclonal antibody that acts as a tumor necrosis factor (TNF) antagonist. It is indicated for the treatment of patients with moderate to severe rheumatoid arthritis who have not responded to more conservative forms of therapy (e.g., NSAIDS). This drug must be used with great caution in patients who have a preexisting infection. Treatment with this drug should be discontinued if the patient develops a serious infection while on the drug. The drug is administered subcutaneously every other week. *(10)*

83. **(E)** Dopamine (Intropin) is a sympathomimetic drug that acts directly on alpha and beta-receptors and produces indirect effects due to release of norepinephrine. Dopamine also dilates renal and mesenteric vessels through a dopamine receptor effect. The hemodynamic effects of dopamine are dose related. At low infusion rates (1–5 mg/kg/min), dopamine increases renal blood flow without much change in cardiac output or total peripheral resistance. In higher doses (5–20 mg/kg/min), cardiac output and heart rate increase, the increase in renal perfusion persists, and total peripheral resistance is variable. At higher infusion rates, renal vasoconstriction occurs, total peripheral resistance rises, and blood pressure increases. Consequently, the infusion rate must be adjusted and monitored carefully to achieve the desired response. *(3)*

84. **(B)** Flumazenil (Romazicon) is a specific benzodiazepine antagonist used to reverse the toxic effects of benzodiazepine intoxication. It should not be used in patients also using tricyclic antidepressants because it may increase the risk of seizures in such patients. *(5:1097)*

85. **(E)** Although there are no reported differences in bioavailability between phenytoin capsules and suspension, this patient's phenytoin level is likely to increase because the milligram-for-milligram conversion is equivalent to an increase in dose. The capsule form of Dilantin is the sodium salt and contains only 92% phenytoin. The suspension is the free acid and contains 100% phenytoin. In this situation, the patient would be going from a daily dose of 276 mg phenytoin (as 300-mg phenytoin sodium) to 300 mg phenytoin. *(3)*

86. **(C)** Fentanyl (Duragesic) patches are effective in treating chronic severe pain. They are applied every 72 h and provide a continuous release of analgesic during that period. PRN treatment is not advisable in treating severe pain because it may cause patient anxiety. Codeine, oral meperidine and acetaminophen are generally not effective enough to control chronic severe pain. *(3)*

87. **(B)** Oprelvekin (Neumega) is a thrombopoietic growth factor that increases the production of platelets in the body. It is used to treat and prevent thrombocytopenia. *(3)*

88. **(D)** Metronidazole (Flagyl) is a drug that has antiprotazoal and antimicrobial action. Patients on this drug should be advised to avoid alcohol because a disulfiram-like reaction may occur. In addition, metronidazole use will darken the urine of most patients. *(3)*

89. **(D)** In general, all insulin products currently available are reasonably stable at room temperature (i.e., 59°–85°F). Traveling diabetics should be advised to avoid prolonged exposure of their insulin to very high temperatures, and told that it is not necessary to refrigerate the vial in use. Insulin vials stored in pharmacies are required to be refrigerated because they may be kept in stock for a long period of time. *(3)*

90. **(D)** Isotretinoin (Accutane) is a vitamin A derivative indicated for the treatment of recalcitrant cystic acne in patients who do not respond to more conservative therapy. Approximately 90% of patients using this product experience cheilitis, a cracking around the margin of the lips. *(3)*

91. **(B)** Fluids employed in TPN are generally very hypertonic and hyperosmotic. Until the technique of subclavian vein catheterization was perfected, it was too irritating and inflammatory to use the usual sites of IV administration. Peripheral veins are seldom used in the administration of hypertonic nutrient solutions because blood flow is insufficient to provide the necessary dilution of the fluid to protect the intima of the vessel. The exception occurs when the slightly hypertonic amino acid solutions containing limited amounts of dextrose are administered. *(3)*

92. **(B)** Dicloxacillin, oxacillin, cloxacillin and nafcillin are beta-lactamase resistant penicillins that would be suitable for the treatment of this patient. Gentamicin is an aminoglycoside and ticarcillin is an extended-acting penicillin. Both are used in treating serious gram-negative infections. *(3)*

93. **(E)** Use of sustained-release nifedipine products, as well as some other sustained-release drug products, may cause the appearance of an empty tablet in the stool. This is the plastic matrix from which the drug diffused and it does not contain the active drug. *(3)*

94. **(A)** Suddenly discontinuing the administration of dextrose solution may cause a rebound hypoglycemia in response to the sudden elimination of the sustained glucose load of the TPN solution. It is best to maintain the patient on a nominal amount of dextrose such as $D_5W$ or to wean the patient slowly from the TPN solution.

(B—incorrect) Hyperchloremic metabolic acidosis may occur during TPN therapy when the total chloride ion content is high. The amino acids in the protein salts are usually chloride or hydrochloride salts. Additional amounts of chloride are obtained when sodium or potassium chlorides are added to the TPN solutions. It may be useful to supply either sodium or potassium as acetate salts.

(C—incorrect) Hyperosmotic nonketotic hyperglycemia is a result of infusing an overload of glucose. Causes include an overly rapid infusion rate, dextrose solutions that are too concentrated, and malfunction of pancreatic secretion of insulin. *(5)*

95. **(D)** Fats provide approximately 9 kcal/g. Fat emulsion products are popularly used in TPN therapy because fat emulsions can be administered safely through peripheral or central veins. Commercial examples of fat emulsion products are Intralipid and Liposyn II or III. Ethanol provides approximately 7 kcal/g, hydrous dextrose provides approximately 3.4 kcal/g and protein provides approximately 3–4 kcal/g. *(3)*

96. **(E)** Tropisetron (Navoban) is a selective 5-HT$_3$ receptor antagonist used to prevent nausea and vomiting associated with cancer chemotherapy. Tropisetron may be administered orally or by IV infusion (given over a 15 min period) or by slow IV injection (for not less than 1 min). Generally an IV dose is administered immediately before chemotherapy is begun (Day 1). This is followed by the use of an oral capsule of the drug each morning upon arising for days 2 through 6. The capsules should be taken with water at least 1 h before any food intake. *(3)*

97. **(D)** Amiloride is a potassium-sparing diuretic with a mechanism of action similar to that of triamterene. Both drugs exert a diuretic effect by promoting the exchange of sodium for potassium in the distal portion of the renal tubule. In contrast to spironolactone, neither of these drugs inhibits aldosterone. Metolazone and chlorthalidone are thiazide-like diuretics. *(3)*

98. **(A)** Treatment of hyperkalemia can be approached by three methods. First, in the presence of ECG changes, calcium should be given to counteract the effects of excess potassium on the heart. Second, bicarbonate or glucose plus insulin can be used to shift potassium rapidly from extracellular to intracellular fluid

compartments. Third, exchange resins (e.g., sodium polystyrene sulfonate) or dialysis can be used to remove potassium from the body. In this case, because there are no symptoms of ECG changes, the rectal administration of sodium polystyrene sulfonate (Kayexalate) (enemas containing 50 g in 70% sorbitol solution) is the most appropriate option. *(5)*

99. **(D)** Dalteparin sodium (Fragmin), ardeparin sodium (Normiflo), and enoxaparin sodium (Lovenox) are low molecular weight heparin products prepared from porcine (pork) heparin. They are administered subcutaneously only. *(3)*

100. **(E)** Miglitol (Glyset) is an alpha-glucosidase inhibitor. Repaglinide (Prandin) lowers blood glucose by stimulating the release of insulin from the pancreas. Rosiglitazone (Avandia) enhances insulin receptor sensitivity. All are indicated for the treatment of type 2 diabetes mellitus. *(3)*

101. **(D)** When administered parenterally, lorazepam (Ativan) is a rapidly acting anticonvulsant with fewer tendencies to produce respiratory depression than the barbiturates. It has become a common choice for initial therapy of status epilepticus. *(6)*

102. **(C)** Chronic (longer than six months) high-dose administration of hydralazine may produce an acute rheumatoid state in approximately 10% of patients taking the drug. A syndrome clinically indistinguishable from disseminated lupus erythematosus develops in a smaller percentage of users. This lupus-like syndrome (fever, arthralgia, splenomegaly, edema, and the presence of lupus erythematosus cells in the peripheral blood) has also been associated with procainamide use. *(6)*

103. **(E)** Vitamin $B_6$ (pyridoxine) use by patients using levodopa may decrease the effectiveness of levodopa by promoting the peripheral decarboxylation of levodopa by dopa-decarboxylase. This is not a problem in patients using levodopa in combination with carbidopa (Sinemet) *(6)*

104. **(A)** Atenolol (Tenormin) blocks beta-adrenergic receptors. It differs from pindolol (Visken) primarily in that it has some preferential effect on beta$_1$-adrenoreceptors, which are located chiefly in the cardiac muscle. This preferential effect is not absolute and, at higher doses, atenolol may also inhibit beta$_2$-adrenoreceptors, which are located chiefly in bronchial and vascular musculature. Although the mechanism of its antihypertensive effect is not known, the drug is indicated in the management of hypertension either alone or in combination with other antihypertensive drugs. *(6)*

105. **(D)** Terazosin (Hytrin) is an alpha$_1$-adrenergic blocker that causes peripheral vasodilation. Side effects of therapy may include a precipitous fall in blood pressure, possibly accompanied by tachycardia and syncope following the first dose. The initial dose of terazosin is usually 1 mg at bedtime and may be increased slowly to 20 mg daily if required. Other *"sin"* drugs, such as doxazosin and prazosin may also produce this first dose effect. *(6)*

106. **(A)** CD4 cells are a type of T lymphocytes whose primary role is to stimulate other cells in the immune response. The lower the level of these cells in the patient's blood, the more susceptible the patient becomes to the development of opportunistic infections such as *Pneumocystis carinii* pneumonia. *(6)*

107. **(E)** Nitroprusside has marked antihypertensive activity when given by IV infusion. It appears to lower blood pressure by relaxing vascular smooth muscle, thereby dilating peripheral arteries and veins. Solutions of nitroprusside must be protected from light. Discolored solutions or those with visible particulate matter should be discarded. Excessive doses may produce symptoms of cyanide poisoning. *(6)*

108. **(D)** Dirithromycin (Dynabac) should not be used to treat bacteremias because its use does not achieve sufficiently high serum levels to provide antimicrobial coverage of the blood stream. *(6)*

109. **(E)** Tobramycin sulfate (Nebcin) is the salt of a weak base and a strong acid. Combining such a drug with alkaline drugs, such as those listed, will result in a chemical incompatibility. *(6)*

110. **(D)** All of the agents listed, except terbinafine, are employed in the treatment of *Helicobacter pylori*–related peptic ulcer disease. Terbinafine (Lamisil) is an antifungal agent used in treating onychomycosis. *(6)*

111. **(C)** Cholestyramine is a basic anion exchange resin. This quaternary ammonium chloride compound exchanges the chloride ion for the negatively charged bile acids, thereby preventing their reabsorption. Cholestyramine binds many organic acids, including warfarin and levothyroxine. *(6)*

112. **(C)** If drug B has a greater affinity (i.e., a higher association constant) for specific protein-binding sites than does drug A, it will have a tendency to displace drug A from these sites. Furthermore, if drug B is given in large doses, the degree of this displacement will increase because there will be a greater amount of drug B competing with drug A for the binding sites. *(6)*

113. **(B)** Tinsaparin (Innohep) is a low molecular weight heparin compound used for the prevention of deep vein thrombosis (DVT). It is only administered by deep subcutaneous injection. *(6)*

114. **(E)** Acetylsalicylic acid (aspirin), dipyridamole (Persantine) and clopidogrel (Plavix) each exhibit antiplatelet action. *(6)*

115. **(C)** Penetration of the cornea by *Pseudomonas aeruginosa* will often lead to destruction of the cornea and interior portions of the eye. Blindness may result. This organism is a common contaminant in water. The need for sterility of ophthalmic products is well recognized. *(6)*

116. **(E)** Boils caused by *Staphylococcus* organisms form in the anterior portion of the external auditory meatus. They are usually self-limiting,

and treatment with antibiotic ointments prevents spreading. *(6)*

117. **(D)** Idoxuridine is an antimetabolite that inhibits the replication of viral DNA with greater selectivity than does that of the host cell. It is used primarily in the treatment of herpes simplex keratitis, a disease of viral origin that can cause blindness. *(6)*

118. **(D)** Although tolnaftate is effective against several types of fungi, it is ineffective against *Candida* organisms. Miconazole, clotrimazole, and amphotericin (Fungizone) are relatively broad-spectrum antifungal agents with activity against some species of *Candida*. *(10)*

119. **(A)** Tolterodine (Detrol) is muscarinic receptor antagonist (anticholinergic) that is used in treating symptoms of overactive bladder, including incontinence, urinary frequency and urgency. *(10)*

120. **(E)** Complications of corticosteroid therapy are usually related to the length of time that they have been administered and the dosage used. Corticosteroids suppress normal tissue responses to infection (increasing susceptibility to infection) and allow further dissemination of existing infections. Because tissue responses to infection are suppressed, the subjective, objective, and laboratory manifestations of infection may be masked. *(6)*

121. **(C)** Although the NSAIDs are structurally different, they all possess similar pharmacological properties and all inhibit prostaglandin synthesis. Furthermore, these drugs produce similar adverse effects, including gastrointestinal (GI) intolerance. Oxaprozin (Daypro) and piroxicam (Feldene) have the longest half-life of the group (approximately 42–80 h) and are recommended to be given on a once-a-day basis. *(10)*

122. **(B)** Adalimumab (Humira) is a monoclonal antibody that is directed against tumor necrosis factor alpha. It is indicated for reducing the signs and symptoms and inhibiting the progression of structural damage in adults with

moderate-to-severe active rheumatoid arthritis who have failed previous treatment with disease-modifying antirheumatic drugs. *(10)*

123. **(D)** Rofecoxib (Vioxx) is a cyclooxygenase-2 (COX-2) inhibitor. It is, therefore, less likely to cause GI upset than most other NSAIDS. *(6)*

124. **(A)** When dispensing isotretinoin (Accutane) to a woman of childbearing potential, the pharmacist should advise the patient of the dangers of becoming pregnant during therapy. In addition, the patient should be advised that the lesions will initially appear worse but then improve and that prolonged exposure to sunlight or sunlamps should be avoided while using the drug. *(6)*

125. **(E)** In the condition known as hypoprothrombinemia, there is a reduction in the levels of prothrombin in the blood. This substance is essential in the blood-clotting mechanism. *(6)*

126. **(B)** Rapid reversal of warfarin-induced hypoprothrombinemia can be accomplished by discontinuing warfarin therapy and, if necessary, the administration of phytonadione (vitamin $K_1$). Phytonadione, when used for this purpose, is best administered IM or SC in a single dose. The dose may be repeated if the patient does not adequately respond within 6–8 h. *(3)*

127. **(E)** Phenazopyridine (Pyridium) is a red dye that commonly causes discoloration of the urine. It is used primarily as a urinary tract analgesic. *(3)*

128. **(C)** Menotropins (Pergonal, Humegon) are hormones that have a moderate follicle stimulating hormone (FSH) and luteinizing hormone (LH) activity. It is administered parenterally to induce ovulation in many patients with amenorrhea and other conditions that cause anovulatory cycles. It may also be used in males to enhance spermatogenesis. It is classified in pregnancy category X. *(3)*

129. **(A)** Amiloride (Midamor) is a potassium-sparing diuretic. Patients should be advised to avoid large quantities of potassium-rich foods because their use with this drug product could cause serious hyperkalemia. *(3)*

130. **(B)** Animal testing of a new drug is completed before the investigational new drug (IND) status is obtained for clinical testing. In phase I of the study, healthy volunteers are tested to determine drug tolerance, dosing schedules, side effects, and pharmacokinetic data. This is followed by phase II, in which actual patients suffering from the disease are tested with the drug. Drug efficacy is observed, and side effects not evident in healthy volunteers may occur. Phase III involves administration of the drug to large numbers of patients by private practitioners. Phase IV is the continuous investigation or monitoring of the drug after marketing. *(3)*

131. **(D)** Hypoparathyroidism usually presents itself as a disorder of calcium metabolism in which serum calcium levels of the patient decrease while levels of phosphate increase in an inversely proportional manner. Low serum calcium levels may precipitate a potentially serious condition known as tetany. To prevent the development of this disorder and to treat the hypoparathyroidism, calcium supplements, such as calcium gluconate, calcium carbonate, or calcium lactate may be prescribed. *(3)*

132. **(A)** Atomoxetine (Strattera) is a nonstimulant medication for ADHD. It acts as a selective norepinephrine reuptake inhibitor and should not be taken within two weeks of using an MAOI. *(3)*

133. **(E)** The hypothyroid state is characterized by marked retardation of mental and physical activity; hoarseness; dry sparse hair; thickening of the skin and subcutaneous tissues; constipation; cold intolerance; anemia; and dry, pale, coarse skin. However, because of the nature of the general symptoms, hypothyroidism is usually recognized and treated before all of the previously mentioned symptoms develop. Patients with hypothyroidism frequently develop enlargement of the thyroid glands (goiter) and may have elevated TSH levels. Hashimoto's disease (autoimmune thyroiditis)

is a common cause of hypothyroidism in adults. *(6)*

**134.** **(C)** Nocturnal enuresis is also called bedwetting. While fairly common in children, it may also continue in some through the teen years and adulthood. A variety of possible causes exist, including psychological, diabetes insipidus, weakness of the bladder sphincter, and others. *(5)*

**135.** **(A)** Fiorinal is the only agent listed that contains aspirin. *(3)*

**136.** **(A)** Hemochromatosis is an iron storage disorder characterized by excessive amounts of iron in parenchymal tissues with resultant tissue damage. Such a condition may be caused by a number of factors, one of which is the prolonged use of excessive doses of iron preparations. *(5)*

**137.** **(B)** Cholestatic hepatitis is a syndrome that may occur when erythromycin estolate is given to susceptible individuals for more than 10–14 days. It is more common after multiple exposures to the drug, although full recovery usually follows discontinuation of the medication. The reaction is unpredictable and is apparently due to individual hypersensitivity. It has not been observed with the use of erythromycin free base or with other derivatives of erythromycin. Because there is no established clinical superiority of the estolate salt, there is little justification for using it in light of the possibility of this potential toxicity. *(3)*

**138.** **(D)** Dornase alfa (Pulmozyme) is a mucolytic agent that liquefies the tenacious respiratory mucus that is often a characteristic of cystic fibrosis. Pancrelipase (Ultrase) is a pancreatic enzyme product indicated for patients with cystic fibrosis. Such a product is useful in this disease because of the common presence of thick mucus plugs in the pancreatic duct, that may block the passage of pancreatic enzymes into the GI tract. *(10)*

**139.** **(B)** Lansoprazole (Prevacid), omeprazole (Prilosec) and pantoprazole (Protonix) reduce gastric acidity by inhibiting the *proton pump* within the gastric mucosa. They are commonly used in the treatment of peptic ulcer disease, gastroesophageal reflux disease (GERD) or pathological hypersecretory conditions. *(3)*

**140.** **(D)** Patients with chronic inflammatory bowel disease may use olsalazine sodium (Dipentum) or mesalamine (Asacol, Pentasa, Rowasa) if they are allergic to sulfa drugs, because these drugs do not contain a sulfa component. Sulfasalazine (Azulfidine) does contain a sulfa component. *(3)*

**141.** **(C)** Ezetimibe (Zetia) is a lipid-lowering compound that selectively inhibits the intestinal absorption of cholestrol. It may be administered alone or it may be administered in combination with an HMG-CoA reductase inhibitor (i.e., a statin drug). *(3)*

**142.** **(D)** Didanosine is a retroviral inhibitor approved for the treatment of HIV infection. Its major adverse reactions include peripheral neuropathy and pancreatitis. Enfuvirtide (Fuseon) is a fusion inhibitor used in treating advanced HIV infection. Ifosfamide is an antineoplastic alkylating agent. *(3)*

**143.** **(E)** Patients with sinus headaches generally experience pain in the periorbital area. Pain is usually greatest on awakening because of the accumulation of fluid in the sinus cavities. *(5)*

**144.** **(C)** Combined drug treatment is usually required because of the rapid development of resistant organisms when a single agent is used. It has also been demonstrated that combined drug therapy enhances the tuberculostatic effects of the individual drugs. For example, a combination of streptomycin and isoniazid is significantly more tuberculostatic than either agent used alone. *(6)*

**145.** **(C)** The color change imparted to urine and sweat is a predictable and harmless side effect. Patients should be told to expect this effect so that they are not alarmed by it. *(3)*

146. **(D)** Ticlopidine (Ticlid) is a platelet aggregation inhibitor used to reduce the risk of thrombotic stroke. While using this drug the patient may be at higher risk of abnormal bleeding. *(3)*

147. **(D)** Mezlocillin (Mezlin) is an extended-spectrum penicillin that is active against both gram-positive and many gram-negative microorganisms. It is particularly useful in treating serious gram negative infections caused by *Pseudomonas* or *Proteus*. *(3)*

148. **(C)** Pseudomembranous colitis is a severe and occasionally fatal complication of antibiotic therapy. One etiology appears to be the presence of an exotoxin produced by overgrowth of *Clostridium difficile* in the bowel. Clindamycin, lincomycin, and ampicillin have been the most commonly implicated antibiotics, although other antibiotics have also been implicated. Treatment is directed against the offending organism and its exotoxin. Oral metronidazole (Flagyl) 250–500 mg three to four times daily for 10 days is most commonly used. *(6)*

149. **(D)** Cushing syndrome is a condition characterized by adrenal hyperplasia caused by overproduction of ACTH by the pituitary gland. Patients with this disease often have obesity, hypertension, and gonadal dysfunction. *(6)*

150. **(B)** The aminoglycosides have activity against a wide range of microorganisms. After parenteral administration, they are excreted unchanged in the urine. Because of their well-established nephrotoxicity and ototoxicity, they are not suitable for long-term treatment of chronic urinary tract infections. *(3)*

151. **(C)** Mycobacterium avium complex (MAC) and *Pneumocystis carinii* pneumonia (PCP) are both infectious complications of HIV. Sudden acute respiratory syndrome (SARS) is a highly transmissible viral disorder that is not specifically related to the presence of HIV. *(6)*

152. **(A)** For the prophylactic treatment of asthma, cromolyn sodium is available in several forms: powder-filled capsules for inhalation; a solution for use with a nebulizer; and an aerosol spray. Cromolyn is used to prevent asthma attacks, not to treat acute attacks. *(3)*

153. **(E)** A major advance in steroid therapy for asthma has been the development of corticosteroid aerosols such as beclomethasone (Vanceril). Like cromolyn (Intal), beclomethasone is a prophylactic agent that must be used regularly. It is not suitable for an acute asthmatic attack. The primary value of steroid therapy by inhalation is to avoid systemic side effects in patients who require steroids for the first time or to permit significant dosage reductions of oral steroids in patients on maintenance therapy. *(3)*

154. **(D)** Vasopressin, which is a purified preparation of the antidiuretic hormone, is used therapeutically in the treatment of diabetes insipidus, a disease of pituitary origin. When administered in any one of a number of available dosage forms (IM, IV, subcutaneous [SC], and nasal insufflation or spray), vasopressin usually reverses the symptom of excessive urination (polyuria), which is the primary symptom of patients suffering from this disease. The initially observed action of the hormone was vasoconstriction, which led to the name vasopressin; this is still the official USP designation. *(3)*

155. **(A)** Lithium carbonate (Lithane, Eskalith) is primarily indicated for treating manic episodes in patients with manic–depressive illness. It is administered orally in daily divided doses of 600 mg to 1.8 g and generally should not be administered with diuretics, because retention of lithium may occur. *(3)*

156. **(A)** The rate of excretion of lithium carbonate is generally independent of urine flow and dietary sodium. However, in the presence of sodium deficiency, the excretion of lithium is markedly decreased and toxic levels can accumulate rapidly. Conversely, high sodium intake enhances lithium excretion. *(3)*

157. **(B)** Glucose-6-phosphate dehydrogenase (G6PD) controls the initial step in the pentose-phosphate pathway, bringing about the oxidation

of glucose-6-phosphate to 6-phosphoglu-conate, which reduces NADP to NADPH. Many oxidant drugs (e.g., primaquine, sul-fisoxazole, probenecid) increase the rate of oxi-dation of glutathione. This increases the intracellular demand for NADPH to maintain glutathione in the reduced form. In patients with a deficiency in erythrocyte G6PD, oxi-dized glutathione accumulates and, by some unknown mechanism, disrupts erythrocyte membrane integrity with subsequent hemoly-sis. *(3)*

158. **(E)** The anticoagulant effect of heparin is quan-tified by measuring the activated partial thromboplastin time (APTT). The usual thera-peutic goal is to prolong the APTT to 2–2.5 times that of the laboratory control. *(6)*

159. **(E)** Because of heparin's brief duration of action, mild hemorrhaging is usually treated by simply withdrawing the drug. In the presence of severe hemorrhage, the use of a specific heparin antagonist (e.g., protamine sulfate) is imperative. If protamine sulfate is required, generally 1 mg of protamine sulfate IV is uti-lized to neutralize 100 units of heparin. After the IV administration of heparin, the quantity of protamine required decreases rapidly with time. Only 0.5 mg of protamine is required to neutralize 100 units of heparin 30 min after IV administration of heparin. *(3)*

160. **(D)** Cimetidine potentiates the effects of oral anticoagulants by decreasing the rate of hepatic metabolism of warfarin. Cimetidine causes a reversible but significant increase in plasma warfarin concentration and, consequently, in the prothrombin time. In this case, it is neces-sary to recognize this interaction and decrease the dose of warfarin or use a safer alternative to cimetidine. *(3)*

161. **(A)** Normal fasting blood sugar values for adults range from 80–120 mg/dL (or 80–120 mg%). When the fasting blood sugar levels exceed 120 mg/dL, diabetes mellitus should be suspected. Levels below 60 mg/dL may sug-gest insulin overdosage, glucagon deficiencies,

and/or hypoactivity of various endocrine glands. *(6)*

162. **(D)** The administration of pharmacological doses (0.4 mg/day or more) of folic acid can stimulate reticulocytosis and improve the anemia associated with vitamin $B_{12}$ deficiency. However, folic acid administration does not prevent the development or progression of the neurologic manifestations of pernicious anemia. *(3)*

163. **(D)** Clomiphene citrate (Clomid) is a nonster-oidal estrogen agonist-antagonist that causes the hypothalamus to release gonadotropin-releasing hormone. This increases the periph-eral concentrations of FSH and LH and promotes ovulation. *(6)*

164. **(E)** Initial therapy of severe hyperkalemia should be the administration of calcium glu-conate since this will rapidly reverse the arrhythmias caused by hyperkalemia. Since calcium administration does not lower potas-sium levels, measures must be taken to lower extracellular levels of potassium. This can be accomplished with the use of insulin, which promotes the passage of potassium into cells. Sodium polystyrene sulfonate (Kayexalate), a cation-exchange resin may also be given orally or rectally to bind potassium in the GI tract. *(5)*

165. **(B)** Angiotensin converting enzyme (ACE) inhibitors such as benazepril and other *pril* drugs may increase serum creatinine levels. Serum creatinine concentration should be checked in all patients within 1 week of start-ing ACE inhibitor therapy, and rechecked if clinical conditions change or medications are changed. ACE inhibitor therapy should be stopped if the serum creatinine concentration increases by more than 1 mg/dL. *(6)*

166. **(E)** Whole blood treated with anticoagulant is centrifuged in a calibrated hematocrit tube. The volume ratio of the packed red blood cells to total blood volume is determined. The hemat-ocrit is normally 39–49 for men and 33–43 for women. It gives some indication of both the

number and size of the red blood cells present in an individual. *(5)*

167. **(E)** A reticulocyte is an immature erythrocyte. *(5)*

168. **(C)** Trimethoprim-sulfamethoxazole (Bactrim, Septra) is an effective combination for the treatment of otitis media. The other choices are either unlikely to be active against organisms that commonly cause otitis media or they are too toxic to use in young children. *(5)*

169. **(E)** Aspirin, ibuprofen, and acetaminophen are capable of reducing elevated body temperature by altering the hypothalamic setpoint. *(3)*

170. **(E)** Clozapine (Clozaril) is an antipsychotic agent that is used to treat patients with severe schizophrenia, who do not respond to standard antipsychotic treatment. The drug is capable of causing agranulocytosis, a potentially life-threatening adverse drug reaction. Patients who are to receive the drug should have a baseline white blood cell and differential count performed before the initiation of treatment. Once therapy has begun, a white blood cell count should be performed every week throughout treatment and for four weeks after the drug has been discontinued. *(3)*

171. **(B)** Zollinger-Ellison syndrome is a condition characterized by gastric acid hypersecretion and recurrent peptic ulceration. It is generally the result of a gastrin-producing tumor. The proton pump inhibitors such as pantoprazole are effective in managing the acid secretion in this condition. *(5)*

172. **(E)** The administration of a drug by intermittent (rather than continuous) IV injection is accomplished over a period of minutes (rather than hours). Stability and/or compatibility problems are less likely to occur because the drug does not remain in contact with a large-volume IV fluid for long periods of time. The potential for thrombophlebitis is reduced because the drug is not in constant contact with the blood vessel tissue at the site of the injection. Finally, the greater concentration gradient produced by a more rapid injection may promote better diffusion of some drugs into tissues. *(3)*

173. **(D)** Vinblastine (Velban), vinorelbine (Navelbine) and other vinca alkaloids such as vincristine (Oncovin) are considered to be mitotic inhibitors. *(5)*

174. **(E)** Aspirin should be avoided during the last trimester of pregnancy. Aspirin exerts a dose-dependent action on uric acid excretion. *(3)*

175. **(A)** Martindale's Extra Pharmacopoeia is probably one of the most comprehensive, international, single-volume references on drugs and drug products. Martindale's is divided into three parts: The first part consists of monographs on drugs and ancillary substances. (Although drugs that are manufactured in the United Kingdom are stressed, generic and proprietary products from many other countries are included.) The monographs include physiochemical data, storage, incompatibilities, uses, doses, and toxic effects. The second part contains a supplementary discussion of new drugs, obsolete drugs, and miscellaneous substances. The third part lists formulas of OTC products sold in the United Kingdom. There is also a directory of worldwide pharmaceutical manufacturers.

176. **(C)** A debriding agent is one that helps to remove necrotic material from a wound. Most are proteolytic or fibrinolytic enzymes. *(5)*

177. **(D)** Ceftriaxone (Rocephin) and cefotaxime (Claforan) are third generation cephalosporins while cefotetan is a second generation cephalosporin. Third generation cephalosporins are more effective in treating CNS infections, such as meningitis, because they penetrate the CNS better than first or second generation agents. *(3)*

178. **(C)** Penciclovir (Denavir) is an antiviral drug that is indicated specifically for the treatment of herpes labialis or cold sores. It is applied topically at the earliest sign of a fever blister and should be applied every 2 h, while awake, for

four days. If applied appropriately, this agent will generally reduce the severity and duration of cold sore symptoms. *(3)*

179. **(B)** Natamycin (Natacyn) is an antibiotic that has antifungal activity. It is used as an intraocular suspension for the treatment of fungal blepharitis, conjunctivitis, and keratitis. *(3)*

180. **(A)** Plantago (psyllium) is a bulk-forming laxative agent. Patients using it should mix the dose with a glass of water or other fluid and drink it down quickly. This should be followed with more fluids. *(3)*

181. **(D)** The relative concentration of different anions and cations varies considerably between intracellular and extracellular fluids of the body. Intracellular body fluids contain high concentrations of potassium (a cation) and phosphate (an anion), whereas extracellular fluid contains high concentrations of sodium (a cation) and chloride (an anion). *(3)*

182. **(B)** Acute toxicity associated with an overdose of the anticholinergic drug atropine sulfate should be treated by the administration of the cholinergic compound physostigmine. *(3)*

183. **(C)** There is a reciprocal relationship between the concentration of calcium and phosphorus in the blood. For example, hypoparathyroidism is characterized by low serum calcium and high serum phosphorus, whereas hyperparathyroidism is characterized by low serum phosphorus and high serum calcium. *(5)*

184. **(D)** Nicotine polacrilex contains nicotine bound to an ion exchange resin in a chewing gum base. It is used to assist smokers in their withdrawal from cigarette use. The drug may cause peripheral vasoconstriction, tachycardia and high blood pressure, so it should be avoided in patients with severe angina. The drug is also classified in pregnancy category X, meaning that it should not be used in pregnant women. *(3)*

185. **(C)** Acetaminophen is metabolized in the liver primarily by conjugation to glucuronide or sulfate metabolites. A small percentage is metabolized by the hepatic cytochrome P450 mixed-function oxidase system to a toxic intermediate metabolite. Normally, this metabolite is preferentially conjugated to glutathione and excreted in the urine. When large doses of acetaminophen are ingested, the glucuronide and sulfate pathways become saturated, and stores of glutathione become inadequate to conjugate the amount of toxic metabolite that is produced. The metabolite binds covalently to hepatocytes and produces hepatic necrosis. *(3)*

186. **(D)** Because the drug was ingested 6 h ago, the likelihood of removing a large amount of drug from this patient's stomach with ipecac syrup is small. Activated charcoal effectively binds acetaminophen if given soon after ingestion, but its use here is also unlikely to be of value because of the elapsed time. *N*-Acetylcysteine serves as a glutathione substitute that effectively binds the toxin and permits it to be excreted in the urine. *N*-Acetylcysteine is given orally or by lavage tube. *(5:78)*

187. **(C)** Because of the poor absorption of sulfasalazine from the GI tract, its localized activity is valuable as one of the first-line treatments for various forms of colitis and enteritis. The drug is available as an oral tablet and as a suspension. *(3)*

188. **(A)** Aspirin allergy in association with asthma is cause for serious concern. Asthma, rhinorrhea, and nasal polyps usually accompany this type of aspirin intolerance, which occurs in about 4–20% of asthmatic patients. These patients appear to exhibit a high degree of cross-reactivity to other NSAIDs, such as meloxicam. *(3)*

189. **(E)** Nonselective beta-adrenergic blocking agents may cause further bradycardia and may cause bronchoconstriction. In addition, the drugs may mask the effects of hypoglycemia, thereby placing type 1 diabetic patients at risk. *(3)*

190. **(B)** Torsemide (Demadex) is a loop diuretic that is capable of producing ototoxicity, which would enhance the similar toxicity produced by gentamicin. *(3)*

191. **(C)** Nitroprusside sodium (Nitropress) is a drug administered by IV infusion in the emergency treatment of acute hypertensive crisis. It causes a rapid fall in blood pressure by reducing both preload and afterload. The degree of blood pressure lowering can be controlled by adjusting the infusion rate of the drug. *(3)*

192. **(D)** Left ventricular failure is associated with bronchial edema, increased airway resistance and dyspnea. In addition, orthopnea (dyspnea that occurs while the patient is in the supine position) also often occurs. *(5)*

193. **(A)** For a healthy adult, values of <200 mg/dL are considered desirable levels of total cholesterol, <190 mg/dL for triglycerides and a value of <130 mg/dL is a desirable level for low density lipoproteins (LDL) cholesterol. Desireable levels may be considerably lower in patients with a history of cardiovascular disease. *(5)*

194. **(A)** Selegeline (Eldepryl) is an MAO-B inhibitor used to treat Parkinson's disease. It may interact with pressor amines such as tyramine in some cheeses, wines, and beers, to produce a hypertensive crisis that may be life threatening. *(3)*

195. **(C)** Frequent urination (polyuria) is a common symptom of diabetes mellitus. *(5)*

196. **(E)** Hyperphosphatemia associated with hypoparathyroidism can be effectively treated by administering calcium salts. Initially, IV calcium administration will correct the hypocalcemia these patients often experience. Oral calcium salts may also be administered to decrease GI absorption of phosphate. The administration of aluminum or magnesium hydroxide will result in GI binding of phosphate, thereby reducing serum phosphate levels. *(5)*

197. **(A)** Sotalol (Betapace) is used primarily for its ability to block beta-adrenergic activity, and is therefore useful in treating patients suffering from ventricular arrhythmias. However, because beta-adrenergic blockade also tends to increase airway resistance, the drug is usually contraindicated for use in patients suffering from asthma or severe allergies. *(3)*

198. **(E)** Bupropion (Wellbutrin) is indicated for the treatment of depression. The product Zyban is used as a smoking deterrent in smoking cessation programs and as an agent which assists narcotic-dependent individuals to become narcotic free. *(3)*

199. **(C)** Tardive (late-occurring) dyskinesia (involuntary muscular movements) is a drug-induced neurologic disorder that appears to be irreversible and unresponsive to drug treatment. It is characterized by involuntary movements of the lips, tongue, or jaw and is commonly observed as a smacking of the lips, rhythmical movement of the tongue, or facial grimaces. This disorder may be due to hypersensitivity of dopaminergic receptors to endogenous dopamine after long-term blockade by antipsychotic drugs.

   (A—incorrect) Akathisia is a feeling of restlessness or a compelling need for movement. *(5)*

200. **(B)** Valsartan (Diovan) is an angiotensin II-receptor antagonist. It is employed in the treatment of hypertension. *(3)*

201. **(A)** Zolpidem (Ambien) is a nonbarbiturate, nonbenzodiazepine hypnotic. *(3)*

202. **(D)** Olsalazine is a salicylate compound that is converted to 5-aminosalicylic acid (mesalamine) in the gut. This agent produces an anti-inflammatory effect in the gut. *(3)*

203. **(A)** Prednisone is approximately four times more potent than hydrocortisone. Because this patient was receiving a total daily dose of 200 mg of hydrocortisone, an equivalent anti-inflammatory dose of prednisone would be 50 mg/day. *(3)*

204. **(D)** Glucocorticoids associated with a lesser degree of mineralocorticoid activity (e.g., dexamethasone, triamcinolone, methylprednisolone, and betamethasone) should be used in patients with conditions such as congestive

heart failure in which sodium retention can be an aggravating factor. Because all glucocorticoids induce potassium loss, regardless of their mineralocorticoid activity, even dexamethasone should be used with caution in this patient. *(3)*

205. **(C)**  At the infusion rate of 50 mg/h, the patient receives a total daily dose of 1200 mg (50 mg/h × 24 h) of aminophylline dihydrate. Because aminophylline dihydrate contains the equivalent of 79% anhydrous theophylline, this patient receives a total daily dose of 948 mg anhydrous theophylline (0.79 × 1200 mg/day). The most practical dose of Theo-Dur would be 900 mg/day given in doses of 300 mg every 8 h. *(3)*

206. **(E)**  None of these agents would be appropriate for the treatment of acute bronchospastic attacks because they are only indicated for the prophylaxis of attacks. *(3)*

207. **(A)**  Choline salicylate (Arthropan) is a liquid salicylate dosage form that has a fishy odor. *(3)*

208. **(C)**  Lanoxicaps contain digoxin in a more bioavailable form than in digoxin tablets. A 20% reduction in dosage is generally required to achieve a comparable therapeutic response with Lanoxin tablets. *(3)*

209. **(A)**  Rifampin is a potent microsomal enzyme inducer and may reduce effectiveness of hormones supplied by oral contraceptive products. *(3)*

210. **(C)**  Bupropion (Zyban) and nicotine (Habitrol, Nicoderm, Nicotrol, ProStep) are products used to aid in smoking cessation programs. *(3)*

# CHAPTER 7

# Patient Profiles

The pharmacist, whether practicing in a community or an institutional setting, must constantly refer to patient profiles for information regarding the medical history of a specific patient. Analysis of profile data requires a strong knowledge base in the pharmacy disciplines already reviewed in this book.

In this section, there are 30 patient medication profiles. Some are related to community pharmacy practice and some to institutional practice.

# Questions

## Community Pharmacy Medication Record

Patient Name: David Rodgers
Address: 1604 Birch Road
Age: 55                    Race: African-American        Height: 5'8"
Sex: M                                                    Weight: 240 lb
History: Mother died of stroke at age 62; father died of MI at age 57

### DIAGNOSIS

| Primary | Secondary |
|---|---|
| 1. hypertension | 1. |
| 2. BPH | 2. |
| 3. | 3. |

### MEDICATION RECORD

| | Date | Rx No. | Physician | Drug & Strength | Quantity | Sig | Refills |
|---|---|---|---|---|---|---|---|
| 1. | 7/21 | 34325 | Jimes | HydroDIURIL 25 mg | 30 | 1 daily | 1 |
| 2. | 8/20 | 34325 | Jimes | refill | 30 | 1 daily | 0 |
| 3. | 9/18 | 37334 | Jimes | HydroDIURIL 25 mg | 30 | 1 daily | 2 |
| 4. | 9/18 | 37335 | Jimes | Diovan 40 mg | 30 | 1 daily | 2 |
| 5. | 10/14 | 37334 | Jimes | refill | 30 | 1 daily | 1 |
| 6. | 11/05 | 60478 | Henry | Proscar 5 mg | 30 | 1 daily | 2 |

### PHARMACIST'S NOTES AND OTHER PATIENT INFORMATION

| Date | Comment |
|---|---|
| 9/24 | Claritin-D # 5 OTC |

**DIRECTIONS (Questions 1a through 1l):** Each of the numbered items or incomplete statements in this section is followed by answers or by completions of the statement. Select the ONE lettered answer or completion that is BEST in each case.

1a. A drug product that is most similar in action to HydroDIURIL is

(A) chlorthalidone (Hygroton)

(B) acetazolamide (Diamox)

(C) torsemide (Demadex)

(D) hydroxyurea (Hydrea)

(E) ethacrynic acid (Edecrin)

**1b.** Which of the following lab tests would be useful in determining the presence of BPH?

(A) HbA1c

(B) TSH

(C) PUD

(D) CPK

(E) PSA

**1c.** Diovan can best be described as a (an)

(A) diuretic

(B) angiotensin II receptor blocker

(C) ACE inhibitor

(D) alpha$_1$-adrenergic blocker

(E) aldosterone blocker

**1d.** When using HydroDIURIL the patient should be advised to

I. take the dose at bedtime

II. restrict the intake of fluids while using the medication

III. take the dose with food or milk

(A) I only

(B) III only

(C) I and II only

(D) II and III only

(E) I, II, and III

**1e.** Proscar can best be described as a (an)

(A) prostaglandin antagonist

(B) antiandrogen

(C) prostaglandin analog

(D) antimitotic agent

(E) alpha$_1$-adrenergic blocker

**1f.** Which of the following is (are) an adverse effect of Proscar?

I. fetal damage

II. hirsutism

III. reflex tachycardia

(A) I only

(B) III only

(C) I and II only

(D) II and III only

(E) I, II, and III

**1g.** The chronic use of HydroDIURIL may result in the development of

I. hypomagnesemia

II. hypercalcemia

III. hypokalemia

(A) I only

(B) III only

(C) I and II only

(D) II and III only

(E) I, II, and III

**1h.** Patients who exhibit hypersensitivity to HydroDIURIL should avoid the use of

(A) aspirin

(B) COMT antagonists

(C) sulfa drugs

(D) MAO inhibitors

(E) selective serotonin reuptake inhibitors

**1i.** The pharmacist should advise Mr. Rodgers to

(A) take the Claritin-D three times a day

(B) avoid the use of Claritin-D

(C) avoid the use of potassium-rich foods

(D) avoid the concomitant use of HydroDIURIL and Diovan

(E) avoid vigorous exercise

**1j.** Which of the following is (are) indicated for the treatment of BPH?

I. Hytrin

II. Flomax

III. Inspra

(A) I only

(B) III only

(C) I and II only

(D) II and III only

(E) I, II, and III

**1k.** A patient is brought to the E.R. and diagnosed as having hypertensive emergency. Which of the following drugs is (are) appropriate for the treatment of this condition?

   I. nitroglycerin IV

   II. diazoxide

   III. nitroprusside

(A) I only

(B) III only

(C) I and II only

(D) II and III only

(E) I, II, and III

**1l.** The best choice for a pregnant woman who needs to be treated for essential hypertension is

(A) telmisartan (Micardis)

(B) hydrochlorothiazide (HydroDIURIL)

(C) epoprostenol (Flolan)

(D) propranolol (Inderal)

(E) methyldopa (Aldomet)

## ■ PROFILE NO. 2

### Community Pharmacy Medication Record

Patient Name: Mona Esperanto
Address: Good Samaritan Home
Age: 84                       Height: 5'4"
Sex: F                         Weight: 185 lb
Allergies: Codeine

### DIAGNOSIS

| Primary | Secondary |
|---|---|
| 1. Osteoarthritis | 1. |
| 2. Angina | 2. |
| 3. | 3. |

### MEDICATION RECORD

| Date | Rx No. | Physician | Drug & Strength | Quantity | Sig | Refills |
|---|---|---|---|---|---|---|
| 1. 4/12 | 34094 | Mouseau | Nitroglycerin 0.4 mg | 100 | prn | 5 |
| 2. 4/12 | 34095 | Mouseau | Vioxx 12.5 mg | 30 | 1 daily | 3 |

### PHARMACIST'S NOTES AND OTHER PATIENT INFORMATION

| Date | Comment |
|---|---|
| 1. 4/21 | Senokot Tablets (OTC)<br>Glucosamine/Chondroitin Capsules (OTC) |

**DIRECTIONS (Questions 2a through 2l): Each of the numbered items or incomplete statements in this section is followed by answers or by completions of the statement. Select the ONE lettered answer or completion that is BEST in each case.**

**2a.** Vioxx is an example of a (an)

   I. COX-2 inhibitor

   II. NSAID

   III. coronary vasodilator

   (A) I only

   (B) III only

   (C) I and II only

   (D) II and III only

   (E) I, II, and III

**2b.** Vioxx should NOT be prescribed for a patient with a

   (A) $CL_{CR} < 25$

   (B) $HR < 60$

   (C) $BP < 100$

   (D) $FPG < 65$

   (E) $HDL < 40$

**2c.** Nitroglycerin sublingual tablets must be

   I. refrigerated

   II. discarded within 30 days after opening the container

   III. packaged in a glass container

   (A) I only

   (B) III only

   (C) I and II only

   (D) II and III only

   (E) I, II, and III

**2d.** Another name for vasospastic angina is

    (A)  Renfeld's angina

    (B)  Pauling's angina

    (C)  Babinski's angina

    (D)  Carlton's angina

    (E)  Prinzmetal's angina

**2e.** Glucosamine/chondroitin is a (an)

    (A)  vasodilator

    (B)  anti-inflammatory

    (C)  cartilage enhancer

    (D)  treatment for hypoglycemia

    (E)  treatment for hyperglycemia

**2f.** After using Vioxx for several weeks, Ms. Esperanto develops GI upset. Which of the following would be helpful in reducing this problem?

    (A)  administer Cytoxan

    (B)  recommmend that Daypro be used instead of Vioxx

    (C)  take the Vioxx on an empty stomach

    (D)  administer Cytotec

    (E)  recommend that Vioxx doses be taken at bedtime

**2g.** Which of the following is (are) NOT an effect associated with the use of nitroglycerin sublingual tablets?

    I.  hypertension

    II.  headache

    III.  a burning sensation under the tongue

    (A)  I only

    (B)  III only

    (C)  I and II only

    (D)  II and III only

    (E)  I, II, and III

**2h.** Which of the following is NOT a dosage form of nitroglycerin?

    (A)  ointment

    (B)  suspension

    (C)  transdermal system

    (D)  transmucosal tablet

    (E)  sustained-release capsule

**2i.** Ms. Esperanto's physician wishes to replace the Vioxx with a different oral analgesic product. Which of the following would be a suitable analgesic for this patient?

    (A)  Parlodel

    (B)  Ultram

    (C)  Ativan

    (D)  Comtan

    (E)  Humira

**2j.** The active ingredient of Senokot can best be described as a (an)

    (A)  amylase inhibitor

    (B)  intestinal lubricant

    (C)  anthraquinone glycoside

    (D)  pyrimidine analog

    (E)  lactase inhibitor

**2k.** An appropriate method for using Nitrolingual Spray is

    (A)  spray 1 or 2 doses onto or under the tongue

    (B)  inhale once p.r.n.

    (C)  inhale 1–2 times p.r.n.

    (D)  inhale 1–2 times three times daily

    (E)  spray once into each nostril

**2l.** When using nitroglycerin sublingual tablets the patient should be advised to avoid the use of

    I.  alcohol

    II.  acetaminophen

    III.  aspirin

    (A)  I only

    (B)  III only

    (C)  I and II only

    (D)  II and III only

    (E)  I, II, and III

# ■ PROFILE NO. 3

## Community Pharmacy Medication Record

Patient Name: Melissa Smith
Address: 165 West Street
Age: 29                                  Height: 5'3"
Sex: F                                   Weight: 120 lb
Allergies: Aspirin

### DIAGNOSIS

| Primary | Secondary |
|---|---|
| 1. Generalized tonic-clonic seizures since age 8 | 1. Constipation |
| 2. | 2. |
| 3. | 3. |

### MEDICATION RECORD

| Date | Rx No. | Physician | Drug & Strength | Quantity | Sig | Refills |
|---|---|---|---|---|---|---|
| 1. 1/2 | 32601 | Mazur | Plan B | 1 | As directed | 0 |
| 2. 2/2 | 34568 | Mazur | Nor Q.D. | 1 | 1 daily | 3 |
| 3. 3/1 | 34568 | Mazur | Refill | | | 2 |
| 4. 3/21 | 35908 | Wilson | Dilantin Kapseals. 0.1 | C | 3 daily | 2 |

### PHARMACIST'S NOTES AND OTHER PATIENT INFORMATION

| Date | Comment |
|---|---|
| 1. 4/2 | Koromex Cream 1 pk (OTC) |
| 2. 4/2 | Centrum Tablets #C (OTC) |
| 2. 4/9 | Colace 100 mg #100 (OTC) |

**DIRECTIONS (Questions 3a through 3q):** Each of the numbered items or incomplete statements in this section is followed by answers or by completions of the statement. Select the ONE lettered answer or completion that is BEST in each case.

**3a.** Nor-QD can best be described as a (an)

(A) vaginal deodorant product
(B) progestin-only oral contraceptive
(C) biphasic oral contraceptive
(D) ovulation inducer
(E) triphasic oral contraceptive

**3b.** Koromex Cream is employed as a

(A) antibacterial
(B) lubricant
(C) antifungal
(D) spermicide
(E) herpes treatment

**3c.** A synonym for generalized tonic-clonic seizures is

(A) Jacksonian seizures
(B) absence seizures
(C) grand mal seizures
(D) status epilepticus
(E) focal seizures

**3d.** Which of the following drugs would be considered to be reasonable alternative drugs to phenytoin for the treatment of this patient's seizures?

    I. lamotrigine
   II. carbamazepine
  III. valproic acid

    (A) I only
    (B) III only
    (C) I and II only
    (D) II and III only
    (E) I, II, and III

**3e.** The Dilantin product prescribed may be administered

    I. in three divided daily doses
   II. as a single daily dose
  III. on a p.r.n. basis

    (A) I only
    (B) III only
    (C) I and II only
    (D) II and III only
    (E) I, II, and III

**3f.** In the course of receiving Dilantin the patient develops gingival hyperplasia. This is a disorder of the

    (A) gums
    (B) cardiac rhythm
    (C) eye
    (D) hematological system
    (E) liver

**3g.** Which of the following is associated with the use of phenytoin?

    (A) pseudomembranous enterocolitis
    (B) myelosuppression
    (C) cheilosis
    (D) first-pass effect
    (E) Michaelis-Menten kinetics

**3h.** A plasma phenytoin determination reveals a plasma concentration of 5 µg/mL. This indicates that

    (A) hepatic impairment may exist
    (B) the patient may not be taking all prescribed doses
    (C) the concentration is within the therapeutic range
    (D) the patient may have renal impairment
    (E) the patient may be taking more doses than prescribed

**3i.** The prescriber should be called because of

    (A) cross-sensitivity between Colace and Dilantin
    (B) carcinogenicity with Dilantin
    (C) reduction in Dilantin effectiveness
    (D) reduction in Nor-QD effectiveness
    (E) improper Dilantin dose prescribed

**3j.** Which of the following is a phenytoin prodrug?

    (A) Mysoline
    (B) Lamictal
    (C) Cerebyx
    (D) Monurol
    (E) Gabitril

**3k.** Which of the following is true of parenterally administered Dilantin?

    I. Dilantin parenteral solutions must be kept refrigerated until just prior to administration.
   II. Precipitation is likely to occur when Dilantin is combined with B-complex with C in an IV admixture.
  III. IM administration should generally be avoided.

    (A) I only
    (B) III only
    (C) I and II only
    (D) II and III only
    (E) I, II, and III

**3l.** Patients receiving Dilantin may develop a morbilliform rash. Morbilliform refers to

    (A) measles-like
    (B) butterfly-shaped

(C) unilateral

(D) acne-like

(E) multicolored

**3m.** Which of the following drugs would be appropriate to use in the treatment of status epilepticus?

I. propofol

II. midazolam

III. lorazepam

(A) I only

(B) III only

(C) I and II only

(D) II and III only

(E) I, II, and III

**3n.** A patient on long-term phenytoin therapy should receive supplements of

(A) ascorbic acid

(B) iron

(C) calcium

(D) folic acid

(E) inositol

**3o.** The active ingredient of Koromex Cream is

(A) hexachlorophene

(B) nonoxynol-9

(C) oxyquinoline sulfate

(D) sodium lauryl sulfate

(E) benzalkonium chloride

**3p.** The active ingredient in Colace is a (an)

(A) nonionic surfactant

(B) coprecipitated laxative

(C) cationic surfactant

(D) osmotic laxative

(E) anionic surfactant

**3q.** An ingredient of Centrum is lycopene. The purpose of this ingredient is to

(A) improve prostate health

(B) reduce the likelihood of osteoporosis

(C) prevent urinary infection

(D) lower blood sugar

(E) prevent hemolysis

# PROFILE NO. 4

## Community Pharmacy Medication Record

Patient Name: David O'Meara
Address: 978 Fannin Road
Age: 72                          Height: 5'10"
Sex: M                           Weight: 191 lb
Allergies:

### DIAGNOSIS

| Primary | Secondary |
|---|---|
| 1. Parkinson's disease | 1. |
| 2. | 2. |
| 3. | 3. |

### MEDICATION RECORD

| Date | Rx No. | Physician | Drug & Strength | Quantity | Sig | Refills |
|---|---|---|---|---|---|---|
| 1. 2/3 | 56445 | Mosely | Sinemet 10/100 | C | 1 t.i.d. | 2 |
| 2. 3/1 | 56445 | Mosely | Refill | | | |
| 3. 3/19 | 59008 | Mosely | Sinemet 25/250 | C | t.i.d. | 2 |
| 4. 3/19 | 59009 | Mosely | Akineton 2 mg | 90 | 1 t.i.d. | 2 |
| 5. 4/15 | 59008 | Mosely | Refill | | | |
| 6. 4/15 | 61122 | Mosely | Comtan 200 mg | 60 | 1 t.i.d. | 3 |

**DIRECTIONS (Questions 4a through 4l):** Each of the numbered items or incomplete statements in this section is followed by answers or by completions of the statement. Select the ONE lettered answer or completion that is BEST in each case.

**4a.** The function of carbidopa in the Sinemet formulation is to

(A) act as a prodrug for levodopa
(B) inhibit peripheral decarboxylation of levodopa
(C) act as an MAO inhibitor
(D) inhibit decarboxylation of levodopa in the CNS
(E) act as a COMT inhibitor

**4b.** Patients receiving levodopa should avoid using vitamin supplements that contain

(A) iron
(B) calcium
(C) folic acid
(D) pyridoxine
(E) cyanocobalamin

**4c.** A patient using Sinemet complains of an appreciable darkening of the urine beginning about three days after starting Sinemet therapy. The pharmacist should tell the patient to

(A) disregard the discoloration because it is not harmful
(B) check the expiration date on the Sinemet container to make sure it has not expired
(C) immediately stop taking the Sinemet and call the prescriber

(D)  avoid the use of acidic foods while on Sinemet

(E)  avoid the use of alkaline foods while on Sinemet

**4d.**  Akineton has been prescribed because of its action as a (an)

(A)  centrally-acting skeletal muscle relaxant

(B)  anticholinergic

(C)  peripheral vasodilator

(D)  memory enhancer

(E)  sedative

**4e.**  Which of the following is NOT employed in the treatment of Parkinson's disease?

(A)  tiagibene (Gabitril)

(B)  selegiline (Eldepryl)

(C)  pergolide (Permax)

(D)  bromocriptine (Parlodel)

(E)  tolcapone (Tasmar)

**4f.**  After several months of being well controlled on Sinemet, the patient experiences a relapse. This is likely due to

(A)  neuroleptic malignant syndrome

(B)  an interaction with Akineton

(C)  the first-pass effect

(D)  the on-off effect

(E)  entero-hepatic cycling

**4g.**  Diplopia is an adverse effect related to the use of levodopa. This can best be described as

(A)  double vision

(B)  a facial tic

(C)  hearing loss

(D)  loss of taste sensation

(E)  a cardiac tachyarrhythmia

**4h.**  When a patient on levodopa is to be switched to Sinemet, which of the following is (are) true?

I.  Permit at least 8 h to elapse between the last dose of levodopa and the first dose of Sinemet.

II.  The daily levodopa dose in the Sinemet should be 25% lower than when levodopa is used alone.

III.  Plasma levodopa levels must be measured each day for the first five days of Sinemet therapy.

(A)  I only

(B)  III only

(C)  I and II only

(D)  II and III only

(E)  I, II, and III

**4i.**  The prolonged use of which of the following drugs is associated with Parkinson-like symptoms?

(A)  citalopram (Celexa)

(B)  raloxifene (Evista)

(C)  chlorpromazine (Thorazine)

(D)  methylphenidate (Ritalin)

(E)  paroxetine (Paxil)

**4j.**  Which one of the following products may be used to provide individual doses of carbidopa?

(A)  Tegretol

(B)  Lodosyn

(C)  Larobec

(D)  Dopar

(E)  Permax

**4k.** An adverse effect associated with the use of Akineton is

(A) aplastic anemia

(B) nyctalopia

(C) the first-dose effect

(D) hyperhidrosis

(E) constipation

**4l.** A patient using selegiline (Eldepryl) for the treatment of Parkinson's disease should be advised to avoid

I. cheese

II. wine

III. nasal decongestants

(A) I only

(B) III only

(C) I and II only

(D) II and III only

(E) I, II and III

# ■ PROFILE NO. 5

## Community Pharmacy Medication Record

Patient Name: Melissa Durgan
Address: 2114 Laughlin Road
Age: 68
Sex: F
Allergies: Pollen, penicillin

Height: 5'4"
Weight: 167 lb

### DIAGNOSIS

| Primary | Secondary |
|---|---|
| 1. Open-angle glaucoma, primary | 1. |
| 2. Emphysema | 2. |
| 3. | 3. |

### MEDICATION RECORD

| Date | Rx No. | Physician | Drug & Strength | Quantity | Sig | Refills |
|---|---|---|---|---|---|---|
| 1. 7/29 | 59083 | Weber | Timoptic-XE 0.25% | 5 mL | gtt 1 os daily | 2 |
| 2. 8/20 | 59083 | Weber | Refill | | | |
| 3. 9/11 | 65002 | Weber | Betagan 0.5% | 10 mL | gtt 1 os b.i.d. | 2 |
| 4. 10/21 | 65002 | Weber | Lumigan 0.03% | 2.5 mL | gtt 1 os daily | 1 |

### PHARMACIST'S NOTES AND OTHER PATIENT INFORMATION

| Date | Comment |
|---|---|
| 1. 9/14 | Orudis-KT (OTC) |
| 2. 10/7 | Visine Allergy Relief (OTC) |

**DIRECTIONS (Questions 5a through 5l):** Each of the numbered items or incomplete statements in this section is followed by answers or by completions of the statement. Select the ONE lettered answer or completion that is BEST in each case.

5a. The primary action of Timoptic-XE in the treatment of glaucoma is as a (an)

    I. mydriatic

   II. cycloplegic

  III. beta-adrenergic blocker

(A) I only

(B) III only

(C) I and II only

(D) II and III only

(E) I, II, and III

5b. Timoptic is most similar in pharmacologic action to

(A) levobetaxolol

(B) acetazolamide

(C) dipivefrin

(D) propofol

(E) carbachol

**5c.** Several weeks after using Timoptic-XE, the patient's intraocular pressure is measured as 14 mmHg. This indicates that

(A) the patient's intraocular pressure is under control
(B) the patient has narrow-angle glaucoma
(C) an error in measurement must have occurred
(D) the dose of Timoptic-XE should be increased
(E) the dose of Timoptic-XE should be decreased

**5d.** The Timoptic-XE dosage form can best be described as a (an)

(A) suspension
(B) emulsion
(C) liposome dispersion
(D) gel-forming solution
(E) microsomal dispersion

**5e.** The use of Timoptic has been reported to produce urticaria in some patients. Another name for urticaria is

(A) hair loss
(B) hives
(C) tooth decay
(D) abnormal hair growth
(E) cold extremities

**5f.** Acetazolamide is sometimes indicated for the treatment of glaucoma. Which of the following best describes the mechanism of action of this drug?

(A) miotic
(B) carbonic anhydrase inhibitor
(C) tocolytic
(D) mydriatic
(E) cycloplegic

**5g.** Which of the following is (are) likely to be adverse effects associated with the use of bimatoprost (Lumigan)?

I. cataracts
II. retinitis pigmentosa
III. conjunctival hyperemia

(A) I only
(B) III only
(C) I and II only
(D) II and III only
(E) I, II, and III

**5h.** Betagan ophthalmic solution contains edetate disodium. Which of the following best describes the function of this agent in this product?

(A) buffer
(B) antibacterial
(C) antifungal
(D) viscosity builder
(E) metal scavenger

**5i.** The patient returns to the pharmacy to purchase more Orudis-KT. If the pharmacy was out of Orudis-KT which of the following products could the pharmacist recommend as the closest substitute?

(A) Datril
(B) Advil
(C) Actron
(D) Aleve
(E) Haltran

**5j.** The Visine Allergy Relief purchased OTC by this patient contains a

(A) beta$_1$ agonist
(B) beta$_2$ agonist
(C) alpha$_1$ agonist
(D) alpha$_2$ agonist
(E) beta$_1$ antagonist

**5k.** The pharmacist should contact the prescriber to discuss the possibility of

(A) blood dyscrasias
(B) respiratory distress
(C) urinary retention
(D) interaction between Timoptic-XE and Betagan
(E) interaction between Timoptic-XE and Lumigan

**5l.** Patients with glaucoma should avoid drugs that are

(A) sympathomimetics
(B) broad-spectrum antimicrobial agents
(C) anticholinergics
(D) potassium depleters
(E) peripheral vasodilators

# ■   PROFILE NO. 6

## Community Pharmacy Medication Record

Patient Name: Carlos Machueta
Address: 701 North Oak Road
Age: 19                          Height: 5'10"
Sex: M                           Weight: 165 lb
Allergies: Penicillin

### DIAGNOSIS

| Primary | Secondary |
|---|---|
| 1. Acne vulgaris—cystic | 1. |
| 2. | 2. |
| 3. | 3. |

### MEDICATION RECORD

| Date | Rx No. | Physician | Drug & Strength | Quantity | Sig | Refills |
|---|---|---|---|---|---|---|
| 1. 6/7 | 45023 | Thomas | Benzac 5 Gel | 45 g | ut dict | 3 |
| 2. 6/22 | 48399 | Wilson | Retin-A Micro | 20 g | Apply p.r.n. | 2 |
| 3. 7/13 | 45023 | Thomas | Refill | | | 2 |
| 4. 8/24 | 45023 | Thomas | Refill | | | 1 |
| 5. 9/17 | 57888 | Wilson | Cleocin T Gel | 30 g | Apply topically | 3 |
| 6. 10/5 | 59778 | Thomas | Accutane  20 mg | 60 | 1 b.i.d. | 5 |

### PHARMACIST'S NOTES AND OTHER PATIENT INFORMATION

| Date | Comment |
|---|---|
| 1. 7/1 | Brasivol Medium |
| 2. 7/30 | Pernox Scrub 60 mL |

**DIRECTIONS (Questions 6a through 6m): Each of the numbered items or incomplete statements in this section is followed by answers or by completions of the statement. Select the ONE lettered answer or completion that is BEST in each case.**

**6a.**   The active ingredient in Benzac is

(A)  budesonide

(B)  benzoyl peroxide

(C)  isotretinoin

(D)  benzyl alcohol

(E)  benzalkonium chloride

**6b.**   Patients using Retin-A should avoid

  I.   use of antimicrobial agents

  II.  having the product come in contact with their eyes

III.  excessive sunlight

(A)  I only

(B)  III only

(C)  I and II only

(D)  II and III only

(E)  I, II, and III

**6c.**   Retin-A liquid contains butylated hydroxytoluene. The function of this ingredient is as a (an)

(A)  antioxidant

(B)  solvent

(C)  abrasive

(D) chelating agent

(E) viscosity builder

**6d.** Retin-A Micro is a product that is only available as a (an)

(A) water-soluble cream

(B) gel

(C) water-insoluble cream

(D) micronized powder

(E) ointment

**6e.** Which of the following adverse effects is associated with the systemic use of Cleocin?

(A) hemorrhagic cystitis

(B) crystalluria

(C) diarrhea

(D) photosensitivity

(E) aplastic anemia

**6f.** The Cleocin-T product contains 10 mg of clindamycin per milliliter and is available in a 30-mL package size. This means that the strength of clindamycin in the solution is

(A) 0.1%

(B) 3%

(C) 1%

(D) 10%

(E) 0.3%

**6g.** Accutane is most closely related to

(A) pantothenic acid

(B) ascorbic acid

(C) ergocalciferol

(D) beta-carotene

(E) cyanocobalamin

**6h.** Which of the following is (are) common adverse effects associated with the use of Accutane?

I. chelitis

II. conjunctivitis

III. hyperlipidemia

(A) I only

(B) III only

(C) I and II only

(D) II and III only

(E) I, II, and III

**6i.** On dispensing Accutane, the pharmacist must provide the patient with a (an)

I. informed consent form

II. "refrigerate" label

III. patient package insert

(A) I only

(B) III only

(C) I and II only

(D) II and III only

(E) I, II, and III

**6j.** Acne can best be described as a (an)

(A) inflammatory response to free fatty acids

(B) allergic response

(C) infection

(D) autoimmune disease

(E) dermatological response to excessive intake of dietary fats

**6k.** Brasivol contains aluminum oxide. This ingredient is employed in this product as a (an)

(A) neutralizing agent

(B) astringent

(C) oxidizing agent

(D) abrasive

(E) desiccating agent

**6l.** Pernox scrub contains salicylic acid. This ingredient is employed in this product as a (an)

(A) antiseptic

(B) keratolytic

(C) antioxidant

(D) buffer

(E) astringent

**6m.** Patients with acne often secrete large amounts of

(A) lactic acid

(B) dihydrotachysterol

(C) pectin

(D) sebum

(E) cerumen

# ■ PROFILE NO. 7

## Community Pharmacy Medication Record

Patient Name: Jennifer Masterson
Address: 42 Placid Lane
Age: 25                              Height: 5'4"
Sex: F                               Weight: 135 lb
Allergies:

### DIAGNOSIS

| Primary | Secondary |
|---------|-----------|
| 1. Asthma | 1. |
| 2. IBS | 2. |
| 3. | 3. |

### MEDICATION RECORD

| Date | Rx No. | Physician | Drug & Strength | Quantity | Sig | Refills |
|------|--------|-----------|-----------------|----------|-----|---------|
| 1. 6/19 | 40098 | Tisch | Singulair 10 mg | 30 | p.r.n. | 2 |
| 2. 7/7 | 40098 | Tisch | Refill | | | 1 |
| 3. 8/1 | 46443 | Tisch | Proventil Aero. | 17 g | p.r.n. | 2 |
| 4. 8/1 | 46444 | Tisch | Vanceril Aerosol | 1 | p.r.n. | 1 |
| 5. 9/22 | 48998 | Tisch | Levsin/SL 0.125 | 60 | p.r.n. | 2 |

### PHARMACIST'S NOTES AND OTHER PATIENT INFORMATION

| Date | Comment |
|------|---------|
| 1. | Patient smokes 2 packs of cigarettes daily. |
| 2. 9/1 | Habitrol Patches 7 mg—1 box OTC |

DIRECTIONS (Questions 7a through 7l): Each of the numbered items or incomplete statements in this section is followed by answers or by completions of the statement. Select the ONE lettered answer or completion that is BEST in each case.

7a. The active ingredient in Singulair is most similar to the active ingredient in

(A) Serevent
(B) Ventolin
(C) Accolate
(D) Intal
(E) Flovent

7b. In an acute asthmatic attack, the patient uses one dose of Singulair and, after 5 min, still has not been relieved. The patient should be advised to

(A) go to the local emergency room immediately
(B) administer a second dose of Singulair if relief is not evident
(C) use the Proventil Aerosol product instead of the Singulair
(D) breathe into a brown bag for 6 min to increase the respiratory concentration of carbon dioxide
(E) inhale steam in order to facilitate the action of the Singulair

**7c.** In reviewing the patient's profile, it is evident that the prescriber needs to be contacted because which of the following is NOT properly prescribed?

    I. Singulair

    II. Vanceril

    III. Levsin

(A) I only

(B) III only

(C) I and II only

(D) II and III only

(E) I, II, and III

**7d.** The Proventil Aerosol product contains
(A) bitolterol
(B) albuterol
(C) ipratropium bromide
(D) terbutaline
(E) zafirlukast

**7e.** When using Proventil Aerosol in an elderly patient, it may be necessary to use a

(A) beta-adrenergic blocking agent with ISA

(B) nasal cannula

(C) spacer device

(D) nebulizer

(E) Busher injector

**7f.** In addition to an aerosol product, Proventil is also available as a (an)

    I. powder for inhalation

    II. oral liquid

    III. oral tablets

(A) I only

(B) III only

(C) I and II only

(D) II and III only

(E) I, II, and III

**7g.** Rotacaps are

(A) capsules that contain a powder for inhalation

(B) oral capsules that must be emptied into food before use

(C) sustained-release capsules

(D) enteric-coated capsules

(E) capsules containing ingredients separated by a semipermeable membrane

**7h.** The active ingredient in Vanceril can best be described as a (an)

(A) respiratory surfactant

(B) leukotriene receptor antagonist

(C) corticosteroid

(D) bronchodilator

(E) anticholinergic

**7i.** When Proventil Aerosol and Vanceril Aerosol have been prescribed to be used at the same time

(A) the Vanceril should be used first

(B) the patient should be advised to rinse her mouth with water immediately before administering the first drug product

(C) the Proventil should be used first

(D) a saline aerosol should be administered first

(E) the prescriber must be contacted to discuss the drug interaction that will occur

**7j.** Which of the following is true of Habitrol Patches?

    I. They are applied for a 24-h period.

    II. They contain the same active ingredient as Nicoderm.

    III. The area to which they are to be applied should be moistened before use.

(A) I only

(B) III only

(C) I and II only

(D) II and III only

(E) I, II, and III

**7k.** An advantage of albuterol over isoproterenol is

(A) availability in a parenteral as well as an inhalation dosage form

(B) more rapid onset of action when inhaled

(C) fewer cardiac effects

(D) no need for refrigeration prior to use

(E) asthmatic control with single daily dosing

**7l.** Vanceril is most similar to

(A) Atrovent

(B) Tornalate

(C) Beclovent

(D) Maxair

(E) Sustaire

■ PROFILE NO. 8

## Community Pharmacy Medication Record

Patient Name: Monica Perez
Address: 404 North Diamond Fork Rd
Age: 68                                    Height: 5'4"
Sex: F                                      Weight: 170 lb
Allergies:

### DIAGNOSIS

| Primary | Secondary |
|---|---|
| 1. Chronic stable angina | 1. |
| 2. Chronic alcoholism | 2. |
| 3. | 3. |

### MEDICATION RECORD

| Date | Rx No. | Physician | Drug & Strength | Quantity | Sig | Refills |
|---|---|---|---|---|---|---|
| 1. 1/14 | 40952 | Krajec | Nitrostat 0.4 mg | C | p.r.n. | 3 |
| 2. 1/30 | 42772 | Krajec | Nitro-Dur 0.1 | 30 | Apply daily | 5 |
| 3. 2/26 | 42772 | Krajec | Refill | | | 4 |
| 4. 3/16 | 42772 | Krajec | Refill | | | 3 |
| 5. 4/7 | 42772 | Krajec | Refill | | | 2 |
| 6. 4/28 | 50632 | Krajec | Nitrolingual Spray | 1 | p.r.n. | 2 |
| 7. 4/28 | 50633 | Krajec | Tranxene 7.5 mg | 30 | 1 t.i.d. | 2 |
| 8. 4/28 | 50634 | Krajec | Persantine 25 mg | 90 | 1 t.i.d. | 3 |

### PHARMACIST'S NOTES AND OTHER PATIENT INFORMATION

| Date | Comment |
|---|---|
| 1. 3/2 | Dristan Tabs (OTC) |

**DIRECTIONS (Questions 8a through 8k): Each of the numbered items or incomplete statements in this section is followed by answers or by completions of the statement. Select the ONE lettered answer or completion that is BEST in each case.**

**8a.** An advantage of Nitrostat over many other sublingual nitroglycerin products is that it is

(A) available in color-coded tablets

(B) less subject to potency loss

(C) more rapidly absorbed

(D) effective when used orally as well as sublingually

(E) longer acting

**8b.** Nitrostat should be dispensed

I. in its original container

II. in quantities not greater than 25 tablets

III. with a "Refrigerate" auxiliary label

(A) I only

(B) III only

(C) I and II only

(D) II and III only

(E) I, II, and III

**8c.** The patient should be advised to apply the Nitro-Dur to

   I. the distal parts of the extremities
  II. only onto the chest close to the heart
 III. a hairless site

  (A) I only
  (B) III only
  (C) I and II only
  (D) II and III only
  (E) I, II, and III

**8d.** When discontinuing therapy with Nitro-Dur

  (A) the dosage and frequency of application should be reduced gradually over a four to six-week period
  (B) the dosage and frequency of application should be reduced gradually over a three-day period
  (C) the number of hours per day that it is applied should be reduced gradually over seven days
  (D) severe nausea and vomiting may occur
  (E) the patient should be advised to take prophylactic aspirin doses for two weeks prior to discontinuation

**8e.** An antianginal product administered by inhalation is

  (A) pentaerythritol tetranitrate
  (B) nitrolingual spray
  (C) erythritol tetranitrate
  (D) isosorbide dinitrate
  (E) amyl nitrite

**8f.** In addition to being employed in the treatment of angina, dipyridamole (Persantine) is also used as a (an)

  (A) antiviral
  (B) antiarrhythmic
  (C) antimalarial
  (D) antihypertensive
  (E) antiplatelet

**8g.** The reason why nitroglycerin products are generally NOT administered orally is because nitroglycerin

  (A) will decompose rapidly in stomach acid
  (B) it can cause GERD
  (C) is decomposed rapidly by pepsin
  (D) is poorly absorbed from the GI tract
  (E) undergoes rapid first-pass deactivation

**8h.** Patients using nitroglycerin should be advised to AVOID the use of

   I. antiplatelet drugs
  II. sildenafil
 III. alcohol

  (A) I only
  (B) III only
  (C) I and II only
  (D) II and III only
  (E) I, II, and III

**8i.** Solutions of nitroglycerin intended for IV administration should be

  (A) refrigerated until 30 min prior to administration
  (B) kept covered with an opaque shield to protect it from decomposition
  (C) warmed for 15 min prior to infusion to dissolve crystalline material
  (D) given only by rapid IV injection
  (E) administered using the administration set provided by the manufacturer

**8j.** When nitroglycerin topical ointment is administered

   I. it should be rubbed into the skin until no further ointment is evident on the skin surface

  II. the area to which it is applied should not be occluded

 III. the dose is measured in inches

(A) I only

(B) III only

(C) I and II only

(D) II and III only

(E) I, II, and III

**8k.** The most rapid onset of action is likely to occur with the use of

(A) Nitro-Dur

(B) Nitrolingual spray

(C) Minitran

(D) Nitrogard

(E) Nitrodisc

# ▪ PROFILE NO. 9

## Community Pharmacy Medication Record

Patient Name: Wilma Tobin
Address: 40610 Via Roma
Age: 59                                    Height: 5'4"
Sex: F                                     Weight: 145 lb
Allergies: Sulfas

### DIAGNOSIS

| Primary | Secondary |
| --- | --- |
| 1. Type I diabetes mellitus | 1. |
| 2. | 2. |
| 3. | 3. |

### MEDICATION RECORD

| Date | Rx No. | Physician | Drug & Strength | Quantity | Sig | Refills |
| --- | --- | --- | --- | --- | --- | --- |
| 1. 9/11 | 29087 | Madison | Humulin R 100 U | 10 mL | 24 U q a.m. | 5 |
| 2. 9/11 | 29088 | Madison | Humulin N 100 U | 10 mL | 30 U mixed with Humulin R q a.m. | 5 |
| 3. 9/11 | 29089 | Madison | B-D Lo-Dose Syringes | 100 | | 5 |
| 4. 9/11 | 29090 | Madison | Glucometer Elite | 1 | As directed | |

### PHARMACIST'S NOTES AND OTHER PATIENT INFORMATION

| Date | Comment |
| --- | --- |
| 1. 9/1 | Theragran M  #100 |
| 2. 9/11 | Glucometer Elite Reagent Strips |
| 3. 9/20 | Sudafed Tablets 60 mg #24 (OTC) |

**DIRECTIONS (Questions 9a through 9o):** Each of the numbered items or incomplete statements in this section is followed by answers or by completions of the statement. Select the ONE lettered answer or completion that is BEST in each case.

**9a.** The term "type 1 diabetes mellitus" is also referred to as

(A)  diabetes insipidus

(B)  insulin-dependent diabetes mellitus

(C)  adult-onset diabetes mellitus

(D)  insulin-resistant diabetes mellitus

(E)  brittle diabetes mellitus

**9b.** Which of the following is (are) true of Humulin R?

I.  It is prepared by recombinant DNA technology.

II.  It is a clear solution.

III.  It is derived from a porcine source.

(A)  I only

(B)  III only

(C)  I and II only

(D)  II and III only

(E)  I, II, and III

**9c.** Which of the following is true of the measurement of the 24 U Humulin R dose?

(A) The patient must withdraw 0.24 mL from the Humulin R vial.

(B) The patient must withdraw 2.4 mL from the Humulin R vial.

(C) The amount the patient must withdraw from the vial depends on the volume of the syringe.

(D) 24 U is an excessive dose and should not be used.

(E) Precise measurement of 24 U cannot be made with an insulin syringe.

**9d.** In examining the patient, the physician notes that the patient complains of polydipsia. This refers to

(A) overgrowth of subcutaneous fat in the area of insulin injection

(B) excessive thirst

(C) excessive weight gain

(D) excessive urination

(E) excessive appetite

**9e.** Which of the following would be considered a normal fasting blood glucose level for this patient?

(A) 90 mg/L

(B) 100 μg/L

(C) 80 μg/dL

(D) 1 μg/mL

(E) 85 mg/dL

**9f.** Which of the following insulins is (are) suitable for administration by IV infusion?

I. aspart

II. lispro

III. regular

(A) I only

(B) III only

(C) I and II only

(D) II and III only

(E) I, II, and III

**9g.** In mixing the insulins prescribed, the patient should be advised

(A) to draw up the Humulin R first

(B) that the mixture may be stored in the syringe for up to one month if kept frozen

(C) that the mixture may be stored in the syringe for up to one month if kept refrigerated

(D) to draw up the Humulin N first

(E) that mixing these insulins is not advisable and the prescriber should be notified

**9h.** Which of the following insulins has the most rapid onset of action?

(A) NPH

(B) Regular

(C) Lispro

(D) Lantus

(E) Semilente

**9i.** Which of the following insulins does NOT have a pH of 7.4?

(A) Aspart

(B) Lispro

(C) Lantus

(D) PZI

(E) NPH

**9j.** To use the Glucometer Elite device properly, patients must also use

I. lancets

II. a tuberculin syringe

III. an alpha-glucosidase inhibitor

(A) I only

(B) III only

(C) I and II only

(D) II and III only

(E) I, II, and III

**9k.** The patient's use of Sudafed tablets may

    (A)  precipitate ketoacidosis

    (B)  increase the patient's insulin requirement

    (C)  increase the chance of lipohypertrophy

    (D)  increase the chance of lipoatrophy

    (E)  decrease the patient's insulin requirement

**9l.** B-D Lo-Dose syringes have a capacity of

    (A)  2 mL

    (B)  5 mL

    (C)  1.0 mL

    (D)  0.25 mL

    (E)  0.5 mL

**9m.** Which of the following antidiabetic products can be classified as a second-generation sulfonylurea?

    I.  Micronase

    II.  Prandin

    III.  Precose

    (A)  I only

    (B)  III only

    (C)  I and II only

    (D)  II and III only

    (E)  I, II, and III

**9n.** A serious potential complication in the use of metformin HCl (Glucophage) in the treatment of diabetes mellitus is

    (A)  metabolic alkalosis

    (B)  pancreatitis

    (C)  lactic acidosis

    (D)  nephropathy

    (E)  thrombocytopenia

**9o.** Which of the following best describes the mechanism of action of rosiglitazone?

    (A)  increases insulin production

    (B)  interferes with glucose absorption in the GI tract

    (C)  promotes glycogenolysis

    (D)  increases insulin receptor sensitivity

    (E)  antagonizes glucagon receptors

# PROFILE NO. 10

## Community Pharmacy Medication Record

Patient Name: Mona Abbatoir
Address: 3304 E. 9th Street
Age: 32                     Height: 5′5″
Sex: F                      Weight: 163 lb
Allergies:

## DIAGNOSIS

| Primary | Secondary |
|---|---|
| 1. Venous thrombosis | 1. |
| 2. Hypothyroidism | 2. |
| 3. | 3. |

## MEDICATION RECORD

| | Date | Rx No. | Physician | Drug & Strength | Quantity | Sig | Refills |
|---|---|---|---|---|---|---|---|
| 1. | 5/3 | 89322 | Coleman | Warfarin 5 mg | 10 | 1 daily | |
| 2. | 5/12 | 90109 | Coleman | Warfarin 7.5 mg | 30 | 1 daily | |
| 3. | 5/21 | 91202 | Coleman | Warfarin 7.5 mg | 30 | 1 daily | 3 |
| 4. | 6/18 | 91202 | Coleman | Refill | | | 2 |
| 5. | 7/15 | 91202 | Coleman | Refill | | | 1 |
| 6. | 8/1 | 94388 | Wilson | Thyrolar – 1/2 | 60 | 1 daily | 5 |
| 7. | 8/29 | 99733 | Waxman | Empirin/Codeine No. 3. | 30 | 1 b.i.d. | |

**DIRECTIONS (Questions 10a through 10l): Each of the numbered items or incomplete statements in this section is followed by answers or by completions of the statement. Select the ONE lettered answer or completion that is BEST in each case.**

**10a.** Warfarin is most closely related chemically to

(A) clopidogrel
(B) alteplase
(C) dicumarol
(D) ticlopidine
(E) heparin

**10b.** Administration of which of the following drugs is likely to decrease warfarin activity in this patient?

I. rifampin
II. phenobarbital
III. cimetidine

(A) I only
(B) III only
(C) I and II only
(D) II and III only
(E) I, II, and III

**10c.** An appropriate antidote for the treatment of warfarin overdose is

(A) EDTA
(B) phytonadione
(C) protamine sulfate
(D) potassium thiosulfate
(E) streptokinase

**10d.** This patient asks the pharmacist for a recommendation for an OTC analgesic for her tennis elbow. Which of the following agents would be appropriate to recommend?

   I.  Advil

  II.  Datril

 III.  Tylenol

(A) I only

(B) III only

(C) I and II only

(D) II and III only

(E) I, II, and III

**10e.** If the pharmacist had no Thyrolar in stock, which of the following could be substituted for it?

(A) Synthroid

(B) Cytomel

(C) Euthroid

(D) Dessicated thyroid

(E) Levoxyl

**10f.** Thyrolar contains which of the following active ingredients?

   I.   methimazole

  II.   thyroglobulin

 III.   liothyronine

(A) I only

(B) III only

(C) I and II only

(D) II and III only

(E) I, II, and III

**10g.** If a radiation dose of 200 mCi of radioactive iodine ($k = 0.23$ h$^{-1}$) is administered to a patient at 8 a.m. in the morning, how long would it take for the amount of radiation emitted by the dose to fall below 25 mCi?

(A) 9 h

(B) 4.6 h

(C) 6 h

(D) 0.23 h

(E) 3 h

**10h.** The use of Thyrolar by this patient is likely to

(A) increase the dosage requirement for warfarin

(B) prevent the oral absorption of warfarin

(C) increase the likelihood of renal damage

(D) decrease the dosage requirement for warfarin

(E) increase the likelihood of hepatic damage

**10i.** In a radiation emergency, which of the following would be appropriate to administer?

(A) potassium iodide

(B) liothyronine

(C) cholestyramine

(D) sodium nitrite

(E) propylthiouracil

**10j.** Thyroid hormone synthesis is controlled by

(A) thyroglobulin releasing cells in the pancreas

(B) oxytocin from the posterior pituitary

(C) FSH from the anterior pituitary

(D) TSH from the anterior pituitary

(E) LH from the anterior pituitary

**10k.** The use of Empirin/Codeine No. 3 by this patient is likely to

(A) increase the action of the Thyrolar

(B) decrease the action of Thyrolar

(C) decrease the action of warfarin

(D) increase the action of warfarin

(E) cause thyroid storm

**10l.** Which of the following laboratory determinations may be used to monitor the patient's progress on warfarin?

(A) APTT

(B) hematocrit

(C) BUN

(D) INR

(E) creatine kinase

# PROFILE NO. 11

## Hospital Pharmacy Medication Record

Patient Name: Maggie Goodsmith
Room Number: 742
Age: 56                          Height: 5'1"
Sex: F                           Weight: 135 lb
Allergies: Aspirin, codeine

### DIAGNOSIS

| Primary | Secondary |
|---|---|
| 1. Chronic UTI | 1. Migraines |
| 2. Conjunctivitis | 2. PMS |
| 3. | |

### LAB TESTS

| Date | Test & Results |
|---|---|
| 1. 7/14 | Urinalysis, pyuria, C&S = $1 \times 10^6$ *E. coli* |
| 2. | |
| 3. | |

### MEDICATION RECORD

| Date | Drug & Strength | Sig |
|---|---|---|
| 1. 7/15 | Cipro 200 mg IV | q12h × 7 days |
| 2. 7/15 | Pyridium 200 mg | 1 t.i.d. |
| 3. 7/23 | TMP-SMX 80 + 400 mg | 1q12h |

### PHARMACIST'S NOTES AND OTHER PATIENT INFORMATION

| Date | Comment |
|---|---|
| 1. 7/25 | Patient discharged with Rx    Septra DS #20 1q12h |

---

DIRECTIONS (Questions 11a through 11n): Each of the numbered items or incomplete statements in this section is followed by answers or by completions of the statement. Select the ONE lettered answer or completion that is BEST in each case.

11a. The term "pyuria" indicates the presence of what substance in the urine?

(A) pyruvate

(B) pyridoxine

(C) pus

(D) red blood cells

(E) pyrogens

11b. *Escherichia coli* may be described as

(A) pneumococci

(B) a systemic fungal organism

(C) gram-positive bacilli

(D) gram-negative bacilli

(E) a virus

**11c.** Which of the following is (are) drugs of choice for the treatment of a UTI caused by *E. coli?*

   I.  trimethoprim-sulfamethoxazole

  II.  ofloxacin

 III.  spectinomycin

(A) I only

(B) III only

(C) I and II only

(D) II and III only

(E) I, II, and III

**11d.** The physician's order for TMP-SMX may be filled using

   I.  Trimox

  II.  Bactrim

 III.  Septra

(A) I only

(B) III only

(C) I and II only

(D) II and III only

(E) I, II, and III

**11e.** Which of the following products are classified as fluoroquinolones?

   I.  Avelox

  II.  Levaquin

 III.  Kantrex

(A) I only

(B) III only

(C) I and II only

(D) II and III only

(E) I, II, and III

**11f.** Patients consuming Septra should be advised to

   I.  drink large amounts of fluids

  II.  maintain a very acidic urine

 III.  avoid the use of folic acid–containing products

(A) I only

(B) III only

(C) I and II only

(D) II and III only

(E) I, II, and III

**11g.** A patient wishes to test her urine to determine the presence of bacteriuria. Which of the following products would be suitable for this purpose?

(A) Ketostix

(B) Azostix

(C) Microstix-3

(D) Diastix

(E) Chemstrip K

**11h.** The Pyridium ordered for this patient can most accurately be classified as a (an)

(A) urinary antiseptic

(B) antimicrobial agent

(C) buffer

(D) antispasmodic

(E) analgesic

**11i.** This patient should be advised that Pyridium may cause

(A) discoloration of the urine

(B) migraines

(C) temporary weight gain

(D) dizziness

(E) temporary infertility

**11j.** Pyridium should not be administered for longer than

(A) 2 days

(B) 5 days

(C) 10 days

(D) 14 days

(E) 30 days

**11k.** Symptoms of premenstrual syndrome (PMS) may include all of the following EXCEPT

(A) backache

(B) cramping

(C) edema

(D) irritability

(E) weight loss

**11l.** Which of the following ingredients is (are) included in over-the-counter (OTC) PMS products?

   I. caffeine

  II. pamabrom

 III. subtilisin

(A) I only

(B) III only

(C) I and II only

(D) II and III only

(E) I, II, and III

**11m.** On 7/28, the physician's office calls concerning the patient's conjunctivitis which is getting worse. The prescriber wants a fluoroquinolone ophthalmic solution. Which of the following products could be suggested?

   I. Tobrex

  II. Levaquin

 III. Ciloxan

(A) I only

(B) III only

(C) I and II only

(D) II and III only

(E) I, II, and III

**11n.** On 8/2, the patient presents a prescription for Ancobon capsules 250 mg. For which one of the following infections is this drug indicated?

(A) *E. coli*

(B) *Candida*

(C) *Streptococcus*

(D) *Staphylococcus*

(E) Pneumonia

# ■ PROFILE NO. 12

## Hospital Pharmacy Medication Record

Patient Name: Harry Lessard
Room Number: 241-2
Age: 64                          Height: 5'11"
Sex: M                           Weight: 188 lb    Estimated surface area = 1.6 m$^2$
Allergies: NK

### DIAGNOSIS

| Primary | Secondary |
|---|---|
| 1. Chronic lymphocytic leukemia | 1. Oral candida |
| 2. | |
| 3. | |

### LAB TESTS

| Date | Test & Results |
|---|---|
| 1. 6/4 | Lymphocytosis 12,000/μL; K = 4.5; Na = 138 |
| 2. 6/10 | Lymphocytosis 8 × 10$^3$/μL; K = 2.6; Na = 128 |

### MEDICATION RECORD

| Date | Drug & Strength | Sig |
|---|---|---|
| 1. 6/4 | Colace 100 mg | 1 or 2 daily |
| 2. 6/4 | Zolpidem 5 mg | 1 h p.r.n. |
| 3. 6/4 | Chlorambucil 14 mg | po b.i.d. |
| 4. 6/4 | D/C chlorambucil | |
| 5. 6/4 | Fludarabine 25 mg/m$^2$ in D$_5$W | daily for 5 days |
| 6. 6/4 | Mycostatin Liq. | q4h for 2 days |
| 7. 6/7 | Mitrolan tabs chew | 1 q4h p.r.n. |

### PHARMACIST'S NOTES AND OTHER PATIENT INFORMATION

6/4 Admissions history—patient has been on a regimen of Leukeran tablets for CLL.

---

**DIRECTIONS (Questions 12a through 12n): Each of the numbered items or incomplete statements in this section is followed by answers or by completions of the statement. Select the ONE lettered answer or completion that is BEST in each case.**

**12a.** Leukeran would be assigned to which one of the following categories of antineoplastic agents?

(A) antimetabolites

(B) alkylating agents

(C) cell cycle–specific agents

(D) antibiotics

(E) hormones

**12b.** How many mg of fludarabine phosphate (Fludara) is needed for the five days of therapy?

(A) 25

(B) 40

(C) 80

(D) 125

(E) 200

**12c.** The patient's body surface area in square meters can best be determined with the use of a

- (A) caliper
- (B) tape measure
- (C) picogram
- (D) nomogram
- (E) micrometer

**12d.** Which one of the following sedatives would be the most appropriate substitute for zolpidem?

- (A) ProSom (estazolam)
- (B) Dalmane (fluazepam)
- (C) Restoril (temazepam)
- (D) Halcion (triazolam)
- (E) Sonata (zalepon)

**12e.** In which age range is acute lymphocytic leukemia (ALL) most prevalent?

- (A) <15 years
- (B) 20–30 years
- (C) 30–50 years
- (D) 50–70 years
- (E) >70 years

**12f.** Chemotherapeutic drugs classified as antimetabolites include

- I. cyclophosphamide
- II. carmustine
- III. methotrexate

- (A) I only
- (B) III only
- (C) I and II only
- (D) II and III only
- (E) I, II, and III

**12g.** Allopurinol is pharmacologically classified as a (an)

- (A) beta-adrenergic agonist
- (B) MAO inhibitor
- (C) xanthine oxidase inhibitor
- (D) antimetabolite
- (E) alkylating agent

**12h.** Patients using allopurinol should be advised to

- (A) drink adequate fluids
- (B) avoid dairy products
- (C) expect urine discoloration
- (D) avoid bruising
- (E) take at least 1 g of vitamin C daily

**12i.** In order to monitor the use of allopurinol, determinations should be made of

- (A) serum potassium
- (B) serum folate
- (C) urinary glucose
- (D) serum uric acid
- (E) urinary 5-HT

**12j.** An appropriate instruction for the use of Mycostatin liquid would be to

- (A) take with a large glass of water
- (B) swish and swallow
- (C) take on an empty stomach
- (D) mix it with fruit juice before administration
- (E) allow product to stand until it thickens

**12k.** If extravasation occurred with the administration of daunorubicin, which of the following would be recommended?

- (A) Inject subcutaneous epinephrine into the area.
- (B) Insert a catheter into the injection site.
- (C) Apply a corticosteroid cream to the injection site.
- (D) Inject sodium bicarbonate solution into the injection site.
- (E) Apply cold compresses to the injection site.

**12l.** Which of the following are serious adverse effects associated with daunorubicin administration?

   I.  ocular degeneration
  II.  nephrotoxicity
 III.  cardiotoxicity

(A) I only
(B) III only
(C) I and II only
(D) II and III only
(E) I, II, and III

**12m.** A new telephone order for "Oral Nilstat" Sig: take as directed" is received. What is the active agent in Nilstat?

(A) nitroglycerin
(B) nystatin
(C) nitrofurantoin
(D) nilomycin
(E) nilstatin

**12n.** Mr. Lessard had been purchasing products from his local health food store. Which of the following ingredients are claimed to be sleep aids?

   I.  melatonin
  II.  L-tryptophan
 III.  ginseng

(A) I only
(B) III only
(C) I and II only
(D) II and III only
(E) I, II, and III

# ■ PROFILE NO. 13

## Hospital Pharmacy Medication Record

Patient Name: Sondra Johnson
Room Number: 406-3
Age: 25                                    Height: 5'3"
Sex: F (NG)                                Weight: 150 lb
Allergies: Pollen, opiates

### DIAGNOSIS

| Primary | Secondary |
|---|---|
| 1. Suspected appendicitis (abdominal pain) | 1. Frequent headaches<br>2. Anemia ? (pallor) |

### LABORATORY TESTS

| Date | Test | Results with (normal ranges) |
|---|---|---|
| 6/4 | Hemo profile | WBC 12,000 /µL (4000–10,000), Hb 8 g/dL (12–16), Hct 24% (36–47), MCH 20 pg (27–32), MCV 20 (82–98), Glucose = 135 mg/dL |

### MEDICATION RECORD

| Date | Physician | Drug & Strength | Sig |
|---|---|---|---|
| 6/4 | Gavin | APAP 325 mg | 1 or 2 po q4h |
|  |  | Colace | 100 mg q a.m. p.r.n. |
|  |  | Alternagel | 15 mL q4h p.r.n. |
|  |  | Ambien | 5 mg hs |

### PHARMACIST'S NOTES AND OTHER PATIENT INFORMATION

| Date | Comment |
|---|---|
| 6/4 | Patient's pain appears to have subsided; still very pale in appearance; complains of increasing frequency of headaches which are relieved by daily use of aspirin (3 to 10 tabs total); has morbid fear of needles, very anxious to leave hospital; BP 105/70 (a.m.)  110/72 (p.m.) |

---

**DIRECTIONS (Questions 13a through 13q):** Each of the numbered items or incomplete statements in this section is followed by answers or by completions of the statement. Select the ONE lettered answer or completion that is BEST in each case.

**13a.** All of the following signs are consistent with a diagnosis of an acute appendicitis EXCEPT

(A) nausea and vomiting

(B) elevated white blood cell counts

(C) high fever

(D) abdominal pain in the lower right quadrant

(E) shift in WBCs to the right

**13b.** When questioned, Ms. Johnson states that she has been very pale and tired for several months. The paleness is likely to be due to which one of the following?

(A) anemia

(B) high white blood cell count

(C) low white blood cell count

(D) polycythemia

(E) drug allergies

**13c.** Ms. Johnson's medical history suggests which of the following?

    I.  type II diabetes

   II.  pernicious anemia

  III.  hypertension

  (A)  I only

  (B)  III only

  (C)  I and II only

  (D)  II & III only

  (E)  I, II, and III

**13d.** A patient with an abnormally elevated number of erythrocytes is described as having

  (A)  aplastic anemia

  (B)  polycythemia

  (C)  macrocytic anemia

  (D)  microcytic anemia

  (E)  sickle cell anemia

**13e.** Before discharging this patient, what drug will the intern likely prescribe for treating the anemia?

  (A)  ferrous sulfate

  (B)  ferric sulfate

  (C)  folic acid + an iron salt

  (D)  iron dextran

  (E)  vitamin $B_{12}$

**13f.** How many milligrams of iron are present in every 300 mg ferrous sulfate tablet? [Ferrous sulfate: $FeSO_4 \cdot 7\ H_2O = 278$; Fe = 56; S = 32; O = 16; H = 1]

  (A)  18

  (B)  35

  (C)  60

  (D)  100

  (E)  300

**13g.** The resident changes the above order of 300 mg ferrous sulfate to ferrous gluconate, which may be less irritating. What strength tablet should be ordered? [Ferrous sulfate: $FeSO_4 \cdot 7\ H_2O = 278$; Ferrous gluconate: $C_{12}H_{22}FeO_{14} \cdot 2\ H_2O = 482$; Fe = 56]

  (A)  100

  (B)  150

  (C)  250

  (D)  300

  (E)  500

**13h.** Which one of the following tests could have been ordered to determine if pernicious anemia was present?

  (A)  Direct Coomb's

  (B)  Indirect Coomb's

  (C)  Total bilirubin

  (D)  Benedict's

  (E)  Schilling

**13i.** In examining her stock of vitamins, the hospital pharmacist notices that the vials of vitamin $B_{12}$ injection have a slightly pink color. What action should she take?

  (A)  store the vials in the refrigerator to prevent further decomposition

  (B)  discard the vials

  (C)  store the vials in a dark place

  (D)  place the vials in warm water until the solution is colorless

  (E)  no action is needed

**13j.** Which one of the following drugs may contribute to the iron deficiency anemia?

  (A)  aspirin

  (B)  ampicillin

  (C)  multivitamins

  (D)  tetracycline

  (E)  vitamin B complex

**13k.** The designation of "NG" in Ms. Johnson's medical history indicates her status with respect to

  (A)  gastric condition

  (B)  health insurance

  (C)  pregnancy

  (D)  presence of HIV

  (E)  possible presence of a sexual transmitted disease such as gonorrhea

**13l.** Based upon Ms. Johnson's blood glucose values, which of the following actions should be taken?

(A) place the patient on a low carbohydrate diet

(B) prescribe insulin

(C) prescribe metformin

(D) prescribe a combination of metformin and insulin

(E) prescribe a low dose of glyburide

**13m.** What is the targeted hemoglobin $A_{1c}$ value for a diabetic patient?

(A) less than 7%

(B) 7 to 10%

(C) greater than 10%

(D) less than 120 mg/dL

(E) less than 200 mg/dL

**13n.** Ms. Johnsons's fear of insulin injections might be relieved if the pharmacist explains that the needle size is likely to be which of the following?

(A) 21G 1/8 in

(B) 21G 1/2 in

(C) 21G 5/8 in

(D) 25G 1 in

(E) 28G 5/8 in

**13o.** Ms. Johnson admits that she will have trouble monitoring her glucose levels if she has to undergo painful finger sticks for blood samples. What is a possible alternative that the pharmacist may suggest to maintain accurate monitoring?

(A) Use the One Touch Fast Take instrument.

(B) Use the Glucometer Elite instrument.

(C) Use any digital glucose monitor but cut the strip in half so that less blood is needed.

(D) Use urine samples in the glucose monitor.

(E) Have someone else perform the finger stick.

**13p.** During her hospital discharge, the patient mentions that both of her parents suffered from macular degeneration. What part of the body does this condition affect?

(A) brain

(B) eyes

(C) heart

(D) kidneys

(E) muscles

**13q.** Which one of the following dietary supplements appears to help slow or prevent the development of macular degeneration?

(A) glucosamine

(B) homocysteine

(C) lutein

(D) selenium

(E) zinc

# ■ PROFILE NO. 14

## Community Pharmacy Medication Record

Patient Name: Patrick Shannon
Address: 456 Park Ave
Age: 68                              Height: 5'10"
Sex: M                               Weight: 180 lb
Allergies: Pollen

### DIAGNOSIS

Primary                              Secondary

1. Obsessive/compulsive disorder     1. Early stages Alzheimer's disease
2. Type II diabetes (under control)  2. Complaints of heartburn (potential of peptic ulcer?)

### MEDICATION RECORD

| Date | Rx No. | Physician | Drug & Strength | Quantity | Sig | Refills |
|------|--------|-----------|-----------------|----------|-----|---------|
| 1/3 | 453078 | T. Lewis | Tofranil 150 mg | 30 | 1 daily | ref #2 |
| 3/2 | 454100 | T. Lewis | Digoxin 0.25 mg | 60 | 1 a.m. | 6 x |
| 4/4 | 455500 | " | Zoloft 100 mg | 30 | 1 daily | 3 x |
| | 455501 | " | Pepcid 20 mg | 90 | 1 t.i.d. | 1 x |
| 4/12 | 456670 | T. Lewis | Nasonex Nasal | 1 bt | 1–2 sprays p.r.n. | 3 x |
| 5/6 | 454100 | | Digoxin | 30 | 1 a.m. | ref #1 |
| 5/8 | 455258 | | Zoloft 25 mg | 30 | 1–2 daily for panic | ref #1 |

### PHARMACIST'S NOTES AND OTHER PATIENT INFORMATION

| Date | Comment |
|------|---------|
| 1/15 | Patient complains of dryness of mouth & other side effects due to Tofranil? Suggest he consult with Dr. Lewis |

**DIRECTIONS (Questions 14a through 14r):** Each of the numbered items or incomplete statement in this section is followed by answers or by completions of the statement. Select the ONE lettered answer or completion that is BEST in each case.

**14a.** Under which one of the following categories would Zoloft be classified?

  (A)  antihyperlipidemic
  (B)  MAOI
  (C)  SSRI
  (D)  tetracyclic antidepressant
  (E)  tricyclic antidepressant

**14b.** Four days after starting therapy with Zoloft, Mr. Shannon complains that he is displeased with the high cost of Zoloft and claims that it is not helping him. The pharmacist should advise him that

  (A)  the drug is less expensive than many others
  (B)  the drug often takes two to four weeks before noticeable improvement occurs
  (C)  it is his imagination that the drug is not working
  (D)  he should be switched to another SSRI
  (E)  he should be switched back to the tricyclic antidepressant previously used

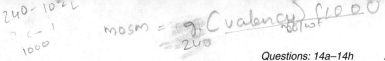

**14c.** The patient shows the pharmacist the results of a cholesterol test performed in a shopping mall health fair. The stated level is 240 mg/dL. What is this value in terms of millimoles per liter [Mol wt cholesterol = 387]

(A) 0.62

(B) 6.2

(C) 62

(D) .062

(E) 0.0062

**14d.** The following week Mr. Shannon brings a copy of his cholesterol screening performed at a medical clinic. The listed levels are

| | |
|---|---|
| Cholesterol | 260 mg/dL |
| Triglycerides | 98 mg/dL |
| HDL | 73 mg/dL |
| VLDL | 19.6 |
| Direct LDL | 114 |
| Chol/HDL ratio | 3.6 |

He is worried that all of the values sound high to him. Which one value is MOST encouraging?

(A) cholesterol

(B) HDL

(C) LDL

(D) triglycerides

(E) VLDL

**14e.** Last year, Mr. Shannon had a prescription filled for one of the "statins" but claims that he stopped taking this medication because of the cost. Which one of the following OTC drugs may be suggested to him for lowering his cholesterol?

(A) aspirin

(B) glucosamine

(C) niacin

(D) thiamine

(E) saw palmetto

**14f.** Mr. Shannon has noticed some increases in his blood pressure measurements but cannot afford expensive heart medicines. The pharmacist should explain that the physician is most likely to initiate therapy for borderline hypertension with which of the following?

(A) ACE inhibitors

(B) calcium channel blockers

(C) diuretics

(D) potassium supplements

(E) direct vasodilators

**14g.** Mr. Shannon requests a bottle of Primatene tablets. When counseling the patient, the pharmacist should advise him that

I. Primatene is available only as a spray product

II. Primatene is a prescription-only product

III. Primatene is intended for the treatment of bronchial asthma not rhinitis

(A) I only

(B) III only

(C) I and II only

(D) II and III only

(E) I, II, and III

**14h.** Which of the following advice should the pharmacist give to Mr. Shannon when dispensing each bottle of Nasonex Nasal Spray?

I. prime each new bottle by pumping about 10 times

II. use in each nostril for most effective activity

III. administer every day to maximize the product's prophylactic activity

(A) I only

(B) III only

(C) I and II only

(D) II and III only

(E) I, II, and III

**14i.** Which of the following is (are) significant advantages of desloratadine (Clarinex)?

    I. significantly lower incidence of drowsiness than Claritin

    II. available in both tablet and oral liquid dosage forms

    III. more potent than fexofenadine (Allegra)

    (A) I only

    (B) III only

    (C) I and II only

    (D) II and III only

    (E) I, II, and III

**14j.** All of the following are classified as second generation $H_1$-receptor antagonist antihistamines EXCEPT

    (A) cetirizine (Zyrtec)

    (B) chlorpheniramine (Chlor-Trimeton)

    (C) desloratadine (Clarinex)

    (D) fexofenadine (Allegra)

    (E) loratadine (Claritin)

**14k.** Which one of the following commercial products could be substituted for Claritin?

    (A) Aleve

    (B) Alavert

    (C) Contac

    (D) Tavist

    (E) Vivarin

**Answer questions 14l through 14o using the following prescription.**

| | |
|---|---|
| Burow's solution | 10 mL |
| salicyclic acid | 4% |
| phenol | 1% |
| white petrolatum qs | 60 g |

Sig: Apply to affected area t.i.d.

**14l.** What is the active ingredient in Burow's solution?

    (A) aluminum acetate

    (B) acetic acid

    (C) aluminum chloride

    (D) calcium hydroxide

    (E) hydrogen peroxide

**14m.** When preparing the above prescription, the pharmacist may wish to include which of the following in the formula?

    I. alcohol

    II. polysorbate 80

    III. Aquaphor

    (A) I only

    (B) III only

    (C) I and II only

    (D) II and III only

    (E) I, II, and III

**14n.** Which one of the following ingredients may be employed in preparing the prescription?

    (A) aspirin

    (B) carbolic acid

    (C) lactic acid

    (D) salicylamide

    (E) thymol

**14o.** The function of salicylic acid in this product is as a (an)

    (A) analgesic

    (B) local anesthetic

    (C) abrasive

    (D) keratolytic

    (E) preservative

**14p.** Today, the patient presents a new prescription for clarithromycin 500 mg #42 Sig: 1 t.i.d. and omeprazole 20 mg #14 Sig: one tablet q a.m. This combination is most likely being used to treat which one of the following conditions?

    (A) *H. pylori*

    (B) *S. aureus*

    (C) otitis media

    (D) community-acquired pneumonia

    (E) SARS

**14q.** Which one of the following drug-drug interactions may occur with Mr. Shannon's therapy?

    (A) decreased levels of digoxin due to the clarithromycin

    (B) increased levels of digoxin due to the clarithromycin

    (C) decreased levels of digoxin due to the omeprazole

    (D) increased levels of digoxin due to the omeprazole

    (E) no reaction with either drug is expected

**14r.** Mr. Shannon is very concerned because his 48-year-old wife is experiencing a constant redness of her cheeks that has lasted for over one month. Which of the following is the MOST likely explanation for this phenomenon?

    (A) chronic alcoholism

    (B) hypertension

    (C) shingles

    (D) rosacea

    (E) menopause

# ■  PROFILE NO. 15

## Community Pharmacy Medication Record

Patient Name: Melissa Tuwold
Address: 766 Avenue D

Age: 9                          Height: 4'9"
Sex: F                          Weight: 72 lb
Allergies: Peanuts, sulfa

### DIAGNOSIS

| Primary | Secondary |
| --- | --- |
| 1. Cystic fibrosis | 1. |
| 2. ADHD | 3. |

### MEDICATION RECORD

| Date | Rx No. | Physician | Drug & Strength | Quantity | Sig | Refills |
| --- | --- | --- | --- | --- | --- | --- |
| 1. 7/4 | 19287 | Castro | Mucomyst | 3 × 30 mL | p.r.n. with nebulizer | 3 |
| 2. 8/22 | 23388 | Castro | Cotazym | 60 | 1 t.i.d. | 5 |
| 3. 9/1 | 27003 | Mason | Ritalin 10 mg | 60 | 1 t.i.d. | 0 |

### PHARMACIST'S NOTES AND OTHER PATIENT INFORMATION

| Date | Comment |
| --- | --- |
| 1. | |
| 2. | |

**DIRECTIONS (Questions 15a through 15i): Each of the numbered items or incomplete statements in this section is followed by answers or by completions of the statement. Select the ONE lettered answer or completion that is BEST in each case.**

**15a.** The cause of cystic fibrosis can best be described as

(A) viral
(B) autoimmune
(C) genetic
(D) bacterial
(E) fungal

**15b.** Which of the following tests are done to diagnose the presence of cystic fibrosis?

(A) OGTT
(B) chemical stress test
(C) sweat test
(D) mucopolysaccharide test
(E) sedimentation rate

**15c.** Mucomyst is generally administered orally for the treatment of

(A) cystic fibrosis
(B) aspirin overdose
(C) drug-resistant tuberculosis
(D) acetaminophen overdose
(E) GERD

**15d.** Children with cystic fibrosis often have difficulty in absorbing

(A) fat
(B) protein
(C) carbohydrate
(D) electrolytes
(E) water-soluble vitamins

**15e.** The patient should be advised to take the Cotazyme

   (A)  an hour before or 2–3 h after meals

   (B)  at bedtime

   (C)  while standing

   (D)  with each meal

   (E)  with an antacid

**15f.** Ritalin contains the same active ingredient as

   I.  Adderall

   II.  Xenical

   III.  Methylin

   (A)  I only

   (B)  III only

   (C)  I and II only

   (D)  II and III only

   (E)  I, II, and III

**15g.** Melissa is having difficulty in remembering to take her Ritalin while she is in school. Which of the following should the pharmacist recommend to alleviate her difficulty?

   (A)  take her entire daily dose in the morning before school

   (B)  take the entire daily dose at bedtime

   (C)  ask her physician to prescribe Concerta

   (D)  ask her physician to prescribe Reglan

   (E)  tell her to take the morning dose with fatty food to slow absorption

**15h.** Which of the following adverse effects is likely to occur when using Ritalin?

   (A)  aplastic anemia

   (B)  tachycardia

   (C)  hypertrichosis

   (D)  bradycardia

   (E)  hemolytic anemia

**15i.** Which of the following drug products are NOT indicated for the treatment of ADHD?

   I.  Orap

   II.  Zyprexa

   III.  Haldol

   (A)  I only

   (B)  III only

   (C)  I and II only

   (D)  II and III only

   (E)  I, II, and III

# ■ PROFILE NO. 16

## Community Pharmacy Medication Record

Patient Name: Joan Lewis
Address: 27 Green St. Apt 4
Age: 32                          Height: 5'4"
Sex: F                           Weight: 120 lb
Allergies: Bee stings, sulfas?

### DIAGNOSIS

| Primary | Secondary |
|---|---|
| 1. Psychotic disorders | 1. Borderline diabetic |
| 2. Mild hypertension | 2. Frequent UTI's |

### PHARMACIST'S NOTES AND OTHER PATIENT INFORMATION

1. Ms. Lewis has had drinking binges resulting in some depression. She now claims that she does not drink any alcohol.

**DIRECTIONS (Questions 16a through 16n): Each of the numbered items or incomplete statements in this section is followed by answers or by completions of the statement. Select the ONE lettered answer or completion that is BEST in each case.**

16a. Ms. Lewis confides in the pharmacist that she thinks that she is "going crazy" because of some of her behavior. She constantly worries about not locking the front door, leaving the stove on, and has a strong desire to rearrange her furniture and kitchen cabinets. What condition should the pharmacist suspect?

(A) Alzheimer's disease
(B) senile dementia
(C) bipolar disorder
(D) OCD
(E) schizophrenia

16b. Which one of the following is commonly employed when initiating treatment for a patient with obsessive-compulsive disorder (OCD)?

(A) long-acting barbiturate
(B) serotonin reuptake inhibitor
(C) lithium carbonate

(D) tricyclic drug
(E) clomipramine

16c. Which one of the following is a brand name product of citalopram?

(A) Celexa
(B) Coreg
(C) Clozaril
(D) Paxil
(E) Serzone

16d. Which of the following drugs is MOST likely to be prescribed for a patient that has a history of panic attacks but with no comorbid major depression?

(A) phenytoin
(B) phenobarbital
(C) lithium carbonate
(D) prazepam
(E) venlafaxine

16e. Ms. Lewis is concerned that one of her tablets lists magnesium stearate as an ingredient. What is the purpose of this chemical?

(A) antioxidant

(B) coating agent

(C) disintegration agent

(D) lubricant

(E) nutritional source of magnesium

**16f.** Ms. Lewis presents a new prescription for a diaphragm. How will the prescriber likely indicate the desired size?

(A) small, medium, or large

(B) 2, 3, or 4 in

(C) 60, 70, or 75 mm

(D) 20, 25, or 30 French

(E) 16, 20, or 25 gauge

**16g.** When dispensing the diaphragm, the pharmacist should suggest concurrent use of a product containing which of the following?

(A) benzalkonium chloride

(B) boric acid

(C) lanolin

(D) mineral oil

(E) nonoxynol-9

**16h.** Ms. Lewis's 4-year-old child, Larry, appears to have behavior abnormalities including hyperactivity, short attention span, and abdominal colic. He also appears to be learning-impaired. Which of the following causes may explain these symptoms?

I. Alzheimer's disease

II. ADHD

III. lead poisoning

(A) I only

(B) III only

(C) I and II only

(D) II and III only

(E) I, II, and III

**16i.** The Centers for Disease Control and Prevention define childhood lead poisoning as when the lead levels in the blood are at 10 μg/dL or higher. What is this concentration in parts per million?

(A) 0.1 ppm

(B) 1 ppm

(C) 10 ppm

(D) 100 ppm

(E) 1000 ppm

**16j.** Which of the following products may be used for the treatment of lead poisoning?

I. BAL

II. succimer

III. Mucomyst

(A) I only

(B) III only

(C) I and II only

(D) II and III only

(E) I, II, and III

**16k.** Ms. Lewis has been experiencing some redness in both eyes. Which one of the following ingredients present in her contact lens products is most likely responsible?

(A) homosalate

(B) polyvinyl alcohol

(C) subtilisin

(D) sodium carboxymethylcellulose

(E) thimerosol

**16l.** Further discussion with Ms. Lewis reveals that she has been preparing pint quantities of her own contact lens soaking solution using salt tablets as the main ingredient. Which one of the following microorganisms presents a specific danger for an eye infection?

(A) *Acanthamoeba*

(B) *E. coli*

(C) *S. aureus*

(D) *Streptococcus*

(E) *Aspergillus niger*

**16m.** Ms. Lewis attempts to purchase the following herbs for her visiting sister, who is pregnant. Which one of the following herbs presents the greatest danger?

    (A)  black cohosh

    (B)  ginger

    (C)  ginkgo biloba

    (D)  St. John's wort

    (E)  milk thistle

**16n.** The sister wants to become updated on necessary vaccines for herself. Because of her pregnancy, which one of the following vaccines should she avoid?

    (A)  influenza

    (B)  hepatitis B

    (C)  pneumococcal

    (D)  smallpox

    (E)  tetanus

# ■ PROFILE NO. 17

## Hospital Pharmacy Medication Record

Patient Name: Lee Albright
Room Number: 604-2
Age: 16                          Height: 5′6″
Sex: M                           Weight: 100 lb
Allergies: None known

### DIAGNOSIS

| Primary | Secondary |
|---|---|
| Sickle cell anemia | General malaise and weakness |

### LABORATORY TESTS

| Date | Test | Results |
|---|---|---|
| 8/15 | Electrolytes | Sodium 145 mEq/L; potassium 3.5 mEq/L; chloride 100 mmol/L; calcium 7 mg/dL; bicarbonate 24 mmol/L; albumin 4 g/dL; BUN 28 mg/dL; glucose 105 mg/dL |
| 8/16 | Serum Cr | 0.8 mg/dL |

### MEDICATION RECORD

| Date | Physician | Drug & Strength | Sig |
|---|---|---|---|
| 8/15 | Dandree | Morphine sulf 0.2 mg/kg SC. STAT then 0.15 mg/kg SC. | q4h p.r.n. for 4 days |
| | | Start $D_5W$/1/2 NS | 1 L q8h |
| | | Colace 100 mg | 1 a.m. as needed |
| | | Zolpidem 5 mg | 1 hs |
| | | Multivitamin | 1 daily |
| 8/16 | Dandree | D/C electrolytes | |
| | | Start standard TPN, 2 L per day at 08:00 & 14:00 with flow rate 125 mL/h if tolerated. | |
| | | Amino acid sol 5% + $D_{50}W$ aa 500 mL NaCl 50 mEq; KCl 40 mEq; | |
| | | MVI Ped 5 mL CaGluconate 8.6 mEq + Trace Metals-5 2 mL | |
| 8/18 | Dandree | Anticipate discharge; convert IV morphine to morphine in PCA unit; arrange visiting nurse coverage | |
| | | p.m.-Discharge with PCA unit containing 100 mL morphine sulfate with flow set at 0.02 mg/kg MS q h for 3 days. | |

### PHARMACIST'S NOTES AND OTHER PATIENT INFORMATION

| Date | Comment |
|---|---|
| 8/16 | Reviewed patient's previous medical history plus present history and complaints; needs further evaluation to determine need for TPN |

**DIRECTIONS (Questions 17a through 17m): Each of the numbered items or incomplete statements in this section is followed by answers or by completions of the statement. Select the ONE lettered answer or completion that is BEST in each case.**

17a. All of the following are methods used to assess the patient's nutritional state EXCEPT

(A) albumin levels

(B) AST levels

(C) anthropometric

(D) proalbumin levels

(E) transferin levels

**17b.** Which of the following diseases is (are) associated with malnutrition?

    I.  Graves

    II.  Kwashiorkor

    III.  Marasmus

  (A)  I only

  (B)  III only

  (C)  I and II only

  (D)  II and III only

  (E)  I, II, and III

**17c.** Which one of the following drugs is most likely to be ordered for the treatment of sickle cell anemia?

  (A)  fluorouracil

  (B)  hydroxyurea

  (C)  iron dextran

  (D)  levothyroxine

  (E)  propylthiouracil

**17d.** Which of the following is true about the prescriber's order for zolpidem?

  (A)  Because it is a benzodiazepine, zolpidem is contraindicated for patients taking morphine.

  (B)  The route of administration, oral or parenteral, must be specified.

  (C)  The drug will duplicate the action of morphine.

  (D)  Administration of the drug should be 2 h before bedtime.

  (E)  None of the above are correct.

**17e.** After the original STAT dose, how many mL of morphine sulfate (10 mg/mL) should be administered per dose?

  (A)  0.15 mL

  (B)  0.7 mL

  (C)  1 mL

  (D)  1.5 mL

  (E)  2.8 mL

**17f.** How many nonprotein kilocalories is the patient receiving per hour if the TPN solution is infused over an 8-h period?

  (A)  100

  (B)  120

  (C)  240

  (D)  800

  (E)  850

**17g.** How many grams of nitrogen are being infused into the patient daily?

  (A)  4

  (B)  8

  (C)  16

  (D)  25

  (E)  50

**17h.** Which of the following methods are appropriate for administering the TPN solutions to Lee Albright?

    I.  through a central catheter

    II.  through a PICC line in the arm

    III.  directly through a peripheral vein

  (A)  I only

  (B)  III only

  (C)  I and II only

  (D)  II & III only

  (E)  I, II, and III

**17i.** Which one of the following equations would enable the pharmacist to estimate the renal creatinine clearance in Mr. Albright?

  (A)  Cockroft-Gault

  (B)  Harris-Benedict

  (C)  Henderson-Hasselbalch

  (D)  Loo-Riegelman

  (E)  Method of least residuals

**17j.** What will be the estimated creatinine clearance rate in this patient?

  (A)  60

  (B)  80

  (C)  100

  (D)  120

  (E)  160

**17k.** Which one of the following types of amino acid formulas is specifically designed for patients under high stress or with liver impairment?

(A) inclusion of homocysteine

(B) increased levels of all nonessential amino acids

(C) increased levels of all of the essential amino acids

(D) higher levels of branched chained amino acids

(E) addition of taurine

**17l.** How many mL of morphine sulfate (10 mg/mL) should be used to fill the PCA device?

(A) 0.14

(B) 2.2

(C) 6.6

(D) 66

(E) 14.4

**17m.** Reasons why the physician may have chosen the employment of a PCA for infusion rather than an elastomeric infusion device include all of the following reasons EXCEPT

(A) can change the dosing while the unit is attached to the patient

(B) patient may remain ambulatory

(C) can program bolus dosing if desired

(D) unit is less expensive to use and maintain

(E) unit can deliver subcutaneous dosing while the elastomeric cannot

# ■ PROFILE NO. 18

## Hospital Pharmacy Medication Record

Patient Name: Anthony Costello
Room Number: 621
Age: 42                                    Height: 5'4"
Sex: M                                     Weight: 132 lb
Allergies: Aspirin, hay fever

### DIAGNOSIS

| Primary | Secondary |
|---|---|
| 1. Hodgkin's disease | 1. Graves' disease |
| 2. | 2. Essential hypertension (under control with diet) |
| 3. | 3. Allergies |

### LAB TESTS

| Date | Test & Results |
|---|---|
| 1. 6/12 | SMA-12 |

### MEDICATION RECORD

| Date | Drug & Strength | Sig |
|---|---|---|
| 1. 6/12 | Propylthiouracil 50 mg | 2 b.i.d. |
| 2. | Mechlorethamine 6 mg/m$^2$ on day 1 | |
| 3. | Procarbazine 100 mg/m$^2$ | |
| 4. | Prednisone 40 mg | 1 daily |
| 5. | Vincristine 2 mg on day 1 | |
| 6. | Lorazepam 2 mg | 1 h.s. p.r.n. |
| 7. | Colace 100 mg | 1 qd |
| 8. | APAP 325 mg | 2 tabs p.r.n. fever |

### PHARMACIST'S NOTES AND OTHER PATIENT INFORMATION

| Date | Comment |
|---|---|
| 1. 6/12 | Start MOPP therapy on 6/14 if blood work results are normal. |

**DIRECTIONS (Questions 18a through 18l): Each of the numbered items or incomplete statements in this section is followed by answers or by completions of the statement. Select the ONE lettered answer or completion that is BEST in each case.**

**18a.** Which of the drugs used by this patient is indicated for the treatment of Graves' disease?

(A) mechlorethamine

(B) prednisone

(C) procarbazine

(D) propylthiouracil

(E) vincristine

**18b.** Which of the following drugs is (are) administered orally during MOPP treatment?

  I. mechlorethamine (Mustargen)

 II. procarbazine (Matulane)

III. prednisone

(A) I only

(B) III only

(C) I and II only

(D)  II and III only

(E)  I, II, and III

**18c.** Which one of the following forms of cancer is LEAST responsive to chemotherapy?

(A)  hepatocellular

(B)  hodgkin's

(C)  ovarian

(D)  prostate

(E)  testicular

**18d.** The nursing staff invites the pharmacist to a meeting for reviewing the SOAP for Mr. Costello. This acronym refers to which one of the following?

(A)  evaluation of his treatment program

(B)  general cleanliness of the patient

(C)  special bathing needs

(D)  special operational procedure for administering chemotherapy

(E)  specific procedures for discharging the patient

**18e.** The intern reports that Mr. Costello is experiencing extravasation of the mechlorethamine (Mustargen). Which one of the following courses of treatment should be initiated?

(A)  Apply warm compresses immediately.

(B)  Infiltrate 1/6 molar sodium thiosulfate into area and apply ice compresses.

(C)  Infiltrate epinephrine 1/1000 into area.

(D)  Infuse heparin sodium 20,000 units into area.

(E)  Withdraw infusion needle and apply compresses of sodium thiosulfate 10% w/v.

**18f.** How many grams of sodium thiosulfate USP are needed to prepare 100 mL of 1/6 molar solution? [Mol wt of $Na_2S_2O_3 \cdot 5 H_2O$ = 248; mol wt of water = 18]

(A)  2.1 g

(B)  4.1 g

(C)  7.5 g

(D)  14.9 g

(E)  24.8 g

**18g.** The pharmacy has only the anhydrous form of sodium thiosulfate. How many grams of this form are needed to obtain a 10% w/v sodium thiosulfate USP solution? [Mol wt of $Na_2S_2O_3 \cdot 5 H_2O$ = 248; mol wt of water = 18]

(A)  3 g

(B)  6.4 g

(C)  13.5 g

(D)  4 g

(E)  0 (because anhydrous form cannot be used)

**18h.** Which one of the following is a serious delayed toxic effect of many chemotherapeutic drugs?

(A)  bone marrow depression

(B)  cardiotoxicity

(C)  nausea and vomiting

(D)  peripheral neuropathy

(E)  respiratory depression

**18i.** By which of the following routes of administration may the 2 mg of vincristine be administered?

I.  into a running IV line

II.  intramuscular injection

III.  intrathecally by syringe

(A)  I only

(B)  III only

(C)  I and II only

(D)  II and III only

(E)  I, II, and III

**18j.** Which of the following agents would be appropriate to administer to a patient on chemotherapy with mechlorethamine?

I.  Epogen (epoetin alfa)

II.  Neupogen (filgrastim)

III.  Plavix (clopidogrel)

(A)  I only

(B)  III only

(C)  I and II only

(D)  II and III only

(E)  I, II, and III

**18k.** The physician orders weekly injections of cyanocobalamin (vitamin $B_{12}$). Which of the following routes of administration are appropriate for this agent?

   I.  subcutaneous
  II.  intramuscular
 III.  intravenous

(A)  I only
(B)  III only
(C)  I and II only
(D)  II and III only
(E)  I, II, and III

**18l.** Mr. Costello requires an antihistamine for the treatment of his allergies. Which of the following is an antihistamine suitable for Mr. Costello's needs?

   I.  Zyrtec (cetirizine)
  II.  Clarinex (desloratadine)
 III.  Allegra (fexofenadine)

(A)  I only
(B)  III only
(C)  I and II only
(D)  II and III only
(E)  I, II, and III

# ■ PROFILE NO. 19

## Hospital Pharmacy Medication Record

Patient Name: Laura Hockford
Room Number: 202B
Age: 52                          Height: 5'10"
Sex: F                           Weight: 140 lb
Allergies: Peanuts

### DIAGNOSIS

| Primary | Secondary |
|---|---|
| 1. CA ovaries | 1. Essential HTN |
| 2. Diabetes | 2. |
| 3. | 3. |

### MEDICATION RECORD

| Date | Drug & Strength | Sig |
|---|---|---|
| 1. 5/2 | HCTZ 50 mg | 1 po qd |
| 2. | Colace 100 mg | 1 every a.m. |
| 3. | Restoril 15 mg | 1 h.s. p.r.n. |
| 4. | Hytrin 2 mg | 1 h.s. |
| 5. 5/4 | Paclitaxel 150 mg/m$^2$, infuse over 24 h followed by Cisplatin 30 mg/m$^2$ | |

### PHARMACIST'S NOTES AND OTHER PATIENT INFORMATION

| Date | Comment |
|---|---|
| 1. 5/4 | Patient declines radiotherapy; drug therapy to be scheduled |
| 2. 5/6 | Anticipate discharge tomorrow, schedule follow-up therapy every 3 weeks for a total of three more sessions with usual blood work. |

DIRECTIONS (Questions 19a through 19m): Each of the numbered items or incomplete statements in this section is followed by answers or by completions of the statement. Select the ONE lettered answer or completion that is BEST in each case.

**19a.** Paclitaxel is available under which of the following tradenames?

I. Tazidime

II. Taxotere

III. Taxol

(A) I only

(B) III only

(C) I and II only

(D) II and III only

(E) I, II, and III

**19b.** Which one of the following procedures is NOT appropriate when dispensing injectable paclitaxel?

(A) storing the solution in PVC bags

(B) storing unopened vials in the refrigerator

(C) dispensing the solution in a glass bottle

(D) administering the solution by infusion through an in-line filter

(E) dispensing a slightly hazy, diluted solution

**19c.** The pharmacist may wish to suggest the addition of dolasetron mesylate to Ms. Hockford's therapy. This drug is used as a (an)

(A) antiemetic
(B) antihistamine
(C) local anesthetic
(D) antidepressant
(E) antivesicant

**19d.** Which of the following statements concerning cisplatin is (are) true?

I. available under the tradename of Paraplatin
II. classified as an alkylating agent
III. often causes nausea and vomiting

(A) I only
(B) III only
(C) I and II only
(D) II and III only
(E) I, II, and III

**19e.** Assuming that the patient's body surface area was determined to be 1.85 m², how many milliliters of paclitaxel injection will be needed if 50 mL multidose vials (6 mg/mL) are available?

(A) 5
(B) 23
(C) 43
(D) 46
(E) 50

**19f.** The literature reports that major side effects for paclitaxel (Taxol) include bone marrow depression, cardiac toxicity, and peripheral neuropathy. Which one of the following chemotherapeutic agents does not cause bone marrow depression?

(A) cytarabine (Cytosar-U)
(B) lomustine (CeeNU)
(C) mitomycin (Mutamycin)
(D) tamoxifen (Nolvadex)
(E) vinblastine (Velban)

**19g.** Which of the following is the best description of peripheral neuropathy?

(A) degenerative state of peripheral nerves
(B) severe, localized headache
(C) inflammation of peripheral veins
(D) numbness of the feet
(E) vasodilation of peripheral blood vessels

**19h.** Adverse effects of chemotherapeutic agents, such as bone marrow depression, pass through three stages—onset, maximum depression, and recovery to normal. Which one of the following terms is used to indicate the time for maximum depression?

(A) climb
(B) lag time
(C) retention time
(D) nadir
(E) suppression time

**19i.** Which of the following suggestions should the pharmacist make to the physician before the start of cisplatin therapy?

I. DC the Hytrin
II. DC the HCTZ
III. Start infusions of 2 L $D_{2.5}W$/1/2NS 12 h before the cisplatin infusion

(A) I only
(B) III only
(C) I and II only
(D) II and III only
(E) I, II, and III

**19j.** On 5/10, Ms. Hockford is readmitted to the hospital. The admitting physician observes weight loss, rales, FUO, N & V, and coughing with a greenish mucus. She orders chest x rays, SMA 16 and blood tests for culture and sensitivity. Which one of the following drugs may be ordered for the diagnosis of FUO?

(A) APAP
(B) biscodyl
(C) diazepam
(D) insulin
(E) IV nitroprusside

**19k.** The pharmacy receives an order for Augmentin 1 g IVMB stat then q6h. For which of the following reasons must the pharmacist consult with the prescriber?

  I. Augmentin is not available as a parenteral dosage form.

  II. The strength ordered is an excessive amount.

  III. The drug is not a broad spectrum antibiotic.

(A) I only
(B) III only
(C) I and II only
(D) II and III only
(E) I, II, and III

**19l.** Culture and sensitivity lab report indicates the following MICs:

Antibiotic A > 4 µg/mL; B = 4 µg/mL; C < 4 µg/mL; D = 8 µg/mL; E < 8 µg/mL

Assuming similar toxicities, which antibiotic is probably the best choice for Ms. Hockford's infection?

(A) antibiotic A
(B) antibiotic B
(C) antibiotic C
(D) antibiotic D
(E) antibiotic E

**19m.** The prescriber is considering using parenteral vancomycin on the patient. Which of the following reactions is (are) likely to occur if a nurse infuses vancomycin too rapidly?

  I. red man syndrome
  II. hypotension
  III. pseudomembranous colitis

(A) I only
(B) III only
(C) I and II only
(D) II and III only
(E) I, II, and III

# ■ PROFILE NO. 20

## Community Pharmacy Medication Record

Patient Name: Catherine Chaudry
Address: 12 Congress St. Fairhaven VT

Age: 35                                    Height: 5'6"
Sex: F                                     Weight: 124 lb
Allergies: Pollen

### DIAGNOSIS

Primary                    Secondary
1. Hypertension            1. High total cholesterol
2. Diabetes                2.
3.

### MEDICATION RECORD

| Date | Rx No. | Physician | Drug & Strength | Quantity | Sig | Refills |
|---|---|---|---|---|---|---|
| 1. 1/5 | 59535 | Lewis | Hytrin 2 mg | 60 | 1 daily | 3 x |
| 2. | 59536 | Collins | Ortho-Tri-Cyclen | 3 pack | 1 q a.m. | 6 mos |
| 3. | 59537 | Lewis | Glyburide 2.5 mg | 60 | 1 qd | 3 x |
| 4. 2/12 | 64012 | Collins | TMP-SMZ, Regular | | 1 q12h for 10d | 1 x |
| 5. 3/5 | 66156 | Lewis | Lipitor 20 mg | 30 | 1 hs | 1 x |
| 6. | 59535 | Lewis | Hytrin 2 mg | 60 | 1 daily | Refill 1/3 |
| 7. | 59537 | | Glyburide 2.5 mg | 60 | 1 qd | Refill 1/3 |

### PHARMACIST'S NOTES AND OTHER PATIENT INFORMATION

| Date | Comment |
|---|---|
| 1. 4/1 | Patient purchased niacin 250 mg |
| 2. | |

**DIRECTIONS (Questions 20a through 20n): Each of the numbered items or incomplete statements in this section is followed by answers or by completions of the statement. Select the ONE lettered answer or completion that is BEST in each case.**

**20a.** To what class of drugs does Hytrin belong?

(A) alpha$_1$-adrenergic blockers

(B) ACE inhibitors

(C) calcium channel blockers

(D) diuretics

(E) angiotensin II-receptor antagonists

**20b.** When the pharmacist originally filled the prescription for Hytrin, he should have warned the patient about the "first-dose" effect. This refers to which of the following?

(A) loss of appetite for 1 to 3 days

(B) hypertension that may occur after the first dose

(C) postural hypotension

(D) drowsiness that diminishes after 2 doses

(E) a flushing of the face

**20c.** Ms. Chaudry is unhappy with the side effects that she attributes to the *Ortho*-Tri-Cyclen. She asks about a drug her mother is taking—Evista which she read was a different type of hormone. Which of the following comments should the pharmacist offer concerning this drug?

    I.  It may be used in premenopausal women to regulate their menstrual cycle.

   II.  It is classified as a selective estrogen receptor modulator.

  III.  Its main intent is for the prevention of osteoporosis in postmenopausal women.

  (A)  I only

  (B)  III only

  (C)  I and II only

  (D)  II and III only

  (E)  I, II, and III

**20d.** The pharmacist could suggest that Ms. Chaudry approach her OB/GYN doctor suggesting a switch from *Ortho*-Tri-Cyclen to which of the following?

  (A)  Microgestin Fe

  (B)  *Ortho*-Evra

  (C)  *Ortho*-Novum

  (D)  *Ortho*-Cyclen

  (E)  Estraderm

**20e.** Ms. Chaudry's husband just returned from a business trip to Canada where he received a prescription written by trade name to treat a peptic ulcer. In which of the following references may the pharmacist locate the generic name of the drug product?

  (A)  *Facts and Comparisons*

  (B)  *Martindale (The Extra Pharmacopeia)*

  (C)  *Merck Index*

  (D)  *PDR*

  (E)  *USP DI*

**20f.** When picking up her prescriptions, the patient mentions that the family is going to the beach and will need a sunscreen lotion with an SPF of 8. All of the following sunscreen agents are suitable EXCEPT

  (A)  benzones

  (B)  homosalate

  (C)  mineral oil + iodine

  (D)  PABA

  (E)  padimates

**20g.** During the past two years, Mr. Chaudry has been treated for schizophrenia. His last stay at a clinic included treatment with fluphenazine decanoate injection 25 mg which he claims was an injection at two week intervals for two months. Upon discharge, which one of the following drugs would most likely be prescribed as an oral medication?

  (A)  divalproex (Depakote)

  (B)  haloperidol (Haldol)

  (C)  metaxalone (Skelaxin)

  (D)  risperidone (Risperdal)

  (E)  quetiapine (Seroquel)

**20h.** What is the best explanation for the administration of the fluphenazine decanoate only once every two weeks?

  (A)  The toxicity of the drug precludes more frequent administration.

  (B)  The injection is a sustained-release dosage form.

  (C)  Schizophrenia is an occasional occurance and does not need more frequent administration.

  (D)  Probably the patient was mistaken and does not remember the daily injections.

  (E)  The drug itself has a very long half-life.

**20i.** Ms. Chaudry's diabetes is under control and she determines her blood glucose levels every other day. At what minimum time interval should a test for glycated hemoglobin be performed?

  (A)  every other day

  (B)  weekly

  (C)  every month

  (D)  every 3 to 6 months

  (E)  every year

**20j.** When picking up her refills, Catherine expresses concern since her mother was just admitted to the hospital with the diagnosis of ascites. Which one of the following best describes this condition?

(A)  a parasite infection

(B)  an accumulation of serous fluid in the peritoneal cavity

(C)  collection of fluid in the lungs

(D)  a fever of unknown origin

(E)  a skin condition caused by mites

**20k.** Catherine's mother also suffers from ankylosing spondylitis. This condition affects which of the following body areas?

(A)  ankles

(B)  knee joints only

(C)  fingers and wrists

(D)  spine and large body joints

(E)  neck

**20l.** Which of the following statements concerning alcohol are true?

I.  Marked mental impairment occurs when blood levels are >100 mg/dL.

II.  Alcohol is oxidized to acetaldehyde in the body.

III.  The metabolism of alcohol follows first-order kinetics exclusively.

(A)  I only

(B)  III only

(C)  I and II only

(D)  II and III only

(E)  I, II, and III

**20m.** A friend suggests the use of Lotrimin Ultra for recurrent athlete's foot. Which one of the following drugs is the active ingredient in this nonprescription product?

(A)  butenafine

(B)  clotrimazole

(C)  miconazole

(D)  tolnaftate

(E)  zinc undecylenate

**20n.** The order for "TMP-SMZ, Regular" may be filled with which of the following?

I.  Bactrim

II.  co-trimoxazole

III.  trimethobenzamide

(A)  I only

(B)  III only

(C)  I and II only

(D)  II and III only

(E)  I, II, and III

# ■ PROFILE NO. 21

## Community Pharmacy Medication Record

Patient Name: Laura Jackson
Address: 12 Comfort Lane
Age: 70                                        Height: 5'4''
Sex: F                                          Weight: 112 lb
Allergies: Sensitive to aspirin, sulfas; limit chocolates

## DIAGNOSIS

Primary                          Secondary
1. Parkinsonism                  1. Mild anemia
2. Glaucoma                      2. Stroke (1 year ago)
3. CHF                           3.

## MEDICATION RECORD

| Date | Rx No. | Physician | Drug & Strength | Quantity | Sig | Refills |
|---|---|---|---|---|---|---|
| 1. 8/4 | 82542 | Puleo | Fe Sulfate 250 mg | 60 | 1 q a.m. | 2x |
| 2. | 82543 | Puleo | Levoxyl 100 μg | 30 | 1 q a.m. | 2x |
| 3. | 82544 | Puleo | Digoxin 0.25 mg | 60 | 1 qd | 1x |
| 4. | 82545 | Puleo | Furosemide 40 mg | 30 | 1 qod | 1x |
| 5. 9/28 | 82543 ref | Puleo | Levoxyl 100 μg | 60 | 1 q a.m. | 1/2 |
| 6. | 87555 ref | Puleo | Fe Sulfate 250 mg | 100 | 2 q a.m. | 2x |
| 7. | 82545 ref | Puleo | Furosemide | 30 | | 1/2 |
| 8. 10/4 | 82544 ref | Puleo | Digoxin | 60 | | 1/1 |
| 9. 10/28 | 82545 ref | Puleo | Furosemide | 30 | | 2/2 |

## PHARMACIST'S NOTES AND OTHER PATIENT INFORMATION

| Date | Comment |
|---|---|
| 1. | Do not use child-resistant closures. |
| 2. | Laura is sometimes confused; explain all medicines to her. Whenever possible, suggest she take medications first thing in the AM with breakfast. |
| 3. | OTCs—Mylanta 15 mL q a.m. and p.m.; Tums 1 or 2 every night; vitamin C 500 mg q a.m. |

**DIRECTIONS (Questions 21a through 21n): Each of the numbered items or incomplete statements in this section is followed by answers or by completions of the statement. Select the ONE lettered answer or completion that is BEST in each case.**

**21a.** Levoxyl was prescribed to control

(A) hypothyroidism
(B) hyperthyroidism
(C) Graves' disease
(D) hyperparathyroidism
(E) hypoparathyroidism

**21b.** If Mrs. Jackson misses a dose of Levoxyl, she should be instructed to

(A) double the following morning's dose
(B) take $1^{1}/_{2}$ tablets the following morning
(C) increase her intake of iodized salt
(D) call her physician for advice
(E) continue with normal dosing the following morning

**21c.** Which of the following drug products contain the same active ingredient as Levoxyl?

    I.  Cytomel

    II.  Thyrolar

    III.  Synthroid

(A) I only

(B) III only

(C) I and II only

(D) II and III only

(E) I, II, and III

**21d.** The pharmacist should question Mrs. Jackson concerning her compliance with which of the following drugs?

    I.  Levoxyl

    II.  furosemide

    III.  digoxin

(A) I only

(B) III only

(C) I and II only

(D) II and III only

(E) I, II, and III

**21e.** For which one of the following reasons may a patient be interested in purchasing a bottle of glucosamine + chondroitin tablets?

(A) relief of arthritis

(B) control of blood sugar

(C) provide proteins (amino acids) for muscles

(D) a dietary supplement to help gain weight

(E) an adaptogen and general energizer

**21f.** Mrs. Jackson's daughter is worried that her mother is showing symptoms of Alzheimer's disease. Which one of the following is the earliest symptom of this disease?

(A) incontinence

(B) inability to learn new skills

(C) loss of recent memory

(D) loss of remote memory

(E) wandering

**21g.** Drugs currently in use for treating Alzheimer's disease include

    I.  selegiline (Eldepryl)

    II.  donepezil (Aricept)

    III.  tacrine (Cognex)

(A) I only

(B) III only

(C) I and II only

(D) II and III only

(E) I, II, and III

**21h.** When questioned about her recent weight loss, Mrs. Jackson admitted that her breakfast and lunch consisted of two pieces of toast and herbal tea sweetened with Equal. The active ingredient in Equal is

(A) lactulose

(B) aspartame

(C) fructose

(D) saccharin

(E) sucrose

**21i.** Factors contributing to Mrs. Jackson's poor blood iron levels may be

    I.  consumption of herbal tea

    II.  antacid consumption

    III.  daily consumption of vitamin C

(A) I only

(B) III only

(C) I and II only

(D) II and III only

(E) I, II, and III

**21j.** For this patient, the evening dose of Tums is probably intended to

(A) decrease gastric secretions

(B) decrease gastroesophageal reflux

(C) prevent osteoporosis

(D) provide magnesium ions

(E) improve the absorption of digoxin

**21k.** Pharmacokinetic changes in the elderly often include increases in

    I. proportional amount of body fat

    II. plasma albumin levels

    III. renal clearance

(A) I only

(B) III only

(C) I and II only

(D) II and III only

(E) I, II, and III

**21l.** Based on the following data, determine how many milliliters of digoxin elixir are needed to replace a daily 0.25-mg dose of digoxin tablets.

| | Strength | "F value" |
|---|---|---|
| Digoxin tablet | 0.25 mg | 0.6 |
| Digoxin elixir | 0.05 mg/mL | 0.75 |

(A) 3 mL

(B) 3.8 mL

(C) 4 mL

(D) 5 mL

(E) 6.4 mL

**21m.** An early sign of digoxin toxicity in Mrs. Jackson is likely to be

(A) hazy vision

(B) hearing impairment

(C) tinnitus

(D) yellowish skin

(E) increased appetite

**21n.** The pharmacist may need to suggest an adjustment in the dosing of digoxin if the patient is placed on

    I. amiodarone

    II. quinidine

    III. verapamil

(A) I only

(B) III only

(C) I and II only

(D) II and III only

(E) I, II, and III

---

■   PROFILE NO. 22

## Hospital Pharmacy Medication Record

Patient Name: Paula Riley
Room Number: ER
Age: 28                          Height: 5'6"
Sex: F                           Weight: 145 lb
Allergies: Penicillin, sulfas

### DIAGNOSIS

| Primary | Secondary |
|---|---|
| 1. Gravid | 1. Colitis |
| 2. Severe cramps | 2. COPD (since childhood) |
| 3. | 3. |

### LAB TESTS

| Date | Test & Results |
|---|---|
| 1. 7/12 | SMA-12 |
| 2. | Blood profile |
| 3. | Blood typing |

### MEDICATION RECORD

| Date | Drug & Strength | Sig |
|---|---|---|
| 1. 7/13 | $D_5W$ 1 L daily | KVO |
| 2. | Terbutaline 25 µg/min then 0.5 mg sc q4h | |
| 3. | Zolpidem 5 mg | 1 h.s. p.r.n. |
| 4. | Colace 100 mg | 1 qd |
| 5. | Advil 200 mg | 1–2 tabs p.r.n. |
| 6. 7/15 | KCl 40 mEq in 1 L $D_5NS$ | Infuse t.i.d. |
| 7. | Barium sulfate | Admin per usual/Dr. Cooper orders |
| 8. 7/16 | Atropine 4 mg + chlorpromazine 12.5 mg | Preop order |

### PHARMACIST'S NOTES AND OTHER PATIENT INFORMATION

| Date | Comments |
|---|---|
| 1. 7/13 | Patient being transfered to room 434b Continue tocolytic therapy. |

---

**DIRECTIONS (Questions 22a through 22n):** Each of the numbered items or incomplete statements in this section is followed by answers or by completions of the statement. Select the ONE lettered answer or completion that is BEST in each case.

**22a.** Terbutaline is being used as a tocolytic agent. The term tocolytic refers to a drug that

    (A)   increases GI tract tone

    (B)   reduces GI tract motility

    (C)   reduces uterine contractility

    (D)   prevents emesis

    (E)   dilates bronchioles

**22b.** Under which one of the following trade names is terbutaline available?

    (A)   Alupent

    (B)   Brethine

    (C)   Hytrin

(D) Proventil

(E) Ventolin

22c. The pharmacist places 2 mL of terbutaline injection (1 mg/mL) into 250 mL of $D_5W$. How many drops per minute will be needed to deliver the terbutaline if the administration set delivers 15 drops to the mL?

(A) 6

(B) 11

(C) 23

(D) 46

(E) 120

22d. Over what period of time will the terbutaline admixture last?

(A) 40 min

(B) 80 min

(C) 100 min

(D) 160 min

(E) 480 min

22e. Which one of the following is the active ingredient in Advil?

(A) aspirin

(B) acetaminophen

(C) ibuprofen

(D) ketoprofen

(E) naproxen

22f. Barium sulfate is best described as a (an)

(A) antacid

(B) antidiarrheal

(C) diagnostic agent

(D) cleansing laxative

(E) protectant against colitis

22g. Which of the following concerning barium sulfate is (are) true?

  I. practically insoluble in water

 II. administered by the oral route

III. administered by the rectal route

(A) I only

(B) III only

(C) I and II only

(D) II and III only

(E) I, II, and III

22h. The purpose of the pre-op atropine is to

(A) relieve the patient's anxiety

(B) reduce secretions

(C) cause vasoconstriction of small blood vessels

(D) constrict the bronchioles

(E) produce a state of "twilight sleep"

22i. The pharmacist should question the atropine/ chlorpromazine order because of

  I. an acid–base reaction between the two ingredients

 II. the combination is irrational

III. the high dose of atropine requested

(A) I only

(B) III only

(C) I and II only

(D) II and III only

(E) I, II, and III

**Questions 22j through 22n: Mrs. Riley is discharged from the hospital on 7/21 with prescriptions for a Foley catheter, ostomy pouches, translucent drain dressings, Valium 2 mg 1 t.i.d. p.r.n., Prinivil 5 mg b.i.d. ProSom 1 mg in a.m., Sonata 5 mg 2 h before bedtime, psyllium 1 dose in a.m., and a multivitamin for pregnancy.**

22j. For which of the following items is a prescription actually needed?

  I. Foley catheter

 II. ostomy pouches

III. translucent drain dressings

(A) I only

(B) III only

(C) I and II only

(D) II and III only

(E) I, II, and III

**22k.** Which of the following is (are) suitable products for the psyllium order?

    I.   Metamucil

    II.  Fibercon

    III.  Mitrolan

    (A)  I only

    (B)  III only

    (C)  I and II only

    (D)  II and III only

    (E)  I, II, and III

**22l.** Mrs. Riley should be counseled to administer the Metamucil by

    (A)  mixing the granules with 8 oz of water, stirring, and drinking immediately

    (B)  mixing the granules with 1 pt of water, stirring, and drinking immediately

    (C)  mixing the granules with 8 oz water, stirring, letting mixture sit for 20 min before drinking

    (D)  swallowing the granules, then drinking 8 oz of water

    (E)  allowing the granules to effervesce in 8 oz of water before drinking

**22m.** Which of the following drugs in Mrs. Riley's discharge orders should be questioned by the pharmacist?

    I.   Prinivil

    II.  ProSom

    III.  Sonata

    (A)  I only

    (B)  III only

    (C)  I and II only

    (D)  II and III only

    (E)  I, II, and III

**22n.** If Mrs. Riley's physician decides to initiate antihypertensive therapy, which one of the following antihypertensive agents is probably the best choice for use during pregnancy?

    (A)  captopril

    (B)  enalapril

    (C)  hydrochlorothiazide

    (D)  methyldopa

    (E)  nifedipine

# ■ PROFILE NO. 23

## Community Pharmacy Medication Record

Patient Name: Lola Woolbright
Address: 7 Evan Road
Age: 31                                    Height: 5'4"
Sex: F                                     Weight: 210 lb
Allergies: Penicillin

### DIAGNOSIS

Primary                          Secondary
1. Vaginal infection             1. Anemia
2. Endometriosis                 2. PMS (painful)
3.                               3. Anxiety
                                 4. Obesity

### MEDICATION RECORD

| Date | Rx No. | Physician | Drug & Strength | Quantity | Sig | Refills |
|------|--------|-----------|-----------------|----------|-----|---------|
| 1. 4/4 | 34765 | Coughlin | Mycelex G | 1 | 1 qn | 1x |
| 2. 4/4 | 34766 | " | Ativan 1 mg | 30 | 1 b.i.d. p.r.n. | 0 |
| 3. 4/4 | 34767 | " | Triphasil 28 | 1 pack | ut dict | 1x |
| 4. 4/27 | 37102 | " | Ativan 1 mg | 30 | 1 b.i.d. p.r.n. | 1x |
| 5. 4/27 | 37103 | " | Xenical 120 mg | 90 | 1 t.i.d. p.r.n. | 1x |
| 5. 4/27 | 37104 | " | Feldene 20 mg | 90 | 1 t.i.d. | 1x |

### PHARMACIST'S NOTES AND OTHER PATIENT INFORMATION

| Date | Comment |
|------|---------|
| 1. 4/7 | Atkins Diet |
| 2. | |

---

**DIRECTIONS (Questions 23a through 23o): Each of the numbered items or incomplete statements in this section is followed by answers or by completions of the statement. Select the ONE lettered answer or completion that is BEST in each case.**

**23a.** The Mycelex G prescription is probably being used to treat

(A) candidiasis
(B) aspergillosis
(C) gonorrhea
(D) genital herpes
(E) syphilis

**23b.** The most common causative microorganism of nongonococcal urethritis is

(A) *Candida cryptococcus*
(B) *Chlamydia trachomatis*
(C) *Klebsiella aerogenes*
(D) *Proteus mirabilis*
(E) *Treponema pallidum*

**23c.** The drug usually considered the first choice to treat all stages of syphilis in a penicillin-allergic individual is

(A) doxycycline
(B) ceftriaxone
(C) fluconazole
(D) erythromycin
(E) ciprofloxacin

**23d.** The drug(s) usually considered as first choice(s) in the treatment of *Chlamydia* infections include

   I.   azithromycin
  II.  gentamicin
 III.  fluconazole

(A) I only
(B) III only
(C) I and II only
(D) II and III only
(E) I, II, and III

**23e.** Ms. Woolbright calls her physician to find out what can be done to avoid unwanted pregnancy since she had unprotected sexual intercourse last night. Which of the following should her physician recommend?

(A) a spermicidal cream
(B) Progestasert
(C) Evra
(D) Plan B
(E) Clomid

**23f.** Which of the following are acceptable lubricants for use with a condom or diaphragm?

   I.   White Vaseline
  II.  Koromex Clear Gel
 III.  K-Y jelly

(A) I only
(B) III only
(C) I and II only
(D) II and III only
(E) I, II, and III

**23g.** Which one of the following products is an intrauterine contraceptive system?

(A) Depo-Provera
(B) Mirena
(C) NuvaRing
(D) Vagisec
(E) Preven

**23h.** Ms. Woolbright's endometriosis is best treated by the use of

(A) Advil
(B) Deltasone
(C) Danocrine
(D) Kytril
(E) Mifeprex

**23i.** The action of Xenical can best be described as a (an)

(A) anxiolytic agent
(B) COMT inhibitor
(C) lipase inhibitor
(D) amylase inhibitor
(E) CNS stimulant

**23j.** Which of the drugs used by this patient does not seem to be properly prescribed?

(A) Triphasil
(B) Ativan
(C) Xenical
(D) Mycelex
(E) Feldene

**23k.** Benzodiazepines are often used to treat generalized anxiety disorders. Which one of the following is NOT a benzodiazepine?

(A) methylphenidate (Ritalin)
(B) chlordiazepoxide (Librium)
(C) alprazolam (Xanax)
(D) clorazepate (Tranxene)
(E) lorazepam (Ativan)

**23l.** The mechanism of action of the benzodiazepines is believed to be

(A) alpha$_1$ blockade
(B) potentiation of the inhibitory neurotransmitter GABA
(C) blockade of dopamine receptor sites
(D) blockade of the reuptake of dopamine
(E) beta-adrenergic blockade

**23m.** The Atkins diet is popularly used. It is based on the consumption of a diet which contains

(A) low fat
(B) low carbohydrate

(C)  mostly citrus fruits

(D)  low protein

(E)  high carbohydrate

**23n.**  If Ms. Woolbright acutely overdosed on her Ativan, which of the following would be appropriate to administer?

(A)  EDTA

(B)  disulfiram

(C)  naloxone

(D)  flumazenil

(E)  naltrexone

**23o.**  Ms. Woolbright is trying to count calories. She reads the labeling of a food product which indicates that each serving of the product contains 3 g of fat, 8 g of carbohydrate, and 1 g of protein. How many calories are in each serving of this product?

(A)  48

(B)  63

(C)  86

(D)  24

(E)  240

# ■ PROFILE NO. 24

## Community Pharmacy Medication Record

Patient Name: Harold White
Address: 869 Elm St.
Age: 3                          Height: 36″
Sex: M                          Weight: 40 lb
Allergies: Chocolate, salicylates

### DIAGNOSIS

| Primary | Secondary |
|---|---|
| 1. Recurrent earaches | 1. Frequent colds |
| 2. Strep. throat | 2. Allergies? |
| 3. Colitis | 3. |

### MEDICATION RECORD

| Date | Rx No. | Physician | Drug & Strength | Quantity | Sig |
|---|---|---|---|---|---|
| 1. 9/2 | 83043 | McLaughlin | Bactrim Susp | 6 oz | 2 tsp b.i.d. |
| 2. 10/6 | 84665 | McLaughlin | Pen Vee K Susp 250 | 200 mL | 1 tsp q.i.d. |
| 3. 11/5 | 86956 | Steen | Cromolyn eye drops | 30 mL | 2 gtts OD t.i.d. |

### PHARMACIST'S NOTES AND OTHER PATIENT INFORMATION

| Date | Comment |
|---|---|
| 1. | |

---

**DIRECTIONS (Questions 24a through 24o): Each of the numbered items or incomplete statements in this section is followed by answers or by completions of the statement. Select the ONE lettered answer or completion that is BEST in each case.**

**24a.** Causative organisms of otitis media include

    I. *Helicobacter pylori*
   II. *Hemophilus influenzae*
  III. *Streptococcus pneumoniae*

(A) I only
(B) III only
(C) I and II only
(D) II and III only
(E) I, II, and III

**24b.** Drugs often used for the treatment of otitis media include

    I. amoxicillin
   II. trimethoprim-sulfamethoxazole
  III. doxycycline

(A) I only
(B) III only
(C) I and II only
(D) II and III only
(E) I, II, and III

**24c.** When asked to suggest a nonprescription product to reduce Harold's fever and headache, the pharmacist could select products containing

    I. aspirin
   II. ibuprofen
  III. acetaminophen

(A) I only
(B) III only

(C) I and II only

(D) II and III only

(E) I, II, and III

**24d.** Chemically, ibuprofen is a derivative of

(A) fibric acid

(B) phenylacetic acid

(C) propionic acid

(D) salicylic acid

(E) xanthines

**24e.** When used to reduce fever, ibuprofen should not be used

(A) for more than 3 days

(B) for more than 10 days

(C) for less than 3 days

(D) for less than 10 days

(E) if the fever is greater than 104°F

**Questions 24f through 24h: The eye drop prescription filled on 11/5 reads as follows:**

> **Rx**
> Cromolyn sodium 2.5%        30 mL
> Dispense a sterile isotonic solution
>
> SIG: Sig: gtt ii OD t.i.d.

**24f.** The pharmacist dilutes the commercially available 4% cromolyn solution with purified water. How many milligrams of sodium chloride are needed to render the solution isotonic, assuming that the 4% solution was isotonic?

(A) 100 mg

(B) 170 mg

(C) 330 mg

(D) 540 mg

(E) 900 mg

**24g.** What pore size filter (in microns) should the pharmacist use to obtain a sterile solution?

(A) 0.22

(B) 0.45

(C) 1.0

(D) 5.0

(E) 10

**24h.** What direction should the the pharmacist place on the prescription label for the Sig of "OD"?

(A) every day

(B) affected eye

(C) left eye

(D) both eyes

(E) right eye

**24i.** Cromolyn solutions are used in the eyes to

I. treat *Pseudomonas* infections

II. relieve glaucoma

III. treat conjunctivitis

(A) I only

(B) III only

(C) I and II only

(D) II and III only

(E) I, II, and III

**24j.** For approximately how many days will the ophthalmic solution last assuming that the product is being used continuously? The dropper delivers 15 drops per 1 mL.

(A) 30

(B) 38

(C) 45

(D) 75

(E) 100

**24k.** Ms. White requests a mild sleep-aid for herself. The pharmacist may suggest an OTC product containing which one of the following ingredients?

(A) loratadine

(B) dimenhydrinate

(C) diphenhydramine

(D) meclizine

(E) ginseng

**24l.** When Ms. White asks how to administer the ophthalmic solution to Harold, the pharmacist may suggest

    I. quickly place the two drops directly onto the cornea

    II. after instillation, gently squeeze inner corner of eye nearest the nose for a minute

    III. place 1 drop into the lower inside lid of the eye then follow with the second drop after a few minutes

    (A) I only

    (B) III only

    (C) I and II only

    (D) II and III only

    (E) I, II, and III

**24m.** Which one of the following tricyclic antidepressants has been used successfully in treating nocturnal enuresis in children?

    (A) amitriptyline (Elavil)

    (B) doxepin (Sinequan)

    (C) imipramine (Tofranil)

    (D) nortriptyline (Pamelor)

    (E) trimipramine (Surmontil)

**24n.** Buildup of cerumen in the ear may be removed with the aid of which of the following OTC products?

    I. Debrox

    II. S.T. 37

    III. Anbesol

    (A) I only

    (B) III only

    (C) I and II only

    (D) II and III only

    (E) I, II, and III

**24o.** The allergist believes that Harold may be sensitive to tartrazine. Tartrazine is present in some pharmaceuticals as a (an)

    (A) antioxidant

    (B) antimicrobial preservative

    (C) antiseptic

    (D) buffer

    (E) coloring agent

# ■ PROFILE NO. 25

## Nursing Home Pharmacy Medication Record

Patient Name: Harold Jacobs
Room Number: 2317
Age: 72                                  Height: 6'1"
Sex: M                                   Weight: 184 lb
Allergies:

### DIAGNOSIS

| Primary | Secondary |
|---------|-----------|
| 1. Borderline hypertension | 1. Recovering alcoholic |
| 2. Gout | 2. Smoker |
| 3. | |
| 4. | |

### MEDICATION RECORD

| Date | Physician | Drug & Strength | Sig | DC'd |
|------|-----------|-----------------|-----|------|
| 1. 2/6 | Waters | Allopurinol 300 mg | 1 daily | 6 mos |
| 2. | Waters | Blocadren 10 mg | b.i.d. | 2 mos |
| 5. 2/8 | Waters/per phone | Mylanta Liq. | 15 mL p.r.n. | |

### PHARMACIST'S NOTES AND OTHER PATIENT INFORMATION

| Date | Comment |
|------|---------|
| 1. 2/9 | Evaluated Mr. Jacobs—Refuses to stop smoking. |

**DIRECTIONS (Questions 25a through 25m):** Each of the numbered items or incomplete statements in this section is followed by answers or by completions of the statement. Select the ONE lettered answer or completion that is BEST in each case.

**25a.** The immediate primary goal(s) for the treatment of acute gout will be to

   I. reduce uric acid levels

   II. administer high doses of an uricosuric agent

   III. relieve the pain of the attack

   (A) I only
   (B) III only
   (C) I and II only
   (D) II and III only
   (E) I, II, and III

**25b.** Drugs of choice for treating acute attacks of gout include

   I. NSAIDs

   II. colchicine

   III. allopurinol

   (A) I only
   (B) III only
   (C) I and II only
   (D) II and III only
   (E) I, II, and III

**25c.** Drugs of choice for controlling hyperuricemia include

   I. prednisone
   II. colchicine
   III. allopurinol

   (A) I only
   (B) III only
   (C) I and II only
   (D) II and III only
   (E) I, II, and III

**25d.** The nursing staff should be advised that the allopurinol

   I. should be consumed with a large amount of fluid
   II. may initially precipitate an attack of gout
   III. must be taken on an empty stomach to assure absorption

   (A) I only
   (B) III only
   (C) I and II only
   (D) II and III only
   (E) I, II, and III

**25e.** Mylanta contains simethicone. This agent acts to

   (A) neutralize excess stomach acid
   (B) inhibit the production of acid in the stomach
   (C) inhibit the production of gastrin in the stomach
   (D) dispel gas in the GI
   (E) bind excessive protease enzyme in the GI tract

**25f.** Simethicone can be found as the major active ingredient in

   I. Tums
   II. Phazyme
   III. Mylicon

   (A) I only
   (B) III only

(C) I and II only
(D) II and III only
(E) I, II, and III

**25g.** A pharmacist wishes to identify a tablet brought into the institution by the patient. Which of the following reference sources does NOT contain a color guide for commercial tablets?

   (A) *USP DI Volume I*
   (B) *USP DI Volume III*
   (C) *Facts and Comparisons*
   (D) *PDR*
   (E) *Red Book*

**25h.** The patient wishes to use minoxidil to reverse his loss of hair. This drug is available in which of the following dosage forms?

   I. topical solution
   II. tablets
   III. topical ointment

   (A) I only
   (B) III only
   (C) I and II only
   (D) II and III only
   (E) I, II, and III

**25i.** Blocadren is most similar in action to

   (A) Avapro
   (B) Mavik
   (C) Benicar
   (D) Cozaar
   (E) Levatol

**25j.** Which one of the the following agents has the MOST lipophilic activity?

   (A) acebutolol
   (B) propranolol
   (C) nadolol
   (D) carvedilol
   (E) bisoprolol

**25k.** Mr. Jacobs shows signs of peripheral neuropathy. This may be caused by a deficiency of

(A) thiamine

(B) riboflavin

(C) inositol

(D) tocopherol

(E) phytonadione

**25l.** Which of the following nutrients is (are) considered to be an antioxidant?

I. phytonadione

II. riboflavin

III. alpha-tocopherol

(A) I only

(B) III only

(C) I and II only

(D) II and III only

(E) I, II, and III

**25m.** A drug that has the tendency to impart an orange color to urine, sweat, and tears is

(A) carbamazepine

(B) isoniazid

(C) verapamil

(D) clindamycin

(E) rifampin

# ■ PROFILE NO. 26

## Community Pharmacy Medication Record

Patient Name: Harold Swersky
Address: 911 Whitebay Road
Age: 51                              Height: 5'11"
Sex: M                               Weight: 175 lb
Allergies:

### DIAGNOSIS

| Primary | Secondary |
|---|---|
| 1. Manic-depressive illness | 1. |
| 2. | 2. |
| 3. | 3. |

### MEDICATION RECORD

| Date | Rx No. | Physician | Drug & Strength | Quantity | Sig | Refills |
|---|---|---|---|---|---|---|
| 1. 8/9 | 78977 | Kramer | Zoloft 50 mg | 30 | 1 daily | 3 |
| 2. 9/4 | 78977 | Kramer | Refill | | | 2 |
| 3. 10/1 | 78977 | Kramer | Refill | | | 1 |
| 4. 10/24 | 80434 | Kramer | Lithotab 300 mg | 60 | 1 t.i.d. | 4 |
| 5. 11/12 | 81773 | Davis | HydroDIURIL 25 mg | 60 | 1 b.i.d. | |
| 6. 11/24 | 82140 | Davis | Azulfidine 500 mg | q.i.d. | 100 | 3 |
| 7. 11/24 | 82141 | Kramer | Wellbutrin 100 mg | b.i.d. | 60 | 3 |

### PHARMACIST'S NOTES AND OTHER PATIENT INFORMATION

| Date | Comment |
|---|---|
| 1. 11/12 | Low-sodium diet, uses Ex-Lax & Mitrolan |

---

**DIRECTIONS (Questions 26a through 26r): Each of the numbered items or incomplete statements in this section is followed by answers or by completions of the statement. Select the ONE lettered answer or completion that is BEST in each case.**

**26a.** Which of the following drugs is most similar in action to Zoloft?

(A) Loxitane

(B) Zofran

(C) Nardil

(D) Celexa

(E) Clozaril

**26b.** Wellbutrin is therapeutically classified as a (an)

(A) antidepressant

(B) antipsychotic

(C) anxiolytic

(D) antimanic

(E) anticonvulsant

**26c.** Wellbutrin contains the same active ingredient as

(A) Cerebyx

(B) Zyban

(C) Lamictal

(D) Habitrol

(E) Sublimaze

**26d.** Patients receiving Lithotab should be advised to

(A) avoid taking the drug at bedtime

(B) avoid taking the drug with milk

(C) consume a low-potassium diet

(D) consume a low-sodium diet

(E) drink 8 to 12 glasses of water per day while on the drug

**26e.** In using lithium products, toxicity commonly occurs when serum lithium levels exceed

(A) 1.5 mEq/L

(B) 1.5 mg/dL

(C) 1.5 mg/L

(D) 15 mg/L

(E) 300 μg/mL

**26f.** The addition of hydrochlorothiazide to the patient's regimen is likely to

(A) increase serum lithium levels

(B) decrease serum lithium levels

(C) decrease the absorption of lithium

(D) increase the absorption of lithium

(E) have no effect on lithium action

**26g.** In monitoring serum lithium levels, blood samples are usually drawn

(A) in the morning

(B) at bedtime

(C) just prior to taking a dose

(D) 1 to 3 h after taking a dose

(E) at the midpoint between two doses

**26h.** Lithotab 300 mg tablets each contain how many milliequivalents (mEq) of lithium? [$Li_2CO_3$ = 74; Li = 7]

(A) 4 mEq

(B) 8 mEq

(C) 16 mEq

(D) 21 mEq

(E) 43 mEq

**26i.** HydroDIURIL can best be described as a (an)

(A) thiazide diuretic

(B) osmotic diuretic

(C) mercurial diuretic

(D) carbonic anhydrase inhibitor

(E) loop diuretic

**26j.** Which one of the following drugs has the greatest potential for causing new memory impairment (anterograde amnesia)?

(A) flurazepam

(B) temazepam

(C) quazepam

(D) estazolam

(E) triazolam

**26k.** Mr. Swersky is having difficulty in falling asleep but does not wake up during the night. Which one of the following is probably the best choice of hypnotic?

(A) estazolam (Prosom)

(B) temazepam (Restoril)

(C) molindone (Moban)

(D) flurazepam (Dalmane)

(E) zolpidem (Ambien)

**26l.** The Azulfidine received by Mr. Swersky is used in the treatment of

(A) respiratory infection

(B) IBS

(C) systemic infection

(D) inflammatory bowel disease

(E) impotence

**26m.** A therapeutic substitute for sulfasalazine is

(A) Bentyl

(B) Buspar

(C) Pentasa

(D) Imodium

(E) Lomotil

**26n.** Mr. Swersky's physician indicates that he wishes to start him on some Nardil. What recommendation would you make to the prescriber about Mr. Swersky's drug regimen?

(A) Have Mr. Swersky discontinue the Zoloft at least 2 weeks before starting Nardil

(B) Immediately discontinue the HydroDIURIL

(C) The dose of Zoloft and Nardil should be at least 4–6 h apart

(D) Lithium will counteract the effect of the Nardil

(E) Nardil is not indicated for this patient

**26o.** Diphenhydramine should not be suggested if an elderly patient is suffering from

 I. incontinence

 II. diarrhea

 III. prostatitis

(A) I only

(B) III only

(C) I and II only

(D) II and III only

(E) I, II, and III

**26p.** A lab test that aids in the diagnosis of cancer of the prostate is

(A) ESR

(B) GGT

(C) PSA

(D) SGOT

(E) PTT

**26q.** Mitrolan is prescribed for the treatment of which of the following disorders?

 I. GERD

 II. diarrhea

 III. constipation

(A) I only

(B) III only

(C) I and II only

(D) II and III only

(E) I, II, and III

**26r.** The active ingredient in Ex-Lax is

(A) calcium polycarbophil

(B) phenolphthalein

(C) methylcellulose

(D) sennosides

(E) bisacodyl

# PROFILE NO. 27

## Community Pharmacy Medication Record

Patient Name: Paula Masterson
Address: 600 No. Bellmore Way—Apt. 24
Age: 64                                    Height: 5'3"
Sex: F                                     Weight: 175 lb
Allergies:

## DIAGNOSIS

| Primary | Secondary |
|---------|-----------|
| 1. Osteoarthritis | 1. |
| 2. | 2. |
| 3. | 3. |

## MEDICATION RECORD

| Date | Rx No. | Physician | Drug & Strength | Quantity | Sig | Refills |
|------|--------|-----------|-----------------|----------|-----|---------|
| 1. 2/27 | 34987 | Garth | Oxaprozin 600 mg | 60 | 2 t.i.d. | 5 |
| 2. 3/15 | 35875 | Garth | Ultram | 40 | 1 q.i.d. | 5 |
| 3. 3/26 | 37091 | Garth | Vioxx 12.5 mg | 30 | 1 daily | |
| 4. 5/29 | 39887 | Garth | Miacalcin | 1 | As directed | |

## PHARMACIST'S NOTES AND OTHER PATIENT INFORMATION

| Date | Comment |
|------|---------|
| 1. 3/6 | Aleve Tablets (OTC) |
| 2. 3/17 | Anacin Tablets |
| 3. 3/17 | Tums Chewable 500 mg |

**DIRECTIONS (Questions 27a through 27l): Each of the numbered items or incomplete statements in this section is followed by answers or by completions of the statement. Select the ONE lettered answer or completion that is BEST in each case.**

**27a.** In dispensing the prescription for oxaprozin, the pharmacist should have dispensed which of the following products?

(A) Bextra

(B) Orudis

(C) Ansaid

(D) Daypro

(E) Lodine

**27b.** Oxaprozin is believed to act by

(A) antagonizing dopamine receptors

(B) stimulating dopamine receptors

(C) inhibiting xanthine oxidase

(D) increasing the production of prostaglandins

(E) decreasing the production of prostaglandins

**27c.** Which of the following statements is (are) true?

   I.   The active ingredient of Aleve is naproxen sodium.

  II.   Advil should be administered two to three times daily.

 III.   Antacids should not be used within 2 h of taking Aleve.

(A) I only

(B) III only

(C) I and II only

(D) II and III only

(E) I, II, and III

**27d.** Tums chewable contains

(A) calcium carbonate

(B) propylene glycol

(C) polyethylene glycol

(D) simethicone

(E) magnesium oxide

**27e.** The pharmacist should advise this patient that Miacalcin should be administered

(A) rectally

(B) by inhalation

(C) sublingually

(D) orally

(E) intranasally

**27f.** When the oxaprozin prescription was filled, the pharmacist should have advised the physician that

(A) it is not available in a 600 mg strength

(B) it is only used on a p.r.n. basis for acute pain

(C) it should not be used for more than 10 days

(D) it is not to be used in patients with osteoarthritis

(E) it should not be administered three times daily

**27g.** Vioxx can best be classified as a (an)

(A) cytoprotectant

(B) COX-2 inhibitor

(C) antimicrobial effective against *H. pylori*

(D) anticholinergic

(E) narcotic agonist-antagonist

**27h.** The product most similar in action to Vioxx is

(A) Enbrel

(B) Lodine

(C) Bextra

(D) Auranofin

(E) Toradol

**27i.** Misoprostol (Cytotec) can best be described as a (an)

   I.   synthetic prostaglandin analog

  II.   inhibitor of gastric acid secretion

 III.   $H_2$-receptor antagonist

(A) I only

(B) III only

(C) I and II only

(D) II and III only

(E) I, II, and III

**27j.** Misoprostol (Cytotec) is contraindicated for use in

(A) the elderly

(B) patients using aspirin

(C) patients with osteoarthritis

(D) pregnant women

(E) patients with hypertension

**27k.** Which of the following is true of Ultram?

   I.   It is an NSAID.

  II.   It is only administered parenterally.

 III.   It works in the CNS.

(A) I only

(B) III only

(C) I and II only

(D) II and III only

(E) I, II, and III

**271.** Which of the following would NOT be appropriate to use in treating this patient's osteoarthritis?

   I. Enbrel

  II. Relafen

 III. Celebrex

(A) I only

(B) III only

(C) I and II only

(D) II and III only

(E) I, II, and III

# ■ PROFILE NO. 28

## Community Pharmacy Medication Record

Patient Name: Miguel Negron
Address: 334 West 33rd St.
Age: 85                           Height: 5'6"
Sex: M                            Weight: 182 lb
Allergies:

### DIAGNOSIS

| Primary | Secondary |
|---|---|
| 1. Hypertension | 1. |
| 2. CHF | 2. |
| 3. | 3. |

### MEDICATION RECORD

| Date | Rx No. | Physician | Drug & Strength | Quantity | Sig | Refills |
|---|---|---|---|---|---|---|
| 1. 6/23 | 90988 | Wilson | Digoxin 0.25 mg | 30 | 1 daily | 3 |
| 2. 6/23 | 90989 | Wilson | Lasix 40 mg | 60 | 1 b.i.d. | 3 |
| 3. 6/23 | 90990 | Wilson | Klorvess 20 mEq | 60 | 1 daily | 3 |
| 4. 8/10 | 90988 | Wilson | Refill | | | |
| 5. 8/10 | 90989 | Wilson | Refill | | | |
| 6. 8/10 | 93889 | Thomas | Amiloride 5 mg tab | 30 | 1 daily in a.m. | 3 |

### PHARMACIST'S NOTES AND OTHER PATIENT INFORMATION

| Date | Comment |
|---|---|
| 1. 7/15 | Baking soda to settle stomach |

**DIRECTIONS (Questions 28a through 28j): Each of the numbered items or incomplete statements in this section is followed by answers or by completions of the statement. Select the ONE lettered answer or completion that is BEST in each case.**

**28a.** Digoxin can be described as an agent that produces a

   I.  positive chronotropic effect
  II.  positive inotropic effect
 III.  vagomimetic effect

(A) I only
(B) III only
(C) I and II only
(D) II and III only
(E) I, II, and III

**28b.** Patients with congestive heart disease who begin using digoxin are likely to experience

(A) classic angina pain
(B) edema
(C) decreased force of cardiac contraction
(D) slowed heart rate
(E) orthostatic hypotension

**28c.** Which of the following drugs is most closely related to digoxin?

(A) amrinone
(B) mexiletine
(C) flecainide
(D) Hytrin
(E) hydralazine

**28d.** Which of the following would be suitable to use in a patient who needs a cardiac glycoside but has severe renal impairment?

(A) amiodarone

(B) disopyramide

(C) digoxin

(D) digitoxin

(E) isradipine

**28e.** If this patient's medication were changed from digoxin tablets to Lanoxicaps, what would be an appropriate equivalent dose?

(A) 2.5 mg

(B) 25 μg

(C) 0.125 mg

(D) 0.25 mg

(E) 200 μg

**28f.** Which of the following are effects associated with digoxin toxicity?

I. diarrhea

II. CNS stimulation

III. thrombocytopenia

(A) I only

(B) III only

(C) I and II only

(D) II and III only

(E) I, II, and III

**28g.** In dispensing Midamor, the pharmacist should recommend to the prescriber that

(A) the dose of digoxin be increased by 50%

(B) the Klorvess be discontinued

(C) the dose of Klorvess be raised by 50%

(D) the dose of digoxin be decreased by 50%

(E) the dose of Klorvess be reduced by 50%

**28h.** Which of the following would be considered to be a normal serum potassium concentration?

(A) 3.9 mEq/L

(B) 9.4 mEq/L

(C) 7.2 mg/dL

(D) 4.4 mg/dL

(E) 120 mEq/L

**28i.** Bumex is most similar to

(A) Diamox

(B) HydroDIURIL

(C) Buprenex

(D) Dyrenium

(E) Demadex

**28j.** The profile for Mr. Negron reveals the possibility of

I. substance abuse

II. potential complexation

III. noncompliance

(A) I only

(B) III only

(C) I and II only

(D) II and III only

(E) I, II, and III

# PROFILE NO. 29

## Community Pharmacy Medication Record

Patient Name: Charles Barkowicz
Address: 11 North Side Road
Age: 19                                      Height: 5'10"
Sex: M                                       Weight: 178 lb
Allergies: Ragweed pollen

### DIAGNOSIS

| Primary | Secondary |
|---|---|
| 1. Bronchial asthma | 1. |
| 2. Head lice | 2. |
| 3. Psoriasis | 3. |

### MEDICATION RECORD

| Date | Rx No. | Physician | Drug & Strength | Quantity | Sig | Refills |
|---|---|---|---|---|---|---|
| 1. 7/9 | 38383 | Toolie | Benadryl 25 mg | 30 | b.i.d. | 1 |
| 2. 7/9 | 38384 | Toolie | RID Shampoo | 2 oz | Apply ut dict | 1 |
| 3. 7/15 | 39439 | Toolie | Diprosone Cream 0.05% | 15 g | Apply as needed | |

### PHARMACIST'S NOTES AND OTHER PATIENT INFORMATION

| Date | Comment |
|---|---|
| 1. 7/9 | Hydrocortisone cream 0.5% (OTC) |

**DIRECTIONS (Questions 29a through 29k):** Each of the numbered items or incomplete statements in this section is followed by answers or by completions of the statement. Select the ONE lettered answer or completion that is BEST in each case.

29a. Benadryl may have been prescribed for this patient as a (an)

   I.   antipruritic

   II.  sedative

   III. antihistamine

   (A) I only

   (B) III only

   (C) I and II only

   (D) II and III only

   (E) I, II, and III

29b. An active ingredient of RID Shampoo is

   (A) lindane

   (B) crotamiton

   (C) piperonyl butoxide

   (D) undecylenic acid

   (E) pyrethrins

29c. In counseling the parent of the patient receiving RID Shampoo, the pharmacist should stress the importance of avoiding

   I.   the use of vitamin A–containing foods

   II.  the use of metallic combs

   III. contact with the eyes

   (A) I only

   (B) III only

   (C) I and II only

(D)  II and III only

(E)  I, II, and III

**29d.** Another name for head lice is

(A)  *Sarcoptes scabiei*

(B)  *Tinea versicolor*

(C)  *Tinea capitis*

(D)  *Pediculus capitis*

(E)  *Pediculus pubis*

**29e.** RID Shampoo is usually administered

(A)  once daily for 3 days

(B)  once daily for 5 days

(C)  once in 7 days

(D)  twice daily for 2 days

(E)  twice daily for 3 days

**29f.** Diprosone Cream contains

(A)  fluoxymesterone

(B)  betamethasone dipropionate

(C)  dexamethasone

(D)  triamcinolone acetonide

(E)  fluocinonide

**29g.** Diprosone Cream should NOT be used in patients with

I.  psoriasis

II.  herpes simplex infection

III.  *Candida* infection

(A)  I only

(B)  III only

(C)  I and II only

(D)  II and III only

(E)  I, II, and III

**29h.** Which of the following products for the treatment of head lice may be purchased over the counter (OTC)?

I.  A-200 Pyrinate

II.  Nix

III.  Eurax

(A)  I only

(B)  III only

(C)  I and II only

(D)  II and III only

(E)  I, II, and III

**29i.** Patients with ragweed allergy should avoid lice remedies that contain

(A)  lindane

(B)  organic solvents

(C)  pyrethrins

(D)  parabens

(E)  pyrogens

**29j.** Scabies is a condition caused by a

(A)  mite

(B)  virus

(C)  flea

(D)  protozoan

(E)  fungus

**29k.** Which of the following products would NOT be indicated for the treatment of psoriasis

I.  coal tar

II.  fluonid cream

III.  EDTA

(A)  I only

(B)  III only

(C)  I and II only

(D)  II and III only

(E)  I, II, and III

# ■ PROFILE NO. 30

## Community Pharmacy Medication Record

Patient Name: Tess Monrow
Address: 755 Avenue M
Age: 28                          Height: 5'4"
Sex: F                           Weight: 105 lb
Allergies:

### DIAGNOSIS

| Primary | Secondary |
|---|---|
| 1. Heroin abuse | 1. PCP |
| 2. AIDS-HIV | 2. |
| 3. | 3. |

### MEDICATION RECORD

| Date | Rx No. | Physician | Drug & Strength | Quantity | Sig | Refills |
|---|---|---|---|---|---|---|
| 1. 5/16 | 39998 | O'Hearn | Norvir 100 mg | 120 | 6 b.i.d. | 2 |
| 2. 5/16 | 39999 | O'Hearn | Retrovir 300 mg | 60 | 1 b.i.d. | 2 |
| 3. 5/16 | 40000 | O'Hearn | Hivid 0.75 mg | 90 | 1 t.i.d. | 2 |
| 2. 7/9 | 48749 | O'Hearn | Pentam 300 | 10 | Bring to office | |

### PHARMACIST'S NOTES AND OTHER PATIENT INFORMATION

| Date | Comment |
|---|---|
| 1. 6/1 | Robitussin DM (OTC) |

---

**DIRECTIONS (Questions 30a through 30l): Each of the numbered items or incomplete statements in this section is followed by answers or by completions of the statement. Select the ONE lettered answer or completion that is BEST in each case.**

**30a.** Which of the following agents would be appropriate to use in treating a patient with acute heroin overdose?

(A) flumazenil
(B) tolazamide
(C) cuprimine
(D) physostigmine
(E) naloxone

**30b.** Another name for heroin is

(A) oxycodone
(B) diacetylmorphine
(C) ethylmorphine
(D) oxymorphone
(E) methylmorphine

**30c.** "PCP" in the profile refers to

(A) phencyclidine
(B) pronounced cardiac pronation
(C) *pneumocystis carinii* pneumonia
(D) postcoronary patient
(E) precancerous psoriasis

**30d.** Another name for Retrovir is

I. zidovudine
II. AZT
III. ribavirin

(A) I only
(B) III only
(C) I and II only
(D) II and III only
(E) I, II, and III

**30e.** Patients receiving Retrovir must be monitored carefully for the development of

(A) pneumothorax
(B) malignant hypertension
(C) edema
(D) hematologic suppression
(E) pulmonary fibrosis

**30f.** Which of the drug products used by this patient is a protease inhibitor?

I. Norvir
II. Retrovir
III. Hivid

(A) I only
(B) III only
(C) I and II only
(D) II and III only
(E) I, II, and III

**30g.** Patients on Retrovir should avoid the use of

(A) acetaminophen
(B) benzodiazepines
(C) penicillins
(D) iron products
(E) vitamin A

**30h.** Pentamidine (Pentam) is available in which of the following dosage forms?

I. capsules
II. aerosol
III. injection

(A) I only
(B) III only
(C) I and II only
(D) II and III only
(E) I, II, and III

**30i.** Patients using Pentam must be monitored for the development of

(A) GI ulceration
(B) *Pseudomonas* infection
(C) kidney failure
(D) liver failure
(E) severe hypotension

**30j.** Which of the following are active ingredients in Robitussin DM?

I. codeine
II. dextromethorphan HBr
III. guaifenesin

(A) I only
(B) III only
(C) I and II only
(D) II and III only
(E) I, II, and III

**30k.** Which of the following are adverse effects associated with the use of Hivid?

I. peripheral neuropathy
II. pseudotumor cerebri
III. hemangioma

(A) I only
(B) III only
(C) I and II only
(D) II and III only
(E) I, II, and III

**30l.** Patents using Norvir should be monitored for clinically significant drug interactions with

I. amiodarone
II. triazolam
III. pimozide

(A) I only
(B) III only
(C) I and II only
(D) II and III only
(E) I, II, and III

# Answers and Explanations

**1a.** **(A)** Chlorthalidone (Hygroton) is a thiazide-like drug that inhibits reabsorption of sodium and chloride in the ascending limb of the loop of Henle and the early distal tubules. Choices (C) and (E) are loop diuretics, choice (B) is a carbonic anhydrase inhibitor, and choice (D) is not a diuretic. *(3)*

**1b.** **(E)** PSA is a protein produced by the cells of the prostate gland. The prostate-specific antigen (PSA) test measures the level of PSA in the blood. When the prostate gland enlarges, PSA levels in the blood tend to rise. Such an elevation can be caused by cancer or benign conditions such as BPH. Generally, a PSA level of 0–4 ng/mL is considered to be normal. Values higher than this level suggest the need for further evaluation to determine the cause of the elevation. *(25)*

**1c.** **(B)** Valsartan (Diovan) is an angiotensin II antagonist. This class of drugs has somewhat fewer adverse effects associated with it than the ACE inhibitors (e.g., nonproductive cough, angioedema). However, like the ACE inhibitors, angiotensin II antagonists are not safe to use during the second and third trimester of pregnancy. *(10)*

**1d.** **(B)** Thiazide diuretics such as HydroDIURIL are best taken in the morning to avoid being awakened during the night because of an urge to void. Patients should also be advised to maintain adequate hydration and to take the drug with food or milk. *(3)*

**1e.** **(B)** Finasteride (Proscar) is an antiandrogen. Since prostate development and size is dependent upon androgen, the use of finasteride will cause a reduction of prostate size. *(3)*

**1f.** **(C)** Finasteride is classified in pregnancy category X. It should, therefore, not be used in women. In addition, since finasteride has antiandrogen effects, it can improve the growth of hair, i.e., it can cause hirsutism, in some men with male-pattern baldness. Finasteride is available as the brand Propecia for this indication. *(3)*

**1g.** **(E)** The use of thiazide diuretics such as hydrochlorothiazide (HydroDIURIL) is associated with the potential for causing hypokalemia, hypomagnesemia, and hypercalcemia. *(3)*

**1h.** **(C)** Thiazide drugs such as hydrochlorothiazide (HydroDIURIL) may exhibit a cross-sensitivity with sulfa drugs. *(3)*

**1i.** **(B)** Mr. Rodgers should be advised to avoid the use of Claritin-D because this product contains pseudoephedrine, a sympathomimetic drug that could cause his blood pressure to rise. *(3)*

**1j.** **(C)** Terazosin (Hytrin) and tamulosin (Flomax) are alpha$_1$-adrenergic blocking agents. They are useful in treating BPH because they relax the smooth muscle of the prostate and of the bladder sphincter, thereby allowing better urine flow. Eplerenone (Inspra) is an aldosterone blocker used in the treatment of hypertension. *(3)*

**1k.** **(E)** Nitroglycerin IV is used to treat hypertensive emergency, particularly when cardiac ischemia is also present. Because of nitroglycerin's propensity to be adsorbed onto PVC plastic, a non-PVC administration set must be used when this product is administered. Diazoxide (Hyperstat) is also used in the treatment of hypertensive emergency. Because it is rapidly protein bound, diazoxide must be administered by IV bolus. Nitroprusside is also used to treat hypertensive emergency. It has a rapid onset of action and is administered by IV infusion. Nitroprusside decreases both preload and afterload and is particularly useful in patients with impaired left ventricular function. Nitroprusside solutions are very easily degraded by light and must be protected from light by using an opaque covering on infusion containers . *(3)*

**1l.** **(E)** Methyldopa (Aldomet) is considered to be the safest antihypertensive agent of those listed. The others may have a higher likelihood of causing fetal damage. *(5)*

# PROFILE NO. 2

**2a.** **(C)** Rofecoxib (Vioxx) is a non-steroidal anti-inflammatory drug (NSAID) that is believed to act by inhibiting prostaglandin synthesis by inhibiting cyclooxygenase-2 (COX-2). As a group, the COX-2 inhibitors are believed to have less GI upsetting effects than COX-1 inhibitors. *(10)*

**2b.** **(A)** A creatinine clearance ($CL_{Cr}$) level of <25 would indicate the presence of severe renal impairment. None of the NSAIDS should be used in such patients because NSAIDS may decrease renal blood flow and may exacerbate renal impairment . *(25)*

**2c.** **(B)** Nitroglycerin sublingual tablets are required by the FDA to be packaged in a glass container with a tight metal cap in order to reduce the loss of drug. The tablets should also be kept in a cool, dry place. *(10)*

**2d.** **(E)** Prinzmetal's angina or vasospastic angina is characterized by spasm of the smooth muscle of the proximal coronary arteries, often leading to an angina attack of long duration. Such attacks often occur at night and without a stress component. *(25)*

**2e.** **(C)** Glucosamine is a drug believed to promote the formation and repair of cartilage. Chondroitin is a substance that is believed to promote water retention and elasticity in cartilage and inhibit enzymes that break down cartilage. These agents are available OTC in many different combinations. *(10)*

**2f.** **(D)** Misoprostol (Cytotec) is a drug that can produce an antisecretory effect in the stomach and can elicit a mucoprotective effect by increasing mucus and bicarbonate production. It is indicated for the prevention of NSAID-induced peptic ulcers and should be used for the duration of NSAID therapy. Misoprostol is categorized as a pregnancy category X drug. *(10)*

**2g.** **(A)** The use of nitroglycerin sublingual tablets may cause a number of effects. Because of its vasodilating effect, nitroglycerin may cause hypotension and headache. Many patients also state that the use of nitroglycerin sublingual tablets produces a slight burning sensation when placed under the tongue. *(10)*

**2h.** **(B)** Nitroglycerin is available in seven different dosage forms, including a sublingual, transmucosal, translingual, transdermal, ointment, IV, and an oral sustained-release form. It is not available as a suspension dosage form. *(3)*

**2i.** **(B)** Tramadol (Ultram) is a centrally-acting analgesic agent that may be useful for this patient. Because of its central action, however, tramadol may cause dizziness, somnolescence, and sweating. *(10)*

**2j.** **(C)** Senokot products contain senna, an anthraquinone which produces a mild stimulant effect on the GI tract. Other laxative products such as aloe and cascara also contain anthraquinones. The advantage of these compounds is that they are not significantly systemically absorbed from the GI, thereby reducing the likelihood of systemic adverse effects. *(3)*

**2k.** **(A)** Nitrolingual spray is a metered-dose aerosol-containing nitroglycerin. It is sprayed onto or under the tongue upon onset of an angina attack. An advantage that this product has over nitroglycerin sublingual tablets is that the pressurized packaging of the nitroglycerin in the nitrolingual spray reduces the likelihood of drug loss by volatility. *(3)*

**2l.** **(A)** When any nitroglycerin products are used, patients should be advised to avoid the use of alcoholic beverages, sildenafil (Viagra), or any other drugs than can cause vasodilation. The combined use of these drugs and nitroglycerin may result in the development of hypotension, dizziness, and/or syncope. *(10)*

## PROFILE NO. 3

**3a.** **(B)** Nor-QD is a progestin-only oral contraceptive product. Such products are somewhat less effective than combination products that contain both an estrogen and progestin. Progestin-only products are taken daily rather than cyclically. *(3)*

**3b.** **(D)** Koromex Cream is a product usually used with a diaphragm. It contains the spermicidal agent nonoxynol-9. *(3)*

**3c.** **(C)** Generalized tonic-clonic seizures have also been referred to as grand mal seizures. Such seizures are characterized by alternating tonic and clonic muscle activity. *(3)*

**3d.** **(D)** Carbamazepine (Tegretol) and valproic acid (Depakene) are anticonvulsants used for the treatment of many convulsive disorders including generalized tonic-clonic seizures. Lamotrigine is indicated for the treatment of partial seizures. *(10)*

**3e.** **(C)** Dilantin Kapseals contain phenytoin sodium extended. This product is suitable for

single daily dosing or divided daily dosing. Products that contain phenytoin sodium, prompt, are suitable only for divided daily dosing. *(3)*

**3f.** **(A)** Gingival hyperplasia is a condition characterized by an overgrowth of gum tissue. Unless quickly treated, this condition can result in tooth loss and further gum disease. *(3)*

**3g.** **(E)** Michaelis-Menten or saturation kinetics is exhibited by some drugs including phenytoin. Such kinetics is characterized by slower metabolism of a drug at high doses than at low doses because of the saturation of metabolic enzymes. *(3)*

**3h.** **(B)** The therapeutic plasma concentration of phenytoin is 10 to 20 µg/mL. A phenytoin plasma concentration of 5 µg/mL several weeks after initiating therapy may indicate inadequate dosing or patient noncompliance. *(3)*

**3i.** **(D)** Phenytoin use may decrease the pharmacologic effect of the Nor-QD by increasing the hepatic metabolism of the progestin in Nor-QD. Because progestin-only products such as Nor-QD tend to be somewhat less effective in preventing pregnancy, this may result in an unwanted pregnancy. *(3)*

**3j.** **(C)** Fosphenytoin (Cerebyx) is a phenytoin ester that is a prodrug of phenytoin. Fosphenytoin causes less irritation at the IV injection site than phenytoin. It can be administered at three times the rate of phenytoin and, unlike phenytoin, is effective when given intramuscularly. Doses of fosphenytoin are stated in phenytoin equivalents (PE). *(10)*

**3k.** **(D)** The IM route for phenytoin sodium is generally avoided because the precipitation of phenytoin at the injection site may be painful and result in erratic absorption. Phenytoin is easily precipitated in the presence of an acidic substance (such as multivitamins) in the IV admixture. The addition of phenytoin sodium to an IV infusion is therefore generally not recommended. *(3)*

**3l.** **(A)** A morbilliform rash is one that resembles that of measles. *(3)*

**3m.** **(E)** The usual drug of choice for the treatment of status epilepticus is lorazepam (Ativan). Other benzodiazepines such as midazolam (Versed) or diazepam (Valium) may also be used. Propofol (Diprivan) is a nonbenzodiazepine anesthetic agent that is also useful in treating status epilepticus. *(3)*

**3n.** **(D)** Patients receiving chronic phenytoin therapy may develop folate deficiency because phenytoin reduces folic acid absorption. Folate supplementation may, therefore, be required in such patients. *(3)*

**3o.** **(B)** Nonoxynol-9 is a surfactant spermicide that is the active ingredient of Koromex Cream. *(3)*

**3p.** **(E)** Docusate sodium, the active ingredient of the stool softener Colace, is an anionic surfactant that promotes the penetration of water into the intestinal contents. This softens the contents and facilitates their evacuation. *(3)*

**3q.** **(A)** Lycopene is a pigment that gives tomatoes their characteristic red color. It has potent antioxidant properties and its use has been shown to reduce the incidence of prostate cancer. This agent has also been shown to reduce the levels of low density lipoproteins (LDL) in the body. *(3)*

## PROFILE NO. 4

**4a.** **(B)** Carbidopa serves as a dopadecarboxylase inhibitor that prevents the peripheral decarboxylation of levodopa and permits a greater proportion of the levodopa dose to enter the brain in its intact form. The use of carbidopa in combination with levodopa permits the use of lower levodopa doses than would be used without carbidopa. *(3)*

**4b.** **(D)** Pyridoxine promotes the peripheral conversion of levodopa to dopamine, thereby decreasing the activity of the administered levodopa. *(3)*

**4c.** **(A)** Darkening of the urine with the use of levodopa or Sinemet is normal and is a product of levodopa metabolism. The patient may disregard it. *(3)*

**4d.** **(B)** Biperiden (Akineton) is an anticholinergic agent used in the treatment of Parkinson's disease. Such agents reduce the incidence and severity of akinesia, rigidity, and tremor in patients with Parkinson's. Anticholinergic drugs are used as adjuncts to levodopa in the treatment of Parkinson's disease. *(3)*

**4e.** **(A)** Tiagibene (Gabitril) is an anticonvulsant. Selegiline (Eldepryl), pergolide (Permax) and bromocriptine (Parlodel) are dopaminergic agents and tolcapone (Tasmar) is a COMT inhibitor used in treating Parkinson's disease. *(3)*

**4f.** **(D)** The on-off effect is a deterioration of levodopa activity which is most prevalent just before the next dose is due. It may be caused by pharmacokinetic issues, altered sensitivity of dopaminergic receptors, or by other alterations in the CNS. The on-off effect can be reduced by reducing the dosing interval used (i.e., give the levodopa more frequently), or by adding an MAO inhibitor such as selegiline (Eldepryl) which will reduce the metabolic breakdown of levodopa. *(3)*

**4g.** **(A)** Diplopia, or double vision, is sometimes experienced by patients receiving levodopa therapy. *(3)*

**4h.** **(A)** When a patient on levodopa is to be switched to Sinemet, at least 8 h must be allowed to elapse from the last dose of levodopa to the first dose of Sinemet in order to decrease the likelihood of toxicity. Because the carbidopa in the Sinemet increases the proportion of intact levodopa that enters the brain, the dose of levodopa administered via Sinemet should be 75–80% less than that administered prior to the initiation of Sinemet therapy. *(3)*

**4i.** **(C)** The prolonged use of phenothiazine drugs such as chlorpromazine (Thorazine) may cause Parkinson-like effects because these drugs act as dopamine antagonists. *(3)*

**4j.** **(B)** Carbidopa is available by itself as Lodosyn. This product should be employed in combination with levodopa to create a dosage combination for patients with Parkinson's disease. *(3)*

**4k.** **(E)** Biperiden (Akineton) is an anticholinergic drug that is used in the treatment of Parkinson's disease. It is believed to work by competitively antagonizing the effects of acetylcholine in the CNS, thereby correcting an imbalance between cholinergic and dopaminergic activity seen in Parkinson patients. Anticholinergic drugs such as biperiden may produce typical anticholinergic adverse effects such as constipation, dry mouth, and urinary retention. *(3)*

**4l.** **(E)** Selegiline (Eldepryl) is a selective irreversible inhibitor of monoamine oxidase (MAO) type B. MAO-B is located primarily in the CNS, and MAO-A is located primarily in the GI tract and in the liver. Therefore, MAO-B inhibitors are less likely to affect the metabolism of tyramine found in cheese and wine, or sympathomimetic agents such as those found in nasal decongestants. While use of moderate doses of selegiline are unlikely to cause such interactions, when higher doses are used the selectivity of selegiline may diminish, thereby causing inhibition of MAO-A. Since the threshold between MAO-A and MAO-B inhibition is not clear, it would be prudent to avoid tyramine-containing foods as well as sympathomimetic drugs when using this drug. *(6)*

## PROFILE NO. 5

**5a.** **(B)** Timolol (Timoptic) acts as a beta-adrenergic blocking agent that reduces the production of aqueous humor in the eye. *(3)*

**5b.** **(A)** Timoptic and levobetaxolol are both beta-adrenergic blocking agents. *(3)*

**5c.** **(A)** Intraocular pressure may vary considerably in the same individual, depending on the

time of day that the measurement is taken as well as many other factors. A measurement of 14 mmHg is well within the normal range of 10 to 20 mmHg. *(3)*

**5d.** **(D)** Timoptic-XE is a sterile ophthalmic solution of timolol maleate. The solution also contains a substance known as Gelrite, which is a purified polysaccharide derived from gellan gum. When the Gelrite solution comes in contact with cations, such as the sodium found in tears, the solution forms a gel which sustains the contact of the timolol with the eye. Eventually the gel is washed away by tears. *(10)*

**5e.** **(B)** Urticaria is a name for hives. These are usually caused by a hypersensitivity reaction and can be manifested as discolored, swollen areas of the body. *(3)*

**5f.** **(B)** Acetazolamide (Diamox) is a carbonic anhydrase inhibitor. Since carbonic anhydrase is an enzyme that promotes aqueous humor production, the use of an inhibitor of carbonic anhydrase will reduce the formation of aqueous humor and reduce intraocular pressure. *(3)*

**5g.** **(B)** Bimatoprost (Lumigan) is a synthetic prostaglandin analog that reduces intraocular pressure by increasing outflow of aqueous humor from the eye. The most common adverse effects associated with this product are conjunctival hyperemia, growth of eyelashes, and ocular pruritis *(10)*

**5h.** **(E)** Edetate disodium is a metal scavenger that binds free metal ions. This is used to reduce the chance of trace metal-catalyzed decomposition reactions. *(3)*

**5i.** **(C)** The active ingredient in Orudis-KT and Actron is ketoprofen. Datril contains acetaminophen. Advil contains ibuprofen. Aleve contains naproxen. Haltran contains ibuprofen. *(3)*

**5j.** **(C)** Visine Allergy Relief contains tetrahydrozoline as its active ingredient. This agent is an imidazoline decongestant that tends to exhibit alpha$_1$ agonist activity. Its use in the eye causes vasoconstriction, relief of "red eyes" and ophthalmic congestion. *(3)*

**5k.** **(B)** The use of a beta-adrenergic blocking agent such as Timoptic-XE or levobunolol (Betagan) by a patient with a history of respiratory illness and breathing difficulty may be hazardous because beta-adrenergic blockers may cause bronchoconstriction. Even the relatively small amount of drug that enters the systemic circulation via an ophthalmic administration has been reported to cause breathing difficulty in susceptible patients. *(3)*

**5l.** **(C)** Anticholinergic drugs may cause mydriasis (pupillary dilation). This is likely to result in increased intraocular pressure. *(3)*

## PROFILE NO. 6

**6a.** **(B)** The active ingredient in Benzac is benzoyl peroxide, an agent that appears to act by providing antibacterial activity, especially against *Propionibacterium acnes*, the predominant organism in acne lesions. *(3)*

**6b.** **(D)** Patients using tretinoin (Retin-A) products should be advised to avoid the use of the product near the eyes, mouth, angles of the nose, and mucous membranes because tretinoin may irritate these tissues. Patients using this product should also be advised to avoid excessive exposure to sunlight and sunlamps because the drug may increase the patient's susceptibility to burning. *(3)*

**6c.** **(A)** Butylated hydroxytoluene, or BHT, is an oil-soluble antioxidant that is commonly employed in food and topical products in order to reduce the likelihood of spoilage. *(3)*

**6d.** **(B)** Retin-A Micro is a gel that contains microspheres containing tretinoin. *(10)*

**6e.** **(C)** The use of clindamycin, the active ingredient of Cleocin, has been associated with the development of diarrhea in some patients. If the diarrhea is severe and/or persistent, the patient's physician should be contacted because such a response may indicate the development of pseudomembranous enterocolitis, a serious and potentially life-threatening condition. *(3)*

**6f.** **(C)** A product that contains 10 mg of drug per milliliter will contain 1000 mg, or 1.0 g/100 mL. This is equivalent to a 1% (w/v) solution of the drug. *(3)*

**6g.** **(D)** Accutane contains isotretinoin as its active ingredient. This is an isomer of retinoic acid, a metabolite of retinol (vitamin A). Beta-carotene is provitamin A. *(3)*

**6h.** **(E)** Many adverse effects are associated with the use of Accutane. Cheilitis, an inflammation around the margins of the lips, is very common. Conjunctivitis (inflammation of the conjunctival lining of the eye) is also a common adverse effect associated with the use of this drug. Hyperlipidemia, sometimes severe, can also occur in patients using Accutane. *(3)*

**6i.** **(B)** Because of the many adverse effects associated with the use of Accutane, a patient package insert must be dispensed by the pharmacist to any patient receiving this drug. *(3)*

**6j.** **(A)** When puberty occurs, the level of sebaceous gland activity increases. This results in an increase in sebum production. When the fats in sebum are converted to free fatty acids by microorganisms such as *Corynbacterium acnes* in the pilosebaceous unit they cause a localized inflammatory response which, in turn, causes the development of the primary lesion of acne, the comedone. *(25)*

**6k.** **(D)** Aluminum oxide is a water-insoluble material that is employed in the Brasivol formulation as an abrasive. When rubbed onto the affected area, the abrasive property is meant to help remove the comedone plugs and allow better drainage of the comedone. *(3)*

**6l. (B)** Salicylic acid is a keratolytic agent, i.e, it helps to remove keratin from the skin surface. This facilitates the opening of plugged comedones and decreases the likelihood of new comedone formation. *(3)*

**6m. (D)** Sebum is a lipid secretion of the sebaceous glands, which are associated with the hair follicle. Sebum acts as a protectant on the skin surface. When the esterified fatty acids of sebum are broken down to free fatty acids by microorganisms, the inflammatory lesion of acne may be formed. *(3)*

## PROFILE NO. 7

**7a. (C)** Montelukast sodium (Singulair) and zafirlukast (Accolate) are both leukotriene antagonists. Salmeterol (Serevent) and albuterol (Ventolin) are selective beta$_2$ agonists, cromolyn (Intal) is a mast cell stabilizer, and fluticasone propionate (Flovent) is a corticosteroid. *(3)*

**7b. (C)** Montelukast sodium (Singulair) is a leukotriene antagonist and is not effective in halting an acute asthma attack. Proventil is a rapidly acting bronchodilator that will be more effective in treating an acute attack. *(3)*

**7c. (C)** Singulair and Vanceril should not be administered on a prn basis. They are only useful for prophylaxis of an asthma attack. Levsin is an antispasmodic product that can be used either prophylactically or to treat an acute attack of IBS. *(3)*

**7d. (B)** The Proventil Aerosol product contains albuterol, a selective beta$_2$ agonist. *(3)*

**7e. (C)** Older and younger patients who have difficulty in coordinating their inhalation of an aerosol may benefit from the use of a spacer device. *(3)*

**7f. (E)** Proventil is available as an aerosol, powder for inhalation, solution for inhalation, tablet, extended-release tablet, and oral liquid dosage forms. *(3)*

**7g. (A)** Rotacaps are a dosage form marketed by GlaxoSmithKline that contain a powder intended for inhalation. It is used with a device called a Rotahaler. *(3)*

**7h. (C)** The active ingredient in Vanceril is beclomethasone dipropionate, a corticosteroid. When administered by inhalation to asthmatic patients, Vanceril reduces the likelihood of future acute asthmatic attacks. Vanceril is not suitable for use during an acute attack. *(3)*

**7i. (C)** When a bronchodilator such as Proventil is to be used with a corticosteroid inhalation such as Vanceril, the patient should be advised to use the bronchodilator at least several minutes before the corticosteroid to promote better passage of the corticosteroid into the lower lung. *(5)*

**7j. (C)** Habitrol patches contain nicotine as their active ingredient. They are applied for a 24-h period. A new site should be used for each application. *(3)*

**7k. (C)** Albuterol is a beta-adrenergic agonist, which is more specific in its action for beta$_2$ receptors in the respiratory tract than for beta$_1$ adrenergic receptors in the heart. Isoproterenol is relatively nonspecific in its effect. Albuterol is therefore less likely to cause unwanted cardiac stimulation than is isoproterenol. *(3)*

**7l. (C)** Both Beclovent and Vanceril are inhalation products containing beclomethasone dipropionate. *(3)*

## PROFILE NO. 8

**8a. (B)** Nitrostat is a nitroglycerin sublingual tablet that has been stabilized with polyethylene glycol in order to decrease the likelihood that volatilization of the nitroglycerin will take place. As a result, Nitrostat has a considerably longer shelf-life than do nonstabilized nitroglycerin tablets. *(3)*

**8b. (A)** Nitrostat, as well as other oral nitroglycerin products, should be dispensed by the pharmacist in its original container because such containers are designed to minimize the loss of nitroglycerin during storage. *(3)*

**8c.** **(B)** Transdermal nitroglycerin patches should be applied onto a hairless site. Site rotation is important with each administration in order to decrease the likelihood of skin irritation. Transdermal patches should not be applied to distal portions of the extremities because these areas do not permit as reliable absorption of the nitroglycerin as do other areas of the body. *(3)*

**8d.** **(A)** When discontinuing therapy with nitroglycerin transdermal systems, gradual reduction of both the dosage and frequency of application over a four- to six-week period is advisable in order to minimize the likelihood of sudden withdrawal reactions. *(3)*

**8e.** **(E)** Amyl nitrite is the only antianginal product administered by inhalation. It is available as a liquid packaged in small glass capsules covered by protective cotton or gauze material. When required, the capsule is crushed and the patient inhales the vapors released. A rapid response is generally evident. Dosage control is, however, a major drawback in the use of this drug. *(3)*

**8f.** **(E)** Dipyridamole (Persantine), in addition to being used in the treatment of angina, is also employed as an antiplatelet agent. It appears to act in this regard by inhibiting cyclic nucleotide phosphodiesterase activity. *(3)*

**8g.** **(E)** Nitroglycerin administered orally undergoes extensive first-pass hepatic deactivation, thereby limiting the usefulness of this route of administration. *(3)*

**8h.** **(D)** The use of alcohol or sildenafil (Viagra) in combination with nitroglycerin may produce a hypotensive response because of the vasodilating action of all of these drugs. The hypotensive response may be manifested as dizziness, fainting, and/or weakness. *(3)*

**8i.** **(E)** Nitroglycerin may be adsorbed onto the polyvinyl chloride (PVC) tubing used in most

IV administration sets. This may result in loss of drug and inadequate dosing. Manufacturers of nitroglycerin for IV use supply non-PVC infusion tubing, which minimizes the adsorption of nitroglycerin. Such special tubing is generally recommended for use with nitroglycerin products. *(3)*

**8j.** **(B)** The dose of nitroglycerin topical ointment is measured in inches. It is applied to the skin with minimal rubbing, and the area to which it has been applied is covered with plastic wrap to facilitate drug absorption, and to prevent staining of clothing. *(3)*

**8k.** **(B)** Nitrolingual spray and sublingual forms of nitroglycerin provide the most rapid onset of action, ranging from 1 to 3 min. Transdermal patches have a 30–60-min onset time. *(3)*

## PROFILE NO. 9

**9a.** **(B)** Patients with type 1 diabetes mellitus are generally insulin dependent. Their disease generally begins early in life and is characterized by little or no insulin production by the pancreas. *(5)*

**9b.** **(C)** Humulin R insulin is human regular insulin that is prepared by recombinant DNA technology. As is the case with all regular insulin products, Humulin is short-acting, and is a clear solution. *(3)*

**9c.** **(A)** The Humulin R insulin contains 100 units of activity per milliliter. Twenty-four units of insulin activity will therefore be contained in 0.24 mL of the product. *(3)*

**9d.** **(B)** Polydipsia refers to excessive thirst. This is frequently seen in type 1 diabetics because of the excessive urination (polyuria) that is associated with the body's attempt to eliminate excessive glucose in the blood. *(3)*

**9e.** **(E)** A fasting blood sugar of 85 mg/dL is well within the normal range of 70–110 mg/dL. *(3)*

**9f.** **(B)** Regular insulin is the only form of insulin suitable for IV infusion. Most of the other forms are suspensions, which would be unsuitable for IV administration. *(3)*

**9g.** **(A)** When mixing two types of insulin, the clear regular insulin is always drawn into the syringe first in order to reduce the likelihood of contamination of the regular insulin with suspended particles of the second insulin. Insulin mixtures may be stored in a prefilled syringe for up to one week with refrigeration. *(3)*

**9h.** **(C)** Lispro Insulin has the most rapid onset of action. Its onset is about 0.25 h as opposed to 0.5–1.0 h for the next most rapid onset insulin, regular. *(3)*

**9i.** **(C)** Insulin glargine (Lantus) is manufactured with a pH of 4. It is, therefore, not compatible with other insulins. Lantus insulin is designed to precipitate when administered subcutaneously and will produce approximately 24 h of action with a single dose. *(3)*

**9j.** **(A)** The Glucometer Elite device requires that a small amount of blood be used to measure the blood glucose level. To obtain this blood, the patient or caregiver must use a lancet device to puncture the skin. *(3)*

**9k.** **(B)** Sudafed tablets contain pseudoephedrine, a sympathomimetic decongestant that is capable of inducing the conversion of glycogen to glucose in the body. This may increase glucose levels in the blood and increase the patient's insulin requirement. *(3)*

**9l.** **(E)** Lo-Dose syringes have a capacity of 0.5 mL. They are useful in situations where a low dose (<50 units) of insulin must be administered. *(3)*

**9m.** **(A)** Gliburide (Diabeta, Micronase), Glimepiride (Amaryl), and glipizide (Glucotrol) are second-generation sulfonylureas. Such agents are administered in lower doses than are first-generation agents and tend to produce somewhat fewer adverse effects than do first-generation agents. *(3)*

**9n.** **(C)** Excessive lactate in the blood results from abnormal conversion of pyruvate into lactate. Lactic acidosis is the result of an increase in blood lactate levels when body buffer systems are overcome. Lactic acidosis may be caused by cardiopulmonary failure, side effects of drugs and toxins, and by various acquired and congenital diseases. Lactic acidosis is a rare but serious complication in the use of metformin HCl that may be fatal in 50% of patients who develop it. *(3)*

**9o.** **(D)** Rosiglitazone (Avandia), unlike many other oral hypoglycemic agents, acts by increasing insulin receptor sensitivity. Most of the other agents work by increasing insulin production by the beta cells of the pancreas. *(3)*

## PROFILE NO. 10

**10a.** **(C)** Both warfarin and dicumarol are oral anticoagulants that interfere with vitamin K–dependent clotting factors. They are both derivatives of 4-hydroxycoumarin. *(3)*

**10b.** **(C)** The administration of rifampin or phenobarbital to a patient stabilized on warfarin is likely to result in decreased warfarin activity because of the ability of these drugs to increase the metabolism of warfarin. Cimetidine is an enzyme inhibitor and would, therefore, likely increase warfarin activity. *(3)*

**10c.** **(B)** Phytonadione (vitamin $K_1$) is a specific antidote for warfarin toxicity. Treatment of hemorrhage caused by oral anticoagulant therapy generally consists of the administration of 10 to 20 mg of phytonadione. *(3)*

**10d.** **(D)** Datril and Tylenol contain acetaminophen, an analgesic/antipyretic that does not appear to displace warfarin from plasma protein–binding sites. Advil contains ibuprofen, an agent that is capable of displacing warfarin from protein-binding sites, thus increasing warfarin activity. *(3)*

**10e.** **(C)** Thyrolar and Euthroid both contain liotrix as their active ingredient. *(3)*

**10f.** **(B)** Thyrolar contains liotrix as its active ingredient. Liotrix is a mixture of liothyronine and levothyroxine in a ratio of 1:4. *(3)*

**10g.** **(A)** 9 h; $t_{50} = 0.693/k = 0.693/0.23 = 3$ h. Therefore, after 3 h 100 mCi would remain, after 6 h 50 mCi would remain, and after 9 h 25 mCi would remain. *(6)*

**10h.** **(D)** Thyrolar and other thyroid hormone products appear to increase the catabolism of vitamin K–dependent clotting factors. This potentiates the action of warfarin and decreases the warfarin dosage requirement. *(3)*

**10i.** **(A)** In a radiation emergency, the administration of potassium iodide would saturate the thyroid with nonradioactive iodide, thereby making it less likely that radioactive iodides created in the emergency would accumulate in thyroid tissue. *(3)*

**10j.** **(D)** Thyroid hormone production in the body is controlled by the level of thyroid-stimulating hormone (TSH) produced by the anterior pituitary. *(3)*

**10k.** **(D)** Empirin/Codeine No. 3 contains aspirin. The aspirin may displace warfarin from protein-binding sites and may increase warfarin activity in the body. *(3)*

**10l.** **(D)** The international normalized ratio (INR) is a measure that takes into consideration the prothrombin time (PT) and the International Sensitivity Index (ISI), which is a measure of the sensitivity of the thromboplastin reagent used to determine the PT. *(3)*

## PROFILE NO. 11

**11a.** **(C)** The term "pyuria" refers to pus in the urine. Such a condition is often associated with a urinary tract infection (UTI). *(27)*

**11b.** **(D)** *E. coli* is a gram-negative bacillus generally associated with the GI tract. It is commonly a causative organism in urinary tract infections

as well as in institutionally borne infections. *(5)*

**11c.** **(C)** Trimethoprim-sulfamethoxazole and ofloxacin products are popular drugs for the treatment of urinary tract infections. Drug-resistant strains may necessitate switching to another antimicrobial agent. *(5)*

**11d.** **(D)** Both Septra and Bactrim are combination products of trimethoprim and sulfamethoxazole that have synergistic action against many microorganisms. The advantage of using such a combination as opposed to single-drug therapy is the ability of this combination to block two consecutive steps used by bacteria to produce tetrahydrofolic acid. Blocking two steps greatly diminishes the likelihood that bacterial resistance will develop. Trimox is one of the brand names for amoxicillin. *(3)*

**11e.** **(C)** Levaquin (levofloxacin) and Avelox (moxifloxacin) are fluoroquinolone drugs. Kanamycin (Kantrex) is an aminoglycoside. *(3)*

**11f.** **(A)** Patients using either Septra or other sulfa drugs should be advised to maintain adequate fluid intake in order to facilitate the urinary antimicrobial action of the product as well as to prevent precipitation of poorly soluble drugs in the urinary tract. Urinary acidification may accelerate the precipitation of sulfa drugs. There is no need for patients to avoid the use of folic acid–containing foods. *(3)*

**11g.** **(C)** Microstix-3 is designed to test for nitrite in the urine. Elevated nitrite levels are indicative of the presence of bacteria in the urine (i.e., bacteriuria). *(3)*

**11h.** **(E)** Phenazopyridine (Pyridium) is an azo dye employed as a urinary analgesic. It has no antiseptic activity. Phenazopyridine is often used to reduce pain in patients with urinary tract infections prior to the successful control of bacteria by antimicrobial agents. *(3)*

**11i.** **(A)** Phenazopyridine (Pyridium) is excreted unchanged into the urine. In doing so, it may cause a red-orange discoloration of the urine. *(3)*

**11j.** **(A)** When used with antimicrobial agents for the treatment of urinary tract infections, Pyridium should not be used for more than two days. This permits Pyridium's analgesic action to be employed during the early period of therapy when the infection is not yet under control. After two days, the infection should be under control and the continued use of Pyridium should not be required. In addition, the use of Pyridium beyond two days would mask pain that might be an indication of the failure of the antimicrobial therapy. *(3)*

**11k.** **(E)** Probably the most common psychological symptom of premenstrual syndrome is tension characterized by irritability and depression, which occur in 70–90% of all women. Weight gain of several pounds may be observed due to water retention. Several OTC products contain mild diuretics to combat this "bloating". *(3)*

**11l.** **(C)** Caffeine in doses of 100–200 mg every 3–4 h is a safe and effective diuretic but may cause sleeplessness. Pamabrom, a derivative of theophylline, is also effective in doses of 50 mg up to four times a day. Pamabrom is the active ingredient in Midol PMS and Pamprin. Subtilisin is an incorrect answer since this chemical is only present in some contact lens products as an enzymatic cleanser. *(2; 3)*

**11m.** **(B)** Two possible choices would be ciprofloxacin (Ciloxan) which is available in a droptainer at a 3.5 mg/mL concentration and ofloxacin (Ocuflox) available as a 0.3% concentration. Both are effective against gram-positive and -negative microorganisms including *P. aeruginosa*. The microbes usually responsible for conjunctivitis are *S. aureus*, *S. epidermis*, and *S. pneumonia*. While Levaquin (levofloxacin) is a fluoroquinolone, it is not available as an ophthalmic solution. Tobrex (tobramycin) is not a fluoroquinolone. *(3)*

**11n.** **(B)** Ancobon (flucytosine) is indicated for candida or cryptococcus infections. It is available as 250 and 500 mg capsules with usual dosing of 50–150 mg/kg each day. The drug should be used cautiously in patients with renal impairment. *(3; 25)*

## PROFILE NO. 12

**12a.** **(B)** Leukeran (chlorambucil) is an alkylating agent that is a cell cycle nonspecific agent. It appears to alkylate DNA by causing breakage of strands and crosslinkages. It is administered orally as 2 mg tablets. *(3; 5)*

**12b.** **(E)** The dose ordered was 25 mg/m² of body surface area (BSA). Since the estimated surface area of this patient is 1.6 m²,

$$1.6 \times 25 \text{ mg} = 40 \text{ mg/day}$$

Since five days of therapy was ordered,

$$40 \text{ mg} \times 5 = 200 \text{ mg total} \qquad (23)$$

**12c.** **(D)** A nomogram is a chart that permits the determination of a patient's body surface area (BSA) in square meters from the patient's known height and weight data. Nomograms are frequently employed in calculating doses for potent agents such as the antineoplastic drugs. *(23)*

**12d.** **(E)** Considering the patient's age, a short acting sedative would be most appropriate. Sonata (zalepon) is a nonbenzodiazepine which is less likely to result in side effects the following day. The other choices are all benzodiazepines—ProSom (estazolam), Dalmane (flurazepam), Halcion (triazolam), and Restoril (temazepam). These drugs or their metabolites have long half-lives in the body. Triazolam appears to cause a higher incidence of anterograde amnesia than the other choices. *(3; 5)*

**12e.** **(A)** Acute lymphocytic leukemia is a common malignancy in children and is rarely observed in persons older than 15. Long-term survival rates of greater than 70% are now obtained with chemotherapy. *(5; 16)*

**12f.** **(B)** One of methotrexate's main uses is in psoriasis therapy. It is available in both oral and parenteral dosage forms. Carmustine (BCNN) inhibits synthesis of DNA and RNA and is classified as an alkylating agent, as is cyclophosphamide. *(3)*

**12g.** **(C)** Allopurinol is a xanthine oxidase inhibitor. Inhibition of xanthine oxidase enzyme results in a reduction in the formation of uric acid, a common metabolite formed in patients being treated with antineoplastic drugs. Allopurinol is, therefore, commonly employed in the prevention or management of hyperuricemia. *(3)*

**12h.** **(A)** When allopurinol therapy is initiated, large quantities of uric acid are mobilized in the body and enter the urinary tract. Without adequate hydration, urates are likely to precipitate in the tract, causing pain and inflammation. *(3)*

**12i.** **(D)** Because allopurinol is employed in managing uric acid levels in the body, the monitoring of serum urate levels will provide a means of determining the success of therapy. *(3)*

**12j.** **(B)** When nystatin (Mycostatin) oral suspension is employed in the treatment of oral candidiasis infection, it is important that sufficient contact time be allowed between the drug and the mucosal surface of the oral cavity. This can be accomplished by having the patient swish the suspension in the mouth for several minutes prior to swallowing it. *(3)*

**12k.** **(E)** Extravasation is the leakage of injection fluid into tissue surrounding the injection site. When this occurs with the use of potent drugs such as daunorubicin, irritation and inflammation commonly occur. Once extravasation has occurred, the application of cold compresses to the injection site will relieve pain and minimize further dissemination of the drug into neighboring tissue. *(13)*

**12l.** **(B)** A serious adverse effect associated with the use of daunorubicin is cardiotoxicity. This is commonly manifested as congestive heart failure (CHF) and requires early diagnosis and aggressive treatment with sodium restriction, diuretics, and digoxin. *(6; 14)*

**12m.** **(B)** Nilstat contains the antifungal agent nystatin, which is used in the treatment of infections due to *Histoplasma capsulatum* and *Candida albicans*. In this patient, the product is probably intended for the prevention and/or treatment of oral thrush due to *Candida*. This problem is a common complication in cancer patients who are immunocompromised. Since there are both oral tablets and a suspension, the pharmacist will have to clarify the order as to whether the oral tablets (500,000 units/tablet) or the oral suspension (100,000 units/mL) is preferred. The usual direction for using the suspension is to take 5 mL and swish in the mouth before swallowing the solution. *(3; 14)*

**12n.** **(C)** Melatonin is an endogenous hormone that may affect human sleep patterns. Tryptophan has been advocated as a sleep aid, but its effectiveness has not been clearly established. *(3)*

## PROFILE 13

**13a.** **(E)** White blood cell counts are valuable in determining the presence of infection in the body. Usually there is a moderate increase in white blood cells especially leukocytes. Counts of 12,000–18,000 cells per microliter (μL) are signs of leukocytosis, which characterizes appendicitis. Some hospitals use the jargon "a shift to the left" to reflect a high neutrophil count since most reports list neutrophils first in the series of white blood cell types. A "shift to the right" indicates a high lymphocyte count. Often in cases of acute appendicitis, the white blood cell count is not elevated. However, if the appendix ruptures, there is a significant danger of septicemia. *(14)*

**13b.** **(A)** Patients suffering from anemia will often have a pale complexion accompanying their feeling of lethargy. While Ms. Johnson has an elevated white blood cell count, that is unlikely to result in paleness. *(14)*

**13c.** **(A)** A blood glucose value of 135 mg/dL is above the targeted maximum value of 120. The patient is also overweight. It is unlikely that she is suffering from pernicious anemia which would have been reflected in a high mean corpuscular volume (MCV). Her low hemoglobin (Hb) values of 4–5 g/dL most likely reflects an iron deficiency. Hypertension is unlikely since her blood pressure values are normal and there is no history of taking antihypertensive drugs. *(14, 16)*

**13d. (B)** Polycythemia vera is a relatively rare disease characterized by an excess of red blood cells which thickens the blood resulting in slower passage through small blood vessels. Bleeding from the gums and a red appearance of the face are common. *(16)*

**13e. (A)** Various iron salts in the reduced forms (ferrous) may be used for iron deficiencies. The sulfates, fumarates, and gluconates are three available forms. It is probably not necessary to subject Ms. Johnson to an intramuscular injection of iron dextran. Vitamin $B_{12}$ is prescribed for pernicious anemia. Folic acid is especially useful in preventing megaloblastic anemia. *(1, 14)*

**13f. (C)**

$$mg \text{ of Fe} = 300 \text{ mg} \times \frac{\text{Atomic wt iron}}{\text{Formula wt ferrous sulfate}}$$
$$= 300 \text{ mg} \times \frac{56}{278}$$
$$= 60.4 \text{ mg} \qquad (1, 23)$$

**13g. (E)** From the previous question, it was determined that 60 mg elemental iron was present in every 300 mg tablet. To obtain 60 mg of iron from the ferrous gluconate, one would calculate

$$\frac{56 \text{ Fe}}{482 \text{ Fe gluconate}} = \frac{60 \text{ mg Fe}}{x \text{ mg Fe gluconate}}$$
$$x = 516 \text{ mg} \qquad (1, 23)$$

**13h. (E)** The Schilling test involves oral administration of a small amount of radioactive vitamin $B_{12}$, followed by urine assay. Intrinsic factor and vitamin $B_{12}$ are then administered. A diagnosis of pernicious anemia may be made if there is an increase in serum vitamin $B_{12}$ when the intrinsic factor is present. *(14)*

**13i. (E)** Unlike epinephrine solutions which may turn a pink or red color due to oxidation, solutions of vitamin $B_{12}$ (cyanocobalamin) may have a slight pink color, which is normal. The

vials need not be destroyed or undergo special storage. *(21)*

**13j. (A)** Constant daily use of large doses of aspirin may increase GI tract irritation with a corresponding increase in bleeding. *(5, 14)*

**13k. (C)** The notation of "G" indicates "gravid" which means pregnant. Nonpregnant females may be designated as "NG" or "nongravid." *(1, 14)*

**13l. (A)** A blood glucose value of 135 suggests that the patient may have type 2 diabetes. Further questioning concerning symptoms such as thirst, frequent urination, and family history may be helpful. Since the patient is overweight, a reasonable strategy will be for self-monitoring of glucose values plus some adjustments in diet. A lower carbohydrate diet coupled with exercise may be sufficient without the use of insulin or oral hypoglycemic drugs. Before discharge the glycosylated hemoglobin (hemoglobin $A_{1C}$) should be determined. This value reflects blood sugar levels for the previous two to three months. *(6, 14)*

**13m. (A)** The hemoglobin $A_{1C}$ indicates whether the patient's blood sugar levels have been under control over the previous two to three months. Normal patients have values less than 7% which is the targeted level for diabetics that are under good control. Values above 9% show poor control and levels above 12% call for more aggressive therapy. Tests for glycosylated hemoglobin should be performed every three to six months. *(6, 14)*

**13n. (E)** Needle sizes are based upon two measurements—the length in inches, and the diameter based upon an arbitrary system in which the smaller the diameter, the larger the number. Since most insulin injections are administered subcutaneously, a short needle of 3/8 to 5/8 in and small gauge of 25 to 27 is used. *(13, 25)*

**13o. (A)** One Touch Fast Take (LifeScan) is a strip and meter that requires drawing of only 1.5 μl of blood from the arm rather than finger, thus the blood sampling is less painful. *(10, 25)*

**13p.** **(B)** Macular degeneration is a condition in which there is deterioration of the macula, which is the central area of the retina. Painless loss of vision occurs. It is more common in the elderly but tends to run in families. *(14, 16)*

**13q.** **(C)** Lutein is a natural carotenoid found in the retina. There is evidence that supplements of lutein may help prevent the development of macular degeneration which is characterized by painless loss of vision. Although the adult daily requirement (ADR) has not been established, suggested levels of lutein are in the range of 1–6 mg. The lutein contents of Ocuvite formulas are 2–6 mg while many multivitamins contain doses of only 250 μg or none of lutein. Lutein is also available as a single entity product. *(1, 14, 25)*

## PROFILE NO. 14

**14a.** **(C)** The generic name for Zoloft is sertraline. The drug is classified as a selective serotonin reuptake inhibitor (SSRI) and is effective for the treatment of obsessive-compulsive disorder (OCD). This condition is characterized by recurrent and persistent ideas, thoughts, and impulses that are often time-consuming and interfere with normal social functioning. Zoloft is available as 25-, 50-, and 100-mg tablets plus an oral concentrate. *(3, 25)*

**14b.** **(B)** Antidepressants often take two weeks or more before significant improvement may be observed. The pharmacist should suggest that the patient continue on therapy for a longer period of time. *(3, 14)*

**14c.** **(B)** 240 mg/dL equals 2400 mg/L or 2.4 g/L.

$$\frac{2.4\ \text{g}}{387\ \text{g/mol}} = 0.0062\ \text{mol or } 6.2\ \text{m mol/L} \quad (23)$$

**14d.** **(B)** Mr. Shannon's high density lipoprotein (HDL) value is desirable when compared to his low density lipoprotein (LDL), triglycerides, and total cholesterol values. Most cholesterol profiles include a LDL/HDL ratio in which a low value is desirable. Another meaningful ratio is the cholesterol/HDL value. In this patient, a ratio of 3.6 is fairly low since the usual range is 4 to 7. Again, a low ratio is desirable. Mr. Shannon's direct LDL is high with a normal range usually considered 0 to 100. *(14, 16)*

**14e.** **(C)** Patients with hyperlipidemia have been successfully treated with daily intake of niacin, especially if the statins do not appear to work well. While niacin is relatively safe, daily doses as high as 3000 mg may be necessary. Side effects of flushing, peptic ulceration and jaundice may occur. *(2)*

**14f.** **(C)** The first approach for reduction of blood pressure should be the combination of diet and diuretics. If the condition does not improve within a couple of months, more aggressive and expensive treatment may be required. *(6, 14)*

**14g.** **(B)** The active ingredients in Primatene Mist and Primatene tablets are epinephrine and guaifenesin. The product is intended for counteracting minor attacks of bronchial asthma by producing bronchodilation. Individuals experiencing asthma attacks should consult with a physician to obtain newer, safer products. Primatene is unlikely to improve Mr. Shannon's allergic rhinitis. *(2)*

**14h.** **(C)** Nasonex Nasal (mometasone furoate) spray is a corticosteroid anti-inflammatory product intended for the treatment of seasonal or perennial allergic rhinitis with dosing of 1 or 2 sprays daily in each nostril. Daily use of this product is not required when pollen counts are low. A new unit must be primed by actuating the pump 10 times before using. If the unit is not used for a week or more, the priming must be repeated. *(10)*

**14i.** **(B)** The adult dose of Clarinex is 5–10 mg once a day while Allegra is dosed as 60 mg twice a day or 180 mg once a day. The incidence of drowsiness of Clarinex is similar to that of Claritin. Actually, desloratadine is the active metabolite of loratadine (Claritin). Dosage forms of Clarinex include regular and rapidly disintegrating tablets (Reditabs). *(2, 3)*

**14j.** **(B)** Chlorpheniramine and diphenhydramine are considered to be "first generation" antihistamines. Although very effective for treatment of allergic rhinitis and urticaria, they cause somnolence and impair psychomotor performance to a greater degree than the newer drugs. The "second generation" antihistamines cause much less sedation because they only poorly penetrate into the brain. *(6, 14)*

**14k.** **(B)** The nonprescription drug product, Alavert, contains the same active ingredient, loratadine, which is present in Claritin. Aleve contains the internal analgesic, naproxen. Contac is a combination product consisting of pseudoephedrine and chlorpheniramine. Tavist contains clemastine fumarate while Vivarin is therapeutically unrelated to the other products. It contains caffeine and is used as a mild stimulant. *(2, 26)*

**14l.** **(A)** Burow's solution contains 5% aluminum acetate. It is used topically as an astringent dressing. Conditions such as athlete's foot, diaper rash, dry skin, and various types of dermatitis such as poison ivy may be treated with this product. *(1)*

**14m.** **(B)** Aquaphor is a good absorbent of liquids such as Burow's solution and will ease its incorporation into the oleaginous petrolatum ointment base. Alcohol should not be included in the formula since it will have a tendency to evaporate and cause migration of the salicylic acid to the surface of the ointment. Polysorbate 80 is a nonionic surfactant which would have no useful purpose in the formula. *(1, 4, 19)*

**14n.** **(B)** Carbolic acid is another name for phenol. Aspirin is acetylsalicylic acid, not salicylic acid. *(1)*

**14o.** **(D)** Salicylic acid is used in topical products as a keratolytic agent, which is an agent that aids in loosening and removing dead skin cells (keratin). *(1, 4)*

**14p.** **(A)** The combination of clarithromycin (Biaxin) and omeprazole 20 mg (Prilosec) is one of the therapies used to eradicate *Helicobacter pylori*.

The duration of therapy is usually 28 days with Biaxin taken during the first 14 days then Prilosec from days 15 through 28. *(14, 18a)*

**14q.** **(B)** In some patients, especially the elderly, digoxin levels may increase when clarithromycin is administered. This is believed to be due to the inhibition of P-glycoprotein by clarithromycin. P-glycoprotein is believed to promote renal clearance of digoxin. *(3, 10, 25)*

**14r.** **(D)** Rosacea is a condition characterized by redness in the cheeks and other areas of the face. Left untreated, the color increases with dilation of small blood vessels. The condition worsens when the patient is exposed to the sun or is under stress. Usually the tetracyclines or metronidazole are used as treatment since there is some evidence of bacterial involvement. *(28: April 2003)*

## PROFILE NO. 15

**15a.** **(C)** Cystic fibrosis is an inherited disease that affects the lungs, digestive system, sweat glands, and male fertility. Its name is derived from the fibrous scar tissue that develops in the pancreas, one of the principal organs affected by the disease. The disease is characterized by the production of thicker than normal mucus in various parts of the body. The organ systems most severely affected by cystic fibrosis are the digestive system and the respiratory system. *(25)*

**15b.** **(C)** While genetic testing can be performed to diagnose cystic fibrosis, the sweat test is one of the easiest and most accurate tests for this disease. People with cystic fibrosis have a higher than normal salt concentration in their sweat. In performing this test, a drug such as pilocarpine is applied to the skin. Then an electric current is applied to the area to enhance pilocarpine absorption. This causes sweating in the area of drug application. By absorbing this sweat and measuring its salt content, the disease can be identified. *(25)*

**15c.** **(D)** While acetylcysteine (Mucomyst) is generally administered by inhalation as a mucolytic agent in treating cystic fibrosis, oral acetylcysteine is considered to be the antidote of choice in treating acetaminophen overdose. Acetylcysteine supplies the sulfhydryl groups that are necessary to provide for normal and safe metabolism of acetaminophen. *(25)*

**15d.** **(A)** From early infancy, children with cystic fibrosis have difficulty in absorbing dietary fats. This is caused by the obstruction of pancreatic and biliary ducts that would otherwise deliver pancreatic lipase and other enzymes that are involved with fat absorption. Such patients, therefore, frequently suffer from steatorrhea, the presence of excessive fat in the stools. *(25)*

**15e.** **(D)** Cotazym is a product that contains pancreatic enzymes such as lipase, amylase, and protease from porcine (pig) origin. It should be taken orally with each meal in order to help digest the food that is being consumed. The product may be administered in a capsule form, or the contents of the capsule may be emptied into food or liquid. *(10)*

**15f.** **(B)** The active ingredient in Ritalin and Methylin is methylphenidate. Adderall contains four different amphetamine salts and Xenical contains orlistat, a lipase inhibitor used for promoting weight reduction. *(3)*

**15g.** **(C)** Concerta is a product that is a sustained-release form of methylphenidate. The method used to provide sustained-release action is an osmotic pump (OROS) system that causes the drug to be released gradually as it passes through the GI tract. *(10)*

**15h.** **(B)** Ritalin contains methylphenidate, an amphetamine-like compound that can cause CNS and cardiac stimulation, resulting in adverse effects such as insomnia, nervousness, loss of appetite, and tachycardia. *(3)*

**15i.** **(E)** None of the choices are indicated for the treatment of ADHD. They are all antipsychotic agents. *(10)*

## PROFILE NO. 16

**16a.** **(D)** OCD (obsessive-compulsive disorder) is a condition characterized by obsessive thoughts and compulsive behavior that hinder everyday functioning. Usually the condition has a gradual onset in early adulthood. Bipolar disorders usually are characterized by unpredictable mood swings from excessive social extroversion to depression. The schizophrenic patient is usually socially withdrawn with periods of delusions or hallucinations. *(14)*

**16b.** **(B)** The SSRIs are usually considered the first-line treatment for OCD patients. Patient response may vary from one product to another. Usual starting doses are 50 mg/day for fluvoxamine and 20 mg for citalopram, paroxetine, or fluoxetine. After a few days of observation, it may be necessary to adjust the dose, usually upward. The tricyclic drug, clomipramine is also effective but has more side effects and presents a greater danger if overdosed. The patient should also be informed that behavioral improvements while taking these drugs may take several weeks. *(14)*

**16c.** **(A)** Celexa is Forest's brand of citalopram. This SSRI is available as 10-, 20-, and 40-mg tablets with the usual daily dose of 20–60 mg. There is also an oral solution (10 mg/5 mL) which allows greater flexibility in dosing. *(10)*

**16d.** **(E)** Venlafaxine (Effexor) is probably the best choice. Dosing of 37.5 mg daily with upward dosing may be necessary. A second mode of therapy may be the use of SSRIs in low doses. Some patients may be given one of the benzodiazepines but this is not considered first-line therapy, especially if the patient's history includes alcoholism or other substance abuse. *(3; 10)*

**16e.** **(D)** Magnesium stearate is a lubricant added to many commercial tablet formulations. It serves as a lubricant to permit better flow of tablet granulations into tablet machines and to reduce the likelihood that compressed tablets will stick in the tablet machine. *(3)*

**16f.** **(C)** Diaphragms are a prescription-only item that are originally fitted by a physician. Their sizes are in millimeters, which refers to the diameter of the diaphragm. *(1; 10; 11)*

**16g.** **(E)** Nonoxynol-9 is a nonionic surface active agent that is classified as a spermicide. Women using a diaphragm as a contraceptive method should coat the unit with a cream or jelly containing nonoxynol-9. The diaphragm should be left in place for 6 h after intercourse. *(1; 10; 11)*

**16h.** **(D)** Larry may be exhibiting signs of Attention Deficit Hyperactivity Disorder (ADHD). Further signs would be impulsive behavior. The young age of the boy precludes the likelihood of Alzheimer's disease, but the symptoms described may also suggest lead poisoning. The pharmacist should query the mother further concerning the possibility that her child has consumed paint chips containing lead. The most serious symptom of lead poisoning is acute encephalopathy. The high toxicity of lead is primarily due to its strong attraction to sulfhydryl (SH) groups found in some proteins. The pharmacist should urge the mother to contact the boy's pediatrician for further evaluation. *(14; 16)*

**16i.** **(A)**

$10\ \mu g = 0.01\ mg = 0.00001\ g$ and $1\ dL = 100\ mL$

$$\frac{0.00001\ g}{100\ mL} = \frac{x\ g}{1,000,000\ mL} \qquad x = 0.1\ ppm \quad (23)$$

**16j.** **(C)** The standard for treating lead poisoning has been intravenous administration of BAL (dimercaprol) followed by disodium calcium edetate. A new therapy is the use of succimer, a drug that contains 2,3-dimercaptosuccinic acid (DMSA), which is administered by the oral route. *N*-Acetylcysteine (Mucomyst) is not effective for this poisoning.

**16k.** **(E)** Although its popularity has decreased, thimerosol has been used in pharmaceutical products such as parenteral and ophthalmic solutions as an antimicrobial preservative. Some people exhibit great sensitivity to this mercury-containing chemical. *(1; 2)*

**16l.** **(A)** *Acanthamoeba* is an opportunistic protozoan with a very resistant cyst. If an eye becomes infected, keratitis may develop. *(2)*

**16m.** **(A)** There is a possibility that black cohosh may cause stimulation of the uterus, which may lead to premature labor. Ginger has been shown to be useful during the first trimester of pregnancy in relieving morning sickness. *(1; 18b)*

**16n.** **(D)** Patients that are pregnant or immunocompromised should avoid any live vaccine. All of the listed vaccines, except smallpox, have been inactivated and present little danger to a pregnant woman. Other live, attenuated vaccines include measles, mumps, rubella, and varicella. *(14; 16)*

## PROFILE NO. 17

**17a.** **(B)** Elevated levels of aspartate aminotransferase enzyme (AST) is an indication that the patient is experiencing a myocardial infarction or a liver disease such as viral hepatitis. Anthropometic assessment consists of physically measuring the patient's muscle mass. Obviously malnourished patients will have less lean muscle which is also reflected in high blood or urine nitrogen levels. Recent unexplained weight loss should have been part of the original patient history. *(14, 16)*

**17b.** **(D)** Kwashiorkor presents as malnutrition with the presence of a fatty liver and edema. Marasmus is a more generalized starvation with a loss of body fat and protein. Graves disease is an incorrect answer since it is related to hyperthyroidism, a hypermetabolic state, psychiatric disturbances, and muscular tremors. This condition may be controlled with drugs such as propylthiouracil, propranolol, or oral iodides. *(14)*

**17c.** **(B)** Sickle cell disease is characterized by anemia with red blood cell hemolysis accompanied by severe pain due to microvascular inclusions. The erythrocytes have a crescent shape. Acute attacks are treated by keeping the patient well hydrated and using oral or parenteral morphine (0.1–0.15 mg/kg) every 3–4 h for the pain. Recent studies have shown that hydroxyurea will increase levels of HbF (fetal hemoglobin) thus, decreasing sickle cell polymerization and erythrocyte sickling. *(3, 14, 16)*

**17d.** **(E)** While the safety and efficacy of zolpidem has not been definitely established, the dose of 5 mg is reasonable as a mild hypnotic or sedative. The drug is marketed under the trade name of Ambien and is available as 5 and 10 mg tablets. Because of its relatively fast onset of action, it is taken at bedtime, not 2 h before. Chemically, zolpidem is not a benzodiazepine. *(25)*

**17e.** **(B)** The original order was for subcutaneous administration of morphine sulfate 0.15 mg/kg of body weight every 4 h when needed.

$$100 \text{ lb} \times 1 \text{ kg}/2.2 \text{ lb} = 46 \text{ kg}$$

$$0.15 \text{ mg/kg} \times 46 \text{ kg} = 6.9 \text{ mg}$$

$$\frac{6.9 \text{ mg}}{x \text{ mL}} = \frac{10 \text{ mg}}{1 \text{ mL}}$$

$$x = 0.69 \text{ or } 0.7 \text{ mL} \qquad (1; 23)$$

**17f.** **(A)** Each 1000 mL of TPN contains 500 mL of 50% dextrose, or 250 g dextrose with a flow rate of 125 mL/h.

$$\frac{250 \text{ g}}{1000 \text{ mL}} = \frac{x \text{ g}}{125 \text{ mL}} \quad x = 31.25 \text{ g of dextrose}$$

Caloric density of dextrose is 3.4 kcal/g. Therefore, 31.25 g × 3.4 kcal/g = 106 kcal *(4, 13)*.

**17g.** **(B)** 1000 mL of 5% amino acid solution will contain 50 g of amino acids. Since the average nitrogen content of amino acids is 16%, 50 g × 16% = 8 g *(4, 13)*

**17h.** **(C)** The prescribed TPN solution is hypertonic. Any solution containing more than 10% glucose should not be administered peripherally because of potential damage to the veins in the arm. Originally administration of these solutions were limited to central catheters, mainly into the subclavian vein, which has a high blood flow. The development of PICC lines (peripherally inserted central catheters) allows the use of veins in the arm since the line is threaded further into the vein to an area with high blood flow. A further advantage of the PICC line is that it may be inserted by health professionals without employing a surgical cutdown for insertion. *(13, 22)*

**17i.** **(A)** The Cockroft-Gault equation is very useful in estimating creatinine clearance. The equation reads:

$$Cl_{Cr} = \frac{(140 - \text{age}) \times \text{body wt}}{72 \, S_{Cr}}$$

where age is in years and weight is in kg

A correction factor of 0.85 is placed before the (140 – age) expression for females. *(5, 17)*

**17j.** **(C)** The serum creatinine value reported on 8/16 was 0.8 mg/dL. The male patient is 16 years old and weighs 100 lb (45.5 kg). Therefore,

$$Cl_{Cr} = \frac{(140 - \text{age}) \times \text{body wt}}{72 \, S_{Cr}}$$

$$CL_{Cr} = \frac{(140 - 16)(45.5 \text{ kg})}{72 \, (0.8)}$$

$$= 98 \text{ mL/min} \qquad (5, 17)$$

**17k.** **(D)** Studies indicate that the branched chain amino acids (BCAA) are more readily assimilated into the body. Formulas with the "BCAAs" are used in stressed patients and those with liver impairment. Commercial products include HepatAmine, FreeAmine HBC, Branch Amine, and Aminosyn-HBC. *(3, 4)*

**17l.** **(C)** The PCA order issued on August 18 reads "0.02 mg morphine sulfate per kilogram of body weight infused each hour for three days."

0.02 mg/kg/h × body wt of 100 lb (46 kg)
= 0.92 mg/h

0.92 mg/h × 24 h × 3 days = 66.2 mg total

$$\frac{10 \text{ mg}}{1 \text{ mL}} = \frac{66.2 \text{ mg}}{x \text{ mL}}$$

$x$ = 6.6 mL of morphine sulfate solution    *(23)*

**17m.** **(D)** Elastomeric devices are used as infusion delivery systems for ambulatory patients in many situations. These disposable pumps such as Baxter's Intermates and Block Medical's Homepumps are convenient and relatively less expensive than PCAs. However, they do not allow extra bolus dosing of analgesics and the flow rate is preset. These devices, as well as PCAs, provide subcutaneous infusion of analgesics as well as other parenteral drugs. *(22)*

## PROFILE NO. 18

**18a.** **(D)** Propylthiouracil is an anti-thyroid drug used in treating Graves' disease since this disease is characterized by hyperthyroidism. *(3)*

**18b.** **(D)** A regimen of chemotherapy known as MOPP is used in the treatment of Hodgkin's disease. Procarbazine (Matulane) and prednisone are given by the oral route on each day of the 14-day schedule. Mechlorethamine (Mustargen) and vincristine (Oncovin) are given intravenously on the first and eighth days of therapy. Combining drugs that have different mechanisms of action increases remission rates and lowers the incidence and severity of side effects. *(3)*

**18c.** **(A)** Hepatocellular, renal cell, and thyroid carcinomas have shown poor responses to presently used chemotherapeutic drugs. Ovarian and prostatic carcinomas are moderately responsive, with palliation and probable prolongation of life. Prolonged survival and probably some cures are expected in patients with testicular cancer and Hodgkin's disease. *(5)*

**18d.** **(A)** The acronym, SOAP, refers to a plan to evaluate a patient's progress. The letters usually refer to Subjective, Objective, Assessment, and Plans. As a group, the health team decides whether the care provided meets the needs of the patient. *(14; 22)*

**18e.** **(B)** Mechlorethamine is a potent vesicant. Serious localized damage may occur if the drug solution seeps into the area surrounding the infusion site. The thiosulfate ion will react with the nitrogen mustard. Ice compresses will relieve the burning sensation and slow the spread of mechlorethamine. Other solutions that have been infused are normal saline and sodium bicarbonate. *(3)*

**18f.** **(B)** A 1-molar solution of sodium thiosulfate will contain 248 g of chemical in 1 L of solution. A one-sixth molar solution will contain 248/6 or 41 g/L or 4.1g/100 ml. *(3)*

**18g.** **(B)** Although the official form of sodium thiosulfate contains five waters of hydration, the correct amount of active ingredient can be obtained by using the anhydrous form. Simply subtract 90 (weight of water in the molecule) from 248 to obtain 158 (the weight of anhydrous sodium thiosulfate), then

| $x$ g | 10 g |
|---|---|
| anhydrous sodium ↔ hydrated sodium |  |
| thiosulfate | thiosulfate |
| mol wt of 158 | mol wt of 248 |

$x$ = 6.4 g    *(1; 23)*

**18h.** **(A)** Many chemotherapeutic drugs, especially the alkylating agents, cause bone marrow depression, which is characterized by low leukocyte counts with increased susceptibility to infections. The term, nadir, indicates the length of time before the deepest depression occurs. For example, the nadir for a given drug may be 7–10 days after the start of therapy, with bone marrow recovery in 14–18 days. *(6; 14)*

**18i.** **(A)** Vincristine as well as the other vinca alkaloids are strong vesicants. The usual method for administration of these drugs is by IV push into the sidearm (Y-site) of a running infusion line.

IM injection would likely result in tissue necrosis at the injection site. Intrathecal administration is contraindicated as there have been several deaths attributed to this procedure. *(6; 14)*

**18j.** **(C)** Epoetin alfa (Epogen) is a stimulant of red blood cell production. Filgrastim (Neupogen) is a stimulant of granulocyte (leukocyte) production. These are used in patients receiving myelosuppressive drugs such as mechlorethamine. Clopidogrel (Plavix) is an inhibitor of platelet aggregation. *(3)*

**18k.** **(C)** Cyanocobalamin injection is a pink-colored solution available in strengths of 100 and 1000 µg/mL. It is administered by either IM or subcutaneous injection, but not IV. The parenteral route offers better bioavailability than oral administration. *(3)*

**18l.** **(E)** Cetirizine (Zyrtec), desloratidine (Clarinex), and fexofenadine (Allegra) are peripherally selective antihistamines. They cause less drowsiness than non-selective agents. *(3)*

## PROFILE NO. 19

**19a.** **(B)** A trade name for paclitaxel is Taxol. Taxotere, is another popular drug for breast cancer with the generic name of docetaxel. Tazidime (ceftazidime) is a cephalosporin antimicrobial agent used for both gram-negative and gram-positive aerobes as well as for anaerobes. *(3; 10)*

**19b.** **(A)** Commercial paclitaxel (Taxol) solution is in a nonaqueous vehicle which, when diluted, may be slightly turbid. Therefore, it is a good technique to infuse the solution using an administration set that has an in-line filter. The admixture should be prepared in a glass bottle not PVC plastic bags which may leach some of the plasticizer, diethylhexyl phthalate (DEHP). Infusion times may be as short as 1 h. *(10)*

**19c.** **(A)** Dolasetron mesylate is available under the tradename of Anzemet. It is used to prevent nausea and vomiting during cancer therapy. Both an injection (20 mg/mL) and tablets (50

and 100 mg) are available. The drug is classified as a 5-HT$_3$–receptor antagonist. *(10)*

**19d.** **(D)** Cisplatin is available as Platinol and Platinol AQ. Paraplatin is a different drug having the generic name of carboplatin. There have been medication errors when these two agents were interchanged with each other. Cisplatin is an alkylating agent used for several types of cancers including ovarian, testicular, and prostate. The incidence of nausea is very high and may be a delayed reaction occurring up to 48 h after the infusion. *(3; 21)*

**19e.** **(D)** The medication order calls for 150 mg/m$^2$ of body surface area, and this patient has a surface area of 1.85 m$^2$. Therefore,

$$\frac{150 \text{ mg}}{1} = \frac{x \text{ mg}}{1.85} \quad x = 278 \text{ mg}$$

Each vial contains 6 mg/mL of drug, thus

$$\frac{6 \text{ mg}}{1 \text{ mL}} = \frac{278 \text{ mg}}{x \text{ mL}} \quad x = 46 \text{ mL} \qquad (23)$$

**19f.** **(D)** Myelosuppression, or suppression of the bone marrow, usually results in a sharp decrease in white blood cells. This may be life-threatening because of the patient's increased susceptibility to infection. The antineoplastic drug, tamoxifen, is a nonsteroidal antiestrogen used in the treatment of breast cancer. Adverse effects of the drug include nausea, vomiting, hot flashes, vaginal bleeding, hypercalcemia, and thrombocytopenia, but the drug is not noted for causing bone marrow depression. Tamoxifen is available as oral tablets under the tradenames of Nolvadex, Nolvadex-D, and Tamofen. Dosage strengths are 10 and 20 mg + a 20 mg enteric-coated tablet to reduce GI tract irritation. *(5; 26)*

**19g.** **(A)** Peripheral neuropathy is a degenerative state of peripheral nerves in which motor, sensory, or vasomotor fibers may be affected. Symptoms may include muscle weakness, numbness, and/or pain. *(16; 27)*

**19h.** **(D)** The dictionary defines "nadir" as the place or time of deepest depression. When discussing drug chemotherapy, the term usually refers to the length of time before maximum bone marrow depression occurs. Many chemotherapeutic drugs, especially the alkylating agents, cause a depression characterized by low leukocyte counts with increased susceptibility to infection. For example, the nadir for a given drug may be 7–10 days after the start of therapy, with bone marrow recovery in 14–18 days. *(3)*

**19i.** **(D)** Patients undergoing therapy with cisplatin should be well hydrated. Usually 1–2 L of solutions containing dextrose and sodium chloride are infused 8–12 h before the cisplatin infusion. Discontinuing the hydrochlorothiazide will also reduce water loss. *(14; 21)*

**19j.** **(A)** FUO refers to the presence of a fever of unknown origin, likely due to a systemic infection. The patient will be placed on a broad spectrum antibiotic until the culture and sensitivity tests indicate the need for a more specific antibiotic. To reduce fever, oral or rectal acetaminophen will likely be prescribed. *(6; 14)*

**19k.** **(A)** Augmentin is available in oral dosage forms including tablets, capsules, and oral suspensions. However, it is not intended for parenteral administration. From the symptoms provided, it appears that Ms. Hockford may have developed a respiratory tract infection. A possible substitute would be ceftriaxone sodium (Rocephin) which has a broad spectrum of action and is dosed at 1 or 2 g daily. *(3; 10)*

**19l.** **(C)** Laboratory culture and sensitivity testing allows identification of antimicrobial activity of common antimicrobial agents against a specific, isolated microorganism. By reviewing the lab report of MICs, one may choose the drug of choice for an infection. Usually the antibiotic with the lowest MIC (minimum inhibitory concentration) should be selected. The targeted peak concentration of the antibiotic is usually 4 to 5 times the MIC. *(1; 14)*

**19m.** **(C)** Vancomycin injection should be infused over a minimum of a 1 h duration. Otherwise, serious hypotension including shock may occur. Also, a rash known as red man syndrome may

occur during or a short time after the infusion has occurred. The rash usually resolves within a few hours. Pseudomembranous colitis may be a result of vancomycin administration but is not an immediate result of rapid infusion. *(3)*

## PROFILE NO. 20

**20a.** **(A)** Hytrin has the generic name of terazosin and is classified as an alpha$_1$-adrenergic blocker. It is indicated for prevention of hypertension either by itself or combined with a diuretic or beta-adrenergic blocking agent. Other drugs in the same class include Cardura, Flomax, and Minipress. *(3)*

**20b.** **(C)** Terazosin is available under the tradename of Hytrin. It and other drugs in its class causes a marked hypotension, especially postural, in patients for the first few doses. Some patients may experience syncope (fainting). *(3)*

**20c.** **(D)** Raloxifene (Evista) is available as 60 mg tablets and is intended for the prevention of osteoporosis in the postmenopausal female. It is classified as a selective estrogen receptor modulator since it has estrogen-like effects on bone but lacks estrogen-like activity on either uterine or breast tissues. It is not intended for the premenopausal woman since it is a pregnancy category X drug. *(3; 10)*

**20d.** **(B)** *Ortho*-Evra is a transdermal drug delivery patch intended as a contraceptive. A patch is applied once weekly for a total of three weeks. Each day, constant amounts of norelgestromin and ethinyl estadiol are released. While the patient may experience some of the adverse effects inherent in the use of hormonal contraceptives, the intensity should be less since there are no "bolus" amounts of drug released at one time. Choice E is incorrect since Estraderm transdermal is intended to moderate the symptoms of menopause. *(3; 10)*

**20e.** **(A)** The buik of *Facts and Comparisons* describes drugs available in the United States. However, it also identifies drugs available in Canada by their generic and trade names. Once the generic name of the drug has been located, comparable products could be located. *Martindale* is another reference book that allows identification of foreign drug products. Its listings are mainly for European drugs. *(1; 3)*

**20f.** **(C)** Iodine dissolved in mineral oil has been used as a topical product because the iodine will impart a darker color to the skin and the mineral oil provides emolliency. However, this combination does not filter out ultraviolet rays and, therefore, provides virtually no protection against sunburn. All of the other choices are approved sunscreen agents. *(1; 2).*

**20g.** **(E)** Haldol, Risperdal, or Seroquel may be tried for schizophrenia. The neuroleptic Seroquel is available as tablets and is considered first-line treatment probably because of the lower incidence of adverse effects. Haldol is available in several dosage forms. Risperdal is available in both tablets and an oral solution. *(10; 16)*

**20h.** **(B)** Fluphenazine is a good choice of a neuroleptic drug for the management of several psychotic disorders. The decanoate and enanthate esters are formulated into oil solvents thus providing a long duration of action—usually two to three weeks. *(1; 14)*

**20i.** **(D)** Glycated hemoglobin (A1c) is formed by a reaction between hemoglobin and glucose and reflects the average glucose level in a patient during the past three- to four-month period. Home testing for A1c is now possible with the development of an OTC test (Metrika A1c Now), which simply requires a blood sample from the finger. Hemoglobin A1c values should ideally be below 7.0. *(2; 10; 14)*

**20j.** **(B)** Ascites refers to an accumulation of serous fluid in the peritoneal cavity First treatment is usually the administration of a diuretic. *(27)*

**20k.** **(D)** Ankylosing spondylitis is a disease of the connective tissue that resembles rheumatoid arthritis. It usually presents as an inflammation of a large joint and spine. Usually symptoms include recurring episodes of back pain. Treatment involves the use of NSAIDs, especially the COX-2 drugs. *(16)*

**20l.** **(C)** Although the depressant effects of alcohol may occur at lower blood levels, mental impairment and loss of motor coordination is obvious in most individuals once blood alcohol levels exceed 0.1%. The major problem with alcohol metabolism is the limited supply of enzymes available for the oxidation. Therefore, alcohol metabolism may be described as mainly following zero-order kinetics with limited amounts metabolized each hour. *(3; 17)*

**20m.** **(A)** Butenafine in Lotrimin Ultra is claimed to possess fungicidal activity rather than just fungistatic properties. Clotrimazole is present in Lotrimin AF cream, lotion, and solution while Lotrimin powder and liquid spray contain miconazole. *(2; 3)*

**20n.** **(C)** TMP-SMZ is the acronym for the combination of trimethoprim and sulfamethoxazole, now referred to as co-trimoxazole. Brand names of this combination include Bactrim and Septra. The product is effective against urinary tract infections, acute otitis media, traveler's diarrhea and chronic bronchitis in adults. The ingredient ratio is 1 part of trimethoprim to every 5 parts of sulfamethoxazole. *(3)*

## PROFILE NO. 21

**21a.** **(A)** Hypothyroidism (myxedema) is characterized by the slowing of body processes because of a deficiency of thyroid hormone. The classic treatment has been thyroid tablets. Today, this drug has been replaced with L-thyroxine (T4), L-thyronine (T3), and liotrix (a mixture of T4 and T3). Levoxyl is levothyroxine sodium (L-thyroxine). Graves' disease is a form of hyperthyroidism. *(5:1247)*

**21b.** **(E)** Omission of a single dose of Levoxyl will not have significant effects on the disease state. *(3)*

**21c.** **(B)** Both Levoxyl and Synthroid are brands of the generic drug levothyroxine. There are a number of strengths of the tablets from 0.025 mg up to 3 mg. Cytomel is a brand of liothyronine and Thyrolar is generically known as liotrix.

**21d.** **(C)** The pharmacist must consider the possibilities of both overusage or underusage of drugs especially by the elderly. The original Levoxyl order on 8/4 was for 30 tablets with directions of one tablet per day, but a refill was not requested until 9/28. Furosemide 40 mg tablets were ordered with the directions of one every other day. Despite the two-month supply provided on 9/28, the patient is requesting a refill on 10/28. Perhaps she is taking a tablet every day rather than every other day. The digoxin appears to be taken on schedule.

**21e.** **(A)** Glucosamine and chondroitin combinations are nonprescription dietary supplements used to improve joint flexibility. Usually doses of 500 mg glucosamine + 400 mg chondroitin are used. *(2; 18a)*

**21f.** **(C)** Although there is some patient-to-patient variation, one of the earliest signs of Alzheimer's disease is the forgetfulness of current events; for example, what one has eaten for lunch. Although gradual, this memory loss becomes progressively worse. *(5)*

**21g.** **(D)** Tacrine (Cognex) and donepezil (Aricept) are cholinesterase inhibitors that have reduced the clinical symptoms of Alzheimer's. Selegiline is available as Eldepryl and is used in the treatment of parkinsonism. *(3)*

**21h.** **(B)** Aspartame and saccharin are artificial sweeteners that are 200 and 400 times sweeter, respectively, than sucrose. These agents are used in many dietary foods and in some pharmaceuticals. The use of saccharin in place of 1 teaspoonful of sugar saves the consumer 33 calories. Aspartame should be avoided in patients with phenylketonuria. *(3)*

**21i.** **(C)** The tannins in teas may react with iron to form insoluble iron tannates. It is well established that many antacids combine with iron, thereby reducing its absorption. *(3)*

**21j.** **(C)** Women, especially postmenopausal women, should increase their intake of calcium to avoid osteoporosis. Tums is available containing 500 mg of calcium carbonate per chewable tablet, 750 mg chewable tablets (Tums E-X) and 1000 mg chewable tablets (Tums Ultra). Although calcium carbonate can be used in the prevention of gastroesophageal reflux (GERD), there are more effective products on the market. The antacid dosing regimen for GERD would be a dose after each meal as well as at bedtime. *(3)*

**21k.** **(A)** Many of the elderly have an increase in the relative amount of fat in their bodies, partially because of dehydration and less activity. The corresponding volume of distribution for lipophilic drugs may increase. Renal clearance rates are often lower in the elderly because of impaired kidney function. The plasma albumin levels are sometimes lower than normal, thereby affecting the amount of protein binding. *(3)*

**21l.** **(C)** If both dosage forms had 100% bioavailability (F value of 1.0), the answer would be 5 mL.

$$\frac{0.05 \text{ mg}}{1 \text{ mL}} = \frac{0.25 \text{ mg}}{x \text{ mL}} \quad x = 5 \text{ mL of elixir}$$

However, the entire dose of the drug is not available as reflected in the "F" values of 0.6 for the tablet and 0.75 for the elixir. Therefore,

$$Q_1 \times C_1 = Q_2 \times C_2$$
$$0.25 \text{ mg} \times 0.6 = x \text{ mg} \times 0.75$$
$$x = 0.2 \text{ mg of digoxin needed}$$

Since the elixir contains 0.05 mg per mL

$$\frac{0.05 \text{ mg}}{1 \text{ mL}} = \frac{0.2 \text{ mg}}{x \text{ mL}} \quad x = 4 \text{ mL of elixir}$$

**21m.** **(A)** Many elderly persons who exhibit digoxin toxicity experience hazy vision rather than the more classic halo and color vision changes that occur in younger patients. Rather than having an increase in appetite, anorexia often occurs. *(3)*

**21n.** **(E)** All of the choices decrease digoxin's volume of distribution and renal clearance rate. When these drugs are used with digoxin, it is often necessary to reduce the digoxin dose by 50%. *(3)*

---

**PROFILE NO. 22**

---

**22a.** **(C)** The term tocolytic refers to a drug that will reduce uterine contractility, thereby preventing premature delivery. *(5:480)*

**22b.** **(B)** Terbutaline is available under the trade names of Brethine and Bricanyl. To inhibit preterm labor, it is administered orally, SC, or IV. However, its greatest market is as a bronchodilator. A second agent that has been very successful for tocolytic therapy is ritodrine (Yutopar), which can be given either orally or IV. *(3)*

**22c.** **(D)** The medication order calls for 25 µg of drug per minute. The pharmacist added 2 mL (2 mg or 2000 mcg) to 250 mL of diluent.

$$\frac{2000 \text{ µg}}{250 \text{ mL}} = \frac{25 \text{ µg}}{x \text{ mL}} \quad x = 3.125 \text{ mL}$$

$$\frac{15 \text{ gtt}}{1 \text{ mL}} = \frac{x \text{ gtt}}{3.125 \text{ mL}} \quad x = 46.8 \text{ drops/min}$$

**22d.** **(B)** The total amount of drug present is 2000 µg in 250 mL. It is being administered at a rate of 25 µg/min or 3.125 mL/min.

$$\frac{250 \text{ mL}}{x \text{ min}} = \frac{3.125 \text{ mL}}{1 \text{ min}} \quad x = 80 \text{ min}$$

**22e.** **(C)** Ibuprofen is available in a number of nonprescription drug products at a strength of 200 mg. It is used as an analgesic, anti-inflammatory, and to reduce fever. *(2)*

**22f.** **(C)** Barium sulfate is used to render the intestinal tract opaque for x rays. A dose of 60–250 g is administered as a suspension. *(3)*

**22g.** **(E)** Barium sulfate is practically insoluble in water; thus, there is little danger of toxicity from systemic absorption of the chemical. It is administered either orally or rectally, depending on the portion of the GI tract to be x-rayed. *(3)*

**22h.** **(B)** Atropine is classified as an antimuscarinic/antispasmodic agent used to inhibit salivation and other excessive secretions during surgery. It may also prevent cholinergic effects such as cardiac arrhythmias, hypotension, and bradycardia during surgery. An alternative drug is glycopyrrolate (Robinul), which may be administered 30 min prior to surgery for action similar to that of atropine. It is also available as oral tablets (1 and 2 mg) to suppress gastric secretions for the treatment of peptic ulcers. *(3)*

**22i.** **(B)** The usual adult dose of atropine is 0.4 mg SC, IM, or even IV. Atropine sulfate and chlorpromazine HCl (Thorazine) will be compatible in a syringe. The purpose of chlorpromazine is to relieve pre-surgical apprehension, and control nausea and vomiting during surgery. *(3)*

**22j.** **(A)** Because of their sizing and use, urinary catheters bear a federal warning concerning dispensing without a prescription. Ostomy pouches are available in several sizes and designs, but the consumer may purchase them, as well as bandages and dressings, without a prescription. *(3)*

**22k.** **(C)** The active ingredient in Metamucil and Fibercon is the bulk-forming laxative psyllium. Some psyllium-containing products contain sucrose as a sweetener. A pharmacist may wish to discourage diabetics away from this type of product to one that contains an artificial sweetener such as aspartame; (e.g., Orange Flavor Metamucil Instant Mix). Mitrolan is an incorrect answer since it and Equalactin contain calcium polycarbophil, another bulk-forming ingredient. *(3)*

**22l.** **(A)** Bulk-forming agents such as Metamucil should be dispersed in water or a flavored liquid such as orange juice, stirred quickly, then swallowed immediately. Otherwise the powder will swell, forming a gel that would be difficult to swallow. Metamucil is also available in a capsule dosage form. *(3)*

**22m.** **(E)** There are several problems for the discharge orders. First, both Prinivil (lisinopril, an ACE inhibitor) and Prosom (estazolam, a benzodiazepine) are pregnancy category D or X drugs and are contraindicated for this patient. Because of its fast onset of action, Sonata (zaleplon) is taken right at bedtime not 2 h before. Since it belongs to pregnancy category C, it would be more appropriate to prescribe a sedative such as Ambien (zolpidem) which is in category B. *(3; 10)*

**22n.** **(D)** The centrally acting beta$_2$-agonist methyldopa (Aldomet) is used as an antihypertensive agent during pregnancy. Other alternatives include labetalol (Normodyne or Trandate) or hydralazine (Apresoline). *(3)*

---

## PROFILE NO. 23

**23a.** **(A)** The active ingredient in Mycelex G is clotrimazole, an antifungal agent effective against *Candida albicans*, which infects the vagina. Mycelex G is available as a vaginal tablet. Many clotrimazole vaginal products are now available OTC. *(10)*

**23b.** **(B)** With the successful treatment of gonorrhea with either fluoroquinolones or cephalosporins, other causes of sexually transmitted urethritis have emerged. More than 50% of cases of nongonorrheal urethritis are caused by the obligate intracellular parasite *Chlamydia*. *(5)*

**23c.** **(A)** Syphilis is usually transmitted by direct contact with an active lesion containing spirochetes. Although there are several stages and types of syphilis, the drug of choice is still parenteral penicillin G, such as 2.4 million units of benzathine penicillin G. For patients allergic to penicillin, doxycycline is generally used. *(5)*

**23d.** **(A)** Infections caused by *Chlamydia* are usually asymptomatic in females, whereas males experience dysuria. Primary treatment will be either doxycycline 100 mg twice a day for 7 days or azithromycin as a single 1000-mg dose. Alternatives include erythromycin 500 mg q.i.d. or ofloxacin 300 mg b.i.d. for 7 days.

Ciprofloxacin has been used but is not as successful as doxycycline. *(5)*

**23e.** **(D)** Plan B is an emergency contraceptive product. It contains a large dose of levonorgestrel, a progestin. When a dose of Plan B is administered within 72 h of unprotected sexual intercourse and a second dose is administered 12 h later, this product is claimed to have a 95% success rate in preventing pregnancy. A spermicidal cream will not likely be effective after intercourse has occurred. Progestasert is an IUD contraceptive device that provides contraceptive action for about one year. Evra is a transdermal contraceptive patch. Clomid is an ovulation stimulant. *(10)*

**23f.** **(D)** White Vaseline or any other petrolatum product is not acceptable as a lubricant for either condoms or diaphragms, because small openings will develop due to the solvent characteristics of petrolatum toward rubber. *(5)*

**23g.** **(B)** Mirena is an intrauterine contraceptive system that releases progestin for up to five years once it has been placed by the physician into the uterus. It can be removed at any time if the patient wishes to become pregnant, or if she wishes to use a different type of contraceptive product. Depo-Provera is a long-acting progesterone product that releases drug for three months after administration. NuvaRing is a vaginal ring that releases hormones for a three-week period and is then removed for a week before a new system is inserted by the patient. Vagisec is a brand of feminine hygiene products. Preven is an emergency contraceptive product. *(10)*

**23h.** **(C)** The testicular hormone danazol (Danocrine) is given orally in 100- to 200-mg doses to treat endometriosis, a condition characterized by menstrual-like bleeding and localized inflammation and pain, usually within the pelvis. A second drug successful in the treatment of endometriosis is nafarelin acetate (Synarel), which is available as an intranasal spray. *(3)*

**23i.** **(C)** Orlistat (Xenical) is a lipase inhibitor used to reduce dietary fat absorption in order to help lose weight. By inhibiting the action of lipase, dietary fats are not absorbed as well and pass out of the body via the colon. If dietary fat restriction is not maintained by the patient, diarrhea and foul smelling stools may result. *(10)*

**23j.** **(E)** Piroxicam (Feldene) is a nonsteroidal anti-inflammatory agent. It has the longest half-life of drugs in this category and should be administered only once daily. The other products have been properly prescribed. *(10)*

**23k.** **(A)** Methylphenidate (Ritalin) is classified as a centrally-acting sympathomimetic agent. It is used in the therapy of attention deficit hyperactivity disorder (ADHD). *(3)*

**23l.** **(B)** The benzodiazepines exert their antianxiety effects by potentiation of the inhibitory neurotransmitter GABA. *(3)*

**23m.** **(B)** The Atkins diet is one which tends to contain low levels of carbohydrate. While it often contains high levels of fat and protein, there is evidence that it may be an effective short-term approach to weight loss. *(3)*

**23n.** **(D)** Flumazenil (Romazicon) is a specific antidote for benzodiazepine overdose. Naloxone and naltrexone are specific opiate antagonists. *(3)*

**23o.** **(B)** An approximation of the caloric content of a product serving can be made by recognizing that fats contribute 9 kcal/g, and protein and fat contribute approximately 4 kcal/g. Therefore, $3 \text{ g} \times 9 \text{ kcal/g} = 27 \text{ kcal}$, $8 \text{ g} \times 4 \text{ kcal/g} = 32 \text{ kcal}$, and $1 \text{ g} \times 4 \text{ kcal/g} = 4 \text{ kcal}$ and $27 + 32 + 4 = 63$. *(3)*

## PROFILE NO. 24

**24a.** **(D)** These two microorganisms are major causes of both otitis media and sinusitis. A third microorganism often implicated is *Moraxella catarrhalis*. *(5)*

**24b.** **(C)** Other appropriate agents are cefixime, cefaclor, azithromycin, etc. Doxycycline is a tetracycline and should not be used in children under 8. *(5)*

**24c.** **(B)** All three drugs possess antipyretic activity. However, Jason is sensitive to salicylates and neither aspirin nor ibuprofen (to which he may also be sensitive) should be dispensed. The newer OTC agents such as naproxen and ketoprofen carry a label warning that they should not be used in young children unless under a physician's supervision. *(3)*

**24d.** **(C)** Ibuprofen is 2-(*p*-isobutylphenyl) propionic acid. *(3)*

**24e.** **(A)** Fever may be the sign of a serious systemic infection. If the fever is masked by the use of an antipyretic, prompt treatment may be delayed. *(3)*

**24f.** **(A)** Amount of cromolyn needed for Rx is $30 \text{ mL} \times 2.5\% = 0.75 \text{ g}$. The amount of the available 4% solution to use:

$$\frac{4 \text{ g}}{100 \text{ mL}} = \frac{0.75 \text{ g}}{x \text{ mL}}$$

$x = 19 \text{ mL}$ (which is already isotonic)

Therefore, the pharmacist must make only the remaining 11 mL isotonic.

$11 \text{ mL} \times 0.9\% \text{ NaCl} = 0.099 \text{ g}$, or 99 mg *(24)*

**24g.** **(A)** Removal of bacteria and fungi from extemporaneously prepared solutions may be accomplished by passage through a 0.20- or 0.22-$\mu$m filter into a sterile container. *(24)*

**24h.** **(E)** "OD" is a Latin abbreviation for the right eye. *(1; 23)*

**24i.** **(B)** Ophthalmic solutions containing cromolyn sodium are effective in the treatment of allergic conjunctivitis. Chronic allergic conjunctivitis patients should also avoid using OTC sympathomimetic decongestants, which may cause rebound vasodilation. *(3)*

**24j.** **(D)** The patient directions on the prescription will read: "2 drops in the right eye three times a day." 2 drops × 3 times a day = 6 drops per day.

$$\frac{6 \text{ gtt}}{x \text{ mL}} = \frac{15 \text{ gtt}}{1 \text{ ml}} \quad x = 0.4 \text{ mL applied per day}$$

Since the bottle contains 30 mL,

$$\frac{0.4 \text{ mL}}{1 \text{ day}} = \frac{30 \text{ mL}}{x \text{ days}} \quad x = 75 \text{ days} \qquad (23)$$

**24k.** **(C)** Diphenhydramine (Benadryl) is a well-known antihistamine exhibiting drowsiness as a major side effect. It is sometimes prescribed as a sleep aid and is available in several commercial OTC sleep-aid products including Compoz, Sominex, and Nytol. *(3)*

**24l.** **(D)** Because of the limited capacity of the eye surface, separating the 2 drops by a few minutes will increase the amount of solution that actually enters and remains in the eye. Blocking the passageway between the eye and nose will reduce the amount of drug lost through the tear duct. *(24)*

**24m.** **(C)** Tofranil (imipramine) in doses of 25 mg 1 h before bedtime reduces the incidence of childhood enuresis. If unsuccessful, the dose may be increased up to 75 mg. *(3)*

**24n.** **(A)** Debrox drops contain carbamide peroxide, which will soften earwax, easing its removal. S.T. 37 is a mouthwash and topical anti-infective with hexylresorcinol as its active ingredient. Anbesol is used in the treatment of cold sores and contains both benzocaine and phenol. *(3)*

**24o.** **(E)** Tartrazine (F.D. & C. Yellow #5) is included in both solid and liquid products. A small fraction of the general population is sensitive to the dye and may respond with typical allergic responses. There appears to be a high incidence of cross sensitivity in individuals sensitive to aspirin and to tartrazine. *(24)*

## PROFILE NO. 25

**25a.** **(B)** Gout is a chronic metabolic disease characterized by hyperuricemia. The uric acid is an end product of protein catabolism. Either uric acid production has increased, or impaired renal clearance is slowing the removal. The immediate concern during an acute attack is to relieve pain. Only after this relief should longer-term therapy be initiated. *(5)*

**25b.** **(C)** To relieve an acute gout attack, an anti-inflammatory drug (NSAID) or colchicine is administered. Colchicine is most effective if given within the first 12–36 h of the acute attack. *(5)*

**25c.** **(B)** Allopurinol (Zyloprim) is the most commonly used agent for long-term control of chronic gout and is the drug of choice for patients that are overproducers of uric acid. Not only does allopurinol inhibit xanthine oxidase, which converts xanthine to uric acid, but allopurinol's metabolite, oxypurinol, also inhibits xanthine oxidase. *(5)*

**25d.** **(C)** Sufficient liquid intake of at least 2 L daily is necessary to prevent formation of urate calculi. Acute attacks of gout may occur on initial therapy; therefore, colchicine therapy should be continued for a few days. Because of possible stomach irritation, it is best to take allopurinol with food. *(3)*

**25e.** **(D)** Simethicone is a defrothicant, i.e., it causes small gas bubbles in the GI to coalesce to form a large bubble that can easily be eliminated. This is useful in treating a patient that is experiencing abdominal pain caused by the accumulation of gas. *(6)*

**25f.** **(D)** Phazyme and Mylicon are OTC products that contain simethicone. They are used to relieve abdominal pain caused by gas. *(3)*

**25g.** **(C)** *Facts and Comparisons* contains information concerning commercial products by listing drugs by similar therapeutic categories. However, it does not present color charts of drug products. All three volumes of the USP DI have color charts. *(3)*

**25h.** **(C)** Minoxidil (Loniten) is available as 2.5 and 10-mg tablets for the treatment of hypertension. Topical 2 and 5% solutions of minoxidil are marketed as Rogaine and Extra Strength Rogaine, respectively, and are indicated for the treatment of alopecia. *(3)*

**25i.** **(E)** Timolol (Blocadren) and penbutolol (Levatol) are beta-adrenergic blocking agents. Irbesartan (Avapro), olmesartan (Benicar), and losartan (Cozaar) are angiotensin II antagonists, and trandolapril (Mavik) is an ACE inhibitor. *(10)*

**25j.** **(B)** Propranolol (Inderal) has the greatest lipophilic activity. It can, therefore, be expected to produce the greatest degree of CNS adverse effects because of its ability to pass through the lipid blood-brain barrier. *(3)*

**25k.** **(A)** Chronic alcoholics may develop thiamine deficiency because alcohol can interfere with the intestinal uptake of thiamine as well as its utilization. Thiamine deficiency can lead to Wernicke-Korsakoff syndrome, which may, in part, be characterized by peripheral neuropathy. *(3)*

**25l.** **(B)** Alpha-tocopherol is a form of vitamin E. This vitamin acts as a lipid-soluble antioxidant. *(6)*

**25m.** **(E)** Rifampin (Rifadin or Rimactane) discolors urine, sweat, and tears. The drug's major use is in the treatment of tuberculosis, usually in combination with isoniazid or pyrazinamide. *(3)*

## PROFILE NO. 26

**26a.** **(D)** Both sertraline (Zoloft) and citalopram (Celexa) are selective serotonin reuptake inhibitors (SSRI) indicated for the treatment of depression. Loxapine (Loxitane) is an antipsychotic agent, ondansetron (Zofran) is an antiemetic, phenelzine (Nardil) as an MAO inhibitor, and clozapine (Clozaril) is an antipsychotic agent. *(3)*

**26b.** **(A)** Bupropion HCl (Wellbutrin) is an aminoketone antidepressant agent and is chemically unrelated to other currently available antidepressant drugs. *(3)*

**26c.** **(B)** Wellbutrin and Zyban both contain bupropion HCl as their active ingredient. Immediate-release bupropion is indicated for the treatment of depression. Sustained-release forms of this drug (Wellbutrin SR and Zyban) are indicated for smoking cessation treatment *(3)*

**26d.** **(E)** Patients using Lithobid should be advised to consume 8–12 glasses of water daily. This will stabilize lithium levels in the blood and prevent lithium toxicity. *(3)*

**26e.** **(A)** Adverse reactions to lithium rarely occur when serum lithium levels are below 1.5 mEq/L. Mild to moderate toxic reactions may occur at a level of 1.5–2.5 mEq/L, and severe toxicity is seen above these levels. *(3)*

**26f.** **(A)** The addition of hydrochlorothiazide to this patient's regimen is likely to increase serum lithium levels because when sodium is depleted from the body, the body will conserve lithium, thereby resulting in lithium accumulation. *(3)*

**26g.** **(C)** Blood samples are drawn just prior to taking a dose, because lithium levels will be steady at that time and will represent the trough value for lithium. *(3)*

**26h.** **(B)**

$$300 \text{ mg} = \frac{(x \text{ mEq})(74)}{2} \quad x = 8 \text{ mEq}$$

**26i.** **(A)** Hydrochlorothiazide (HydroDIURIL) is an example of a thiazide diuretic. *(3)*

**26j.** **(E)** Triazolam (Halcion) is an ultrashort hypnotic with a half-life of 2–3 h. It is the least likely of any of the benzodiazepines to produce a morning hangover; however, it does produce short-term amnesia in some patients. *(3)*

**26k.** **(E)** Ambien and Halcion both have an onset of action of less than 30 min and half-lives of

2–5 h. Thus, a patient will fall asleep quickly, and the drug wears off before waking. Prosom and Restoril have an onset of 1 to 2 h with half-lives of 10 to 20 h. *(3)*

**26l.** **(D)** Azulfidine (sulfasalazine) is used in the treatment of inflammatory bowel disease and ulcerative colitis. Usually 1–2 g of drug is needed daily. *(3)*

**26m.** **(C)** Sulfasalazine (Azulfidine) is usually administered for ulcerative colitis in doses of 500 mg q.i.d. Mesalamine (Pentasa, Rowasa, Asacol) may also be used. It is a topical anti-inflammatory agent that is an active metabolite of sulfasalazine. *(3)*

**26n.** **(A)** Phenelzine (Nardil) is an MAO inhibitor. Because the use of an MAO inhibitor in combination with a serotoninergic drug such as fluoxetine, fluvoxamine, paroxetine, sertraline, or venlafaxine can cause serious adverse effects such as hypertensive crisis, it is important to discontinue the Zoloft at least two weeks before the Nardil is started. *(3)*

**26o.** **(B)** Anticholinergic action such as that caused by diphenhydramine or doxylamine include constipation and urinary retention. A major symptom of prostatitis is restricted urinary flow. *(3)*

**26p.** **(C)** PSA refers to the prostate-specific antigen, which as a glycoprotein product is almost exclusively produced by prostate epithelial cells. Routine determination of PSA allows comparison of newer values to the individual's baseline value. Increases indicate the possibility of prostate cancer. *(3)*

**26q.** **(D)** Mitrolan tablets contain calcium polycarbophil, which possesses both laxative and antidiarrheal properties. It quickly binds water in the GI tract and forms a gel, which provides a bulking effect. *(3)*

**26r.** **(D)** For many years Ex-Lax contained phenolphthalein as its active ingredient. Because phenolphthalein has been suspected of being a carcinogen, Ex-Lax and many other products containing phenolphthalein were reformulated.

Ex-Lax now contains 15 mg of sennosides, also a stimulant laxative. *(3)*

## PROFILE NO. 27

**27a.** **(D)** Daypro is the brand name of oxaprozin. All of the choices are nonsteroidal anti-inflammatory drugs (NSAIDS). *(3)*

**27b.** **(E)** NSAIDS have analgesic and antipyretic action, which appears to be related to their ability to inhibit cyclooxygenase activity and prostaglandin synthesis. *(3)*

**27c.** **(C)** Aleve is a nonprescription brand of naproxen sodium. This drug is usually administered two to three times daily. Antacids may be taken with naproxen sodium to increase its GI tolerance. *(3)*

**27d.** **(A)** Tums chewable contains calcium carbonate. The product has become popular not only as an antacid but as a source of calcium for individuals who are attempting to reduce their chance of developing osteoporosis. *(3)*

**27e.** **(E)** Miacalcin contains salmon calcitonin as its active ingredient. It is used primarily in reducing bone resorption in postmenopausal women. It is administered intranasally as a spray, generally alternating nostrils each day. *(10)*

**27f.** **(E)** Oxaprozin (Daypro) is a relatively long-acting NSAID that requires only a single daily 1200 mg dose for most patients. *(3)*

**27g.** **(B)** Rofecoxib (Vioxx) is an NSAID that is an inhibitor of cyclooxygenase-2 (COX-2). Most other NSAIDS are COX-1 inhibitors and are, therefore, more likely to cause GI upset and bleeding. *(3)*

**27h.** **(C)** Valdecoxib (Bextra) and rofecoxib (Vioxx) are both COX-2 inhibitors. The usual dose of Bextra in the treatment of arthritis is 10 mg once daily. *(10)*

**27i.** **(C)** Misoprostol is a synthetic prostaglandin analog that has both antisecretory activity and mucosal protective properties. It is employed primarily in preventing NSAID-induced gastric ulcers. *(3)*

**27j.** **(D)** Misoprostol (Cytotec) is contraindicated for use during pregnancy and is classified as a pregnancy category X drug by the US Food and Drug Administration. *(3)*

**27k.** **(B)** Tramadol (Ultram) is a centrally-acting analgesic agent that can be administered every 4 to 6 h in treating pain. Because it acts centrally, patients should be advised to expect central adverse effects such as dizziness and fatigue. *(10)*

**27l.** **(A)** Etanercept (Enbrel) is a drug product that is used parenterally in the treatment of rheumatoid arthritis. It is not indicated for the treatment of osteoarthritis. *(3)*

## PROFILE NO. 28

**28a.** **(D)** Digoxin is a cardiac glycoside that produces a negative chronotropic effect (slowed heart rate), a positive inotropic effect (greater force of contraction), and a vagomimetic effect on the heart. *(3)*

**28b.** **(D)** Most patients using digoxin will experience a slowed heart rate (negative chronotropic effect). *(3)*

**28c.** **(A)** Amrinone (Inocor), although not a digitalis glycoside, is a positive inotropic agent. *(3)*

**28d.** **(D)** Digitoxin is a cardiac glycoside suitable for use in patients with renal impairment because it is primarily cleared by the liver. Digoxin is cleared primarily by the kidneys. *(3)*

**28e.** **(E)** Lanoxicaps are liquid-filled capsules that contain a solution of digoxin in polyethylene glycol. Because the digoxin is already in solution, the Lanoxicap dosage form provides greater bioavailability of digoxin than is achieved from digoxin tablets. A dose of 0.25 mg (250 µg) of digoxin from a tablet dosage form is equivalent to 0.2 mg (200 µg) from the Lanoxicap dosage form. *(3)*

**28f.** **(A)** Digoxin toxicity is characterized by nausea and vomiting, diarrhea, disorientation, and ventricular tachycardia. *(3)*

**28g.** **(B)** If amiloride (Midamor) is substituted for Lasix in this patient's regimen, the patient should no longer receive the potassium supplement Klorvess because amiloride is a potassium-sparing diuretic, and the administration of the combined agents would likely result in hyperkalemia. *(3)*

**28h.** **(A)** Normal serum potassium concentration is 3.5–5.0 mEq/L. When the serum level of potassium is below this range, the patient is said to be hypokalemic. If above this range, the patient is said to be hyperkalemic. *(5)*

**28i.** **(E)** Torsemide (Demadex) and bumetanide (Bumex) are both loop diuretics. Dyrenium is a potassium-sparing diuretic, and Diamox is a carbonic anhydrase inhibitor. *(3)*

**28j.** **(B)** The patient appears to be noncompliant because he received a month's supply of digoxin but did not get a refill until about one and half months later. *(3)*

## PROFILE NO. 29

**29a.** **(E)** Diphenhydramine (Benadryl) is an ethanolamine antihistamine with both sedative and antipruritic properties. *(3)*

**29b.** **(E)** Pyrethrins, one of the active ingredients in RID, is a parasite neurotoxin that is used for the treatment of human lice and scabies. *(3)*

**29c.** **(B)** When RID Shampoo is used, it is essential that the product does not come in contact with the eyes because it can cause significant irritation. RID should not be used on the face or on open cuts or excoriated areas of the body. *(3)*

**29d.** **(D)** The term *"pediculus"* refers to lice. *Pediculus capitis* refers to head lice, whereas *Pediculus pubis* refers to pubic lice. *Sarcoptes* scabiei is the organism that causes scabies. The term *"Tinea"* refers to a type of fungal organism. *(3)*

**29e.** **(C)** RID Shampoo is generally administered once. After working it thoroughly into the shampooed and dried hair, it remains in place for 10 min and is then worked into a lather with water. It is then rinsed well from the hair, and the hair is towel-dried and combed to ensure the removal of any remaining nit shells. Retreatment may occur after seven days if there is still evidence of living lice at that time. *(3)*

**29f.** **(B)** Diprosone Cream contains 0.05% betamethasone dipropionate in a hydrophilic emollient base. *(3)*

**29g.** **(D)** Diprosone Cream, or any other potent corticosteroid topical product should not be used on areas of the skin that are infected by bacteria, fungi, or a virus because the corticosteroid will inhibit the body's defense mechanisms and potentially cause spreading of the infection. Corticosteroids are useful in the treatment of psoriasis because they slow down the rate of skin cell replication. *(3)*

**29h.** **(C)** Both Nix (permethrin) and A-200 Pyrinate (pyrethrins, piperonyl butoxide, and petroleum distillate) are available for OTC use. Eurax (crotamiton) is available only by prescription. *(3)*

**29i.** **(C)** Pyrethrin-containing products should be avoided by people with ragweed allergy because pyrethrins are plant derivatives that may precipitate a hypersensitivity reaction in such patients. *(3)*

**29j.** **(A)** Scabies is a skin condition caused by the mite *Sarcoptes scabiei*. The mite burrows into the skin and causes severe itching and excoriation of the affected area. Lindane and crotamiton are effective drugs for the treatment of scabies. *(3)*

**29k.** **(B)** Treatment of psoriasis is generally aimed at reducing the rate of skin cell turnover and

reducing pruritis, which can lead to scratching that would exaserbate the disease. Coal tar products and corticosteroids such as Fluonid Cream will slow down skin cell replication. EDTA is a chelating agent. *(3)*

## PROFILE NO. 30

**30a.** **(E)** Naloxone is a pure narcotic antagonist that, when administered parenterally, rapidly reverses the effects of opioid narcotic agents such as heroin. Because it has no agonist action of its own, there is no danger in administering this agent to an unconscious patient even if the source of drug toxicity is unknown. *(3)*

**30b.** **(B)** Heroin is diacetylmorphine. Codeine is methylmorphine, whereas dionin is ethylmorphine. *(3)*

**30c.** **(C)** *Pneumocystis carinii* pneumonia (PCP) is a condition seen commonly in AIDS patients. It is an opportunistic infection that emerges when the immune system of a patient is suppressed by disease or drugs. *(3)*

**30d.** **(C)** Zidovudine or azidothymidine (AZT) is a nucleoside reverse transcriptase inhibitor (NRTI) antiviral agent commonly used in the management of patients with HIV infection who have evidence of impaired immunity. The drug is available by the brand name Retrovir. *(3)*

**30e.** **(D)** Patients on Retrovir are at risk of developing granulocytopenia or anemia that may require discontinuation of the medication or blood transfusions. It is therefore important to monitor the patient's hematologic status closely while on Retrovir therapy. *(3)*

**30f.** **(A)** Ritonavir (Norvir) is the only choice that is a protease inhibitor. The other choices are reverse transcriptase inhibitors. *(3)*

**30g.** **(A)** Acetaminophen use may competitively inhibit the glucuronidation of zidovudine (Retrovir). This may increase the likelihood of granulocytopenia developing with the use of Retrovir. *(3)*

**30h.** **(D)** Pentamidine isethionate (Pentam 300, NebuPent) is an agent that is useful in the treatment of *Pneumocystis carinii* pneumonia. It is available as an injectable product that may be administered intravenously or intramuscularly, and as an aerosol solution administered by inhalation using a nebulizer. *(3)*

**30i.** **(E)** Patients receiving pentamidine must be monitored for a variety of serious adverse effects, including sudden, severe hypotension that may occur after a single parenteral dose. Other adverse effects include hypoglycemia, bronchospasm, and cough. *(3)*

**30j.** **(D)** Robitussin DM is an OTC product used for the treatment of cough. It contains guaifenesin, an expectorant, and dextromethorphan HBr, a cough suppressant. *(3)*

**30k.** **(A)** Zalcitabine (Hivid) is a nucleoside reverse transcriptase inhibitor (NRTI) that may cause severe peripheral neuropathy in up to as many as one-third of patients with advanced HIV disease being treated with this drug. This reaction may be manifested as numbness and painful burning in distal extremities *(10)*

**30l.** **(E)** Ritonavir (Norvir) is protease inhibitor that has been found to be a potent inhibitor of cytochrome P450 3A (CYP3A) both in vitro and in vivo. Drugs that are extensively metabolized by this enzyme and are involved in significant first-pass metabolism may be most severely affected. This interaction can increase the AUC of these drugs by more than three-fold, thereby necessitating a corresponding reduction in the dose of these interacting drugs. All of the drugs listed have this potentially serious drug interaction with Ritonavir. *(3)*

# Frequently Dispensed Drugs

The candidate should be familiar with commonly prescribed drug products. If given the generic name, he/she should be able to identify the following information:

1. brand or tradename
2. commonly available dosage forms
3. strengths available
4. general pharmacological category or use
5. names of other drug products with identical or similar ingredients

While it is impossible to memorize all of the above information for all commercially available products, those products most frequently dispensed are most likely to be included on the NAPLEX. The list on the following pages represents compilations from "Top 200 Drugs" lists published every year in several pharmacy journals. Being acquainted with the tradename and generic names of these drugs will be a good starting point for answering questions. It is not necessary to learn the company name for individual products, but this information is provided since many pharmacists associate certain products with their manufacturer by picturing the package which often has a distinctive color. Those drugs marketed by several companies are shown with a number designating the number of tradenames associated with the generic name.

Other useful information is the brief description of pharmacological categories, common dosage forms, and strengths. Again it is impossible to memorize all of this information, but familiarity with some will be useful. Note especially when a product is available in a sustained-release dosage form or as an injectable.

This table is also useful when reviewing pharmacology for the NAPLEX. If the candidate is not familiar with a specific drug, review it in one of the standard references such as the Remington, Facts and Comparisons, or even the PDR. At the same time, investigate closely related drugs so that you can picture how each drug fits into its specific category. Abbreviations used in the table include:

## Companies

| | |
|---|---|
| A&H | Allen & Hanbury's |
| BMS | Bristol-Myers Squibb |
| B-W | Burroughs Wellcome |
| ESI | Elkins-Sinn Inc |
| G-W | Glaxo Wellcome |
| GSK | GlaxoSmithKline |
| M-J | Mead Johnson |
| P-D | Parke-Davis |
| P-G | Proctor & Gamble |
| P&U | Pharmacia & Upjohn |
| R-PR | Rhone-Poulenc |
| SKB | Smith Kline Beecham |
| SW | Sanofi-Synthelabo |

Note: Company names change frequently

## Drug Abbreviations

| | |
|---|---|
| APAP | acetaminophen |
| ASA | aspirin |
| HCTZ | hydrochlorothiazide |
| HC | hydrocortisone |
| NSAID | nonsteroidal anti-inflammatory drug |
| PE | phenylephrine |

**TABLE OF FREQUENTLY DISPENSED DRUGS**

| Generic Name | Tradename & Company | Category or Use | Dosage Forms & Strengths |
|---|---|---|---|
| Acetaminophen + codeine | Tylenol with Codeine (McNeil) Empracet with Cod. (G-W) + generic | analgesic | APAP 300 mg with 7.5, 15, 30, or 60 mg Cod. |
| Acyclovir sodium | Zovirax (B-W) | treatment of herpes | injection vial (600 mg), cap. 200 mg; oint 5%; tab (800 mg); suspension |
| Albuterol | Proventil (Schering) Ventolin (Glaxo) Volmax + generic | bronchodilator | tab (2 & 4 mg); repetabs; inhalation aerosol; syrup; nebulizer solution; extended release tabs (4 and 8 mg) |
| Alendronate sodium | Fosamax (Merck) | treat & prevent osteoporosis & Paget's disease | tab (5, 10, & 40 mg) |
| Allopurinol | Zyloprim (B-W) + generic | treatment of gout (hyperuricemia) | tab (100 & 300 mg) |
| Alprazolam | Xanax (Upjohn) + generic | anxiolytic | tab (0.25, 0.5, & 1 mg) |
| Amitriptyline HCl | Elavil (Merck) + generic | antidepressant | tab (10, 25, 50, 75, 100, 150 mg); injection |
| Amlodipine | Norvasc (Pfizer) | antihypertensive [Ca channel blocker] | tab (2.5, 5, & 10 mg) |
| Amlodipine + benazepril | Lotrel (Ciba-Geigy) | same | 2.5 mg +10 mg |
| Amoxicillin [5] | Amoxil (GSK) Trimox (Apothecon) Larotid (GSK) Polymox (Apothecon) Wymox (Wyeth) | broad spectrum antibiotic | cap (250, 500 mg); suspensions |
| Amoxicillin + clavulanate K | Augmentin (Beecham) | broad spectrum antibiotic | tab (250 & 500 mg + 125 mg clavulanate); 875 mg tab; suspensions; Augmentin BID 875 mg pediatric use, take q12h with food |
| Amphetamine salts | Adderall XR (Shire) | CNS stimulant | Mixed amphetamine salt mixture including the saccharate, aspartate, sulfate, and dextroamphetamine sulfate salts totaling 5, 7.5, 10, 12.5, 15, 20, & 30 mg; also XR totaling 10, 20, & 30 mg |
| Ampicillin | Omnipen (Wyeth) Principen (Squibb) Polycillin (Bristol) Totacillin (GSK) | broad spectrum antibiotic | cap (250 & 500 mg); and suspensions |
| Atorvastatin calcium | Lipitor (P-D) | antihyperlipidemic | tab (10, 20, & 40 mg) |
| Atenolol | Tenormin (ICI) + generic | antihypertensive [beta-adrenergic blocking agent] | tab (50 & 100 mg) |
| Azithromycin | Zithromax (Pfizer) | antibiotic [macrolide] | tab (250 mg); can be taken with food; available in a Z-pak |
| Benazepril HCl | Lotensin (Novartis) | antihypertensive (ACE inhibitor) | tab (5, 10, 20, & 40 mg) |
| Benzonatate | Tessalon (Forest Labs) | relief of cough | Perle (100 mg), capsule (200 mg) |

*(continued)*

## TABLE OF FREQUENTLY DISPENSED DRUGS (cont.)

| Generic Name | Tradename & Company | Category or Use | Dosage Forms & Strengths |
|---|---|---|---|
| Bisoprolol fumarate + HCTZ | Ziac (Lederle) | antihypertensive | tab (2.5, 5, or 10 mg + 6.25 mg HCTZ) |
| Budesonide | Rhinocort<br>Rhinocort Aqua<br>Pulmicort Turbuhaler (AstraZeneca) | intranasal steroid<br>anti-inflammatory<br>intranasal steroid | aerosol for nasal use respiratory inhalant, |
| Bupropion HCl | Zyban | aid in smoke cessation | SR (100 & 150 mg) |
| Buspirone HCl | Buspar (M-J) | antianxiety | tab (5 & 10 mg); 15 mg as a Dividose |
| Butalbital + APAP + caffeine | Esgic (Forest Labs)<br>Esgic + generic | analgesic (tension headache & migraine) | cap (50/325/40 mg) (50/500/40 mg) |
| Calcitonin-salmon | Miacalcin (Sandoz)<br>Calcimar (R-PR) | postmenopausal osteoporosis | nasal spray |
| Captopril | Capoten (BMS) | antihypertensive | tab (12.5, 25, 50, & 100 mg) |
| Carbidopa/levodopa | Generic | antiparkinson | tabs of several strengths (10 + 100 mg up to 50 + 200 mg) |
| Carisoprodol | Soma (Wallace) generic | skeletal muscle relaxant | tab (350 mg) |
| Carvedilol | Coreg (GlaxoSK) | antihypertensive | tab (3.125, 6.25, 12.5, & 25 mg) |
| Cefprozil | Cefzil (Bristol) | antibiotic | tab 250 & 500 mg; suspension |
| Cefuroxime | Ceftin (G-W)<br>Zinacef (Glaxo-SF) | antibiotic | tablet; oral suspension; injection (frozen sol.) & (powder for reconstitution & inj.) |
| Celecoxib | Celebrex (P&U) | NSAID | capsule (100 & 200 mg) |
| Cetirizine HCl | Zyrtec (Pfizer) | antihistamine | tab (5 & 10 mg); syrup (5 mg/5 mL) |
| Cephalexin HCl | Generic<br>Keftab (Biovail) | antibiotic | tabs & capsules (250 & 500 mg); suspension |
| Cephalexin | Keflex (Lilly) | same | same |
| Cimetidine | Tagamet (SKB) + generic | prevent and treat peptic ulcer | tab (200, 400, 800 mg) |
| Ciprofloxacin | Cipro (Bayer) | broad spectrum antibiotic | tab (250, 500, 750 mg); injection solution |
| Citalopram | Celexa (Forest) | antidepressant | tab (20 & 40 mg) |
| Clarithromycin | Biaxin (Abbott) | macrolide antibiotic | Filmtab (250 & 500 mg); suspension |
| Clonidine HCl | Catapres (Boehringer) | antihypertensive | tab (0.1, 0.2, & 0.3 mg); transdermal patches |
| Clonazepam | Klonopin (Roche) | treat petit mal | tab (0.5, 1, & 2 mg) |
| Clopidogrel | Plavix (BMS) | inhibits platelet aggregation | tab (75 mg) |
| Cyclobenzaprine | Flexeril (Merck) + generic | skeletal muscle relaxant | tab (10 mg) |
| Desloratadine | Clarinex (Schering-Plough) | antihistamine | tab (5 mg) |
| Desogestrel/ethinyl estradiol | Apri (Barr)<br>Mircette (Organon)<br>Ortho-Cept (Ortho-McNeil) | oral contraceptive | tab (0.15 mg + 30 μg) |
| Dexamethasone + tobramycin | TobraDex (Alcon) | ophthalmic steroid and antibiotic | Suspension (0.1 + 0.3%); ointment |

*(continued)*

# TABLE OF FREQUENTLY DISPENSED DRUGS (cont.)

| Generic Name | Tradename & Company | Category or Use | Dosage Forms & Strengths |
|---|---|---|---|
| Dextroamphetamine salts | Adderall (Shire) | attention deficit disorder, obesity | tab (5 mg) |
| Dextromethorphan & guaifenesin | Trocal (Roberts) | antitussive and expectorant | lozenges |
| Diazepam | Valium (Roche) | antianxiety | tab (2, 5, & 10 mg) |
| Diclofenac | Generic<br>Voltaren (Novartis)<br>Voltaren XR | anti-inflammatory | tab (25, 50, & 75 mg); extended release tab (100 mg); ophthal. drops 0.1% |
| Digoxin | Lanoxin (B-W) | cardiovascular agent | tab (0.125, 0.25, & 0.5 mg); pediatric elixir; injection |
| Diltiazem | Cardizem (Marion)<br>Dilacor XR (R-PR)<br>Tiazac (Forest)<br><br><br>Cartia XT (Andrx) | antianginal agent (calcium channel blocker) | tab (30, 60, 90, & 120 mg); SR cap (60, 90, &120 mg); sust. release (180 mg); extended release caps (120, 180, 240, 300, 360, & 420 mg)<br>cap (120, 180, 240, & 300 mg) |
| Divalproex | Depakote (Abbott)<br><br><br>Depakote ER | anticonvulsant | delayed release tabs (125, 250, & 500 mg); sprinkle caps (125)<br>extended release (500 mg) |
| Donepezil | Aricept (Pfizer) | treat mild-moderate dementia (Alzheimer's) | tab (5 & 10 mg) |
| Doxazosin | Cardura (Roerig) | antihypertenive | tab (1, 2, 3, & 8 mg) |
| Doxycycline | Vibramycin (Pfizer)<br>Vibratab<br>Doryx (P-D) | antibiotic | cap and tab (50 & 100 mg); suspension; injection |
| Efavirenz | Sustiva (Dupont Merck) | antiviral | cap (50, 100, 200 mg) |
| Enalapril | Vasotec<br>Vaseretic (Merck) | antihypertensive | tab (2.5, 5, 10, & 20 mg); tab 5 or 10 mg + HCTZ (12.5 or 25 mg) |
| Esomeprazole | Nexium (AstraZeneca) | treatment of GERD | delayed release cap (20 & 40 mg) |
| Estradiol | Estraderm<br>Transdermal (Ciba)<br>Climara (Berlex)<br>Vivelle (Ciba-Geigy) | moderate symptoms of menopause | transdermal patches (4 and 8 mg) |
| Estradiol | Estrace (BMS) + generic | same and to treat atrophic vaginitis | tab (1 & 2 mg); vaginal cream |
| Estrogens esterified + methyltestosterone | Estratest (Solvay) | estrogen/androgen combination | tab (1.25 & 2.5 mg) |
| Estrogens + medroxyprogesterone | Prempro (Wyeth) [1 card]<br>Prempro<br>Premphase (Wyeth) [2 blister cards] | prevent and manage osteoporosis<br>same—low dose formula menopause symptoms | tab (0.625 mg + 2.5 mg)<br>tab (0.45 + 1.5 mg) |
| Estrogens mixed | Premarin (Wyeth) | replacement therapy in menopause and post-menopause | tab (0.3, 0.625, 1.25, & 2.5 mg) |
| Ethinyl estradiol + desogestrel | Ortho-Cept<br>Desogen (Organon)<br>Ortho-Tri-Cyclen | oral contraceptive | tab (30 µg + 0.15 mg) |

*(continued)*

# TABLE OF FREQUENTLY DISPENSED DRUGS (cont.)

| Generic Name | Tradename & Company | Category or Use | Dosage Forms & Strengths |
|---|---|---|---|
| Ethinyl estradiol + levonorgestrel | Alesse 28 (Wyeth)<br>Triphasil 21 (Wyeth)<br>Trivoral-28 (Watson) | oral contraceptive | tab (0.02 + 0.1 mg) |
| Ethinyl estradiol + norethindrone | Loestrin 21 (P-D)<br>Loestrin Fe I/20<br>Ovcon 35; 50 (M-J) | monophasic oral<br>contraceptives | tab<br>(+ 75 mg ferrous fumarate) |
| Famciclovir | Famvir (GSK) | management of<br>herpes zoster (shingles) | tab (125, 250, & 500 mg) |
| Famotidine | Generic<br>Pepcid, Pepcid AC (Merck) | treatment of peptic ulcer<br>($H_2$-receptor antagonist) | tab (20 & 40 mg); suspension |
| Felodipine | Plendil (Astra-Merck) | antihypertensive (calcium<br>channel blocker) | extended release tab (2.5,<br>5, & 10 mg) |
| Fenofibrate | Tricor (Abbott) | antihyperlipidemic | cap (67, 134, & 200 mg) |
| Fentanyl | Duragesic<br>Sublimaze (Janssen) (Abbott) | narcotic analgesic | transdermal patch (25, 50, 75,<br>100 µg/ h); injection,<br>transmucosal |
| Fexofenadine | Allegra (Hoechst) | antihistamine | cap (60 mg) |
| Finasteride | Proscar (Merck) | androgen inhibitor<br>(shrink prostate) | tab (5 mg) |
| Fluconazole | Diflucan (Roerig) | antifungal | tab (50, 100, 150, & 200 mg);<br>pwd for susp.;<br>injection |
| Fluticasone | Flovent (G-W) | corticosteroid | 44, 110, & 200 µg aerosol |
|  | Flonase | seasonal and perennial<br>allergic rhinitis | nasal spray |
| Fluoxetine | Prozac (Lilly)<br>+ generic | antidepressant | pulvules (10, 20, & 40 mg)<br>liquid; cap (90 mg) |
| Fluvastatin | Lescol (Novartis) | antihyperlipidemic | cap (20 & 40 mg) |
| Folic acid | Generic | treat megaloblastic anemia | tab (0.4, 0.8, & 1 mg);<br>injection (5 mg/mL) |
| Fosfomycin | Monurol (Forest) | treat UTIs | granules (packet of 3) |
| Fosinopril sodium | Monopril (B-M Squibb) | antihypertensive; congestive<br>heart failure  (ACE inhibitor) | tab (10, 20, & 40 mg) |
| Furosemide | Lasix (Hoechst) + generic | diuretic | tab (20, 40, & 80 mg);<br>oral sol.; injection |
| Gabapentin | Neurontin (P-D) | anticonvulsant | cap (100, 300, & 400) |
| Gatifloxacin | Tequin (BM Squibb) | antibiotic | tab (200 & 400 mg); injection |
| Gemfibrozil | Lopid (P-D)<br>Gemco (Upsher-Smith) | antihyperlipidemic | tab (600 mg);  cap (300 mg) |
| Gentamicin HCl | Garamycin (Schering)<br>+ generic | broad spectrum antibiotic | ointment, cream, ophthalmic<br>sol. & ointment; injection |
| Glimepiride | Amaryl (Hoechst-Marion) | antidiabetic | tab (1, 2, & 4 mg) |
| Glipizide | Glucotrol (Roerig) | antihyperglycemic | tab (5 & 10 mg); + XL |
| Glyburide | Micronase (Upjohn)<br>DiaBeta (Hoechst)<br>Glynase (Upjohn) + generic | antidiabetic | tab (1.25, 2.5, & 5 mg);<br>Prestab (3 & 6 mg) |
| Granisetron | Kytril (SKB) | prevent nausea and vomiting | tab (1 mg) |
| Haloperidol | Haldol (McNeil) | antipsychotic | tab (1, 2, 5, & 10 mg);<br>oral liquid;  injection |

*(continued)*

343

## TABLE OF FREQUENTLY DISPENSED DRUGS (cont.)

| Generic Name | Tradename & Company | Category or Use | Dosage Forms & Strengths |
|---|---|---|---|
| Hydrochlorothiazide [HCTZ] | Esidrex (Ciba)<br>HydroDIURIL (Merck) + generic | antihypertensive; diuretic | tab (25 & 50 mg) |
| Hydrocodone bitartrate + APAP | Vicodin (Knoll)<br>Lortab (Russ)<br>Lorcet Plus + generic | narcotic, analgesic;<br>antitussive | tab of 5 mg + 500 mg<br>ES = 7.5 mg + 750<br>tab of 2.5 mg + 750 |
| Hydrocodone + ibuprofen | Vicoprofen (Knoll) | analgesic + NSAID | tab (7.5 + 200 mg) |
| Indinavir sulfate | Crixivan (Merck) | antiviral agent | cap (200 & 400 mg) |
| Insulin isophane (all are OTC) | Humulin (Lilly)<br>Novolin (Novo Nordisk) | control of diabetes | pure, 50/50 & 70/30 mixtures |
| Insulin lispro | Humalog (Lilly) | antidiabetic | injection |
| Insulin, human 70/30 | Humulin 70/30 (Lilly) | antidiabetic | injection |
| Insulin, human NPH | Humulin N (Lilly) | antidiabetic | injection |
| Ipratropium Br + albuterol | Combivent (Boehringer) | bronchodilator (secondary<br>treatment of COPD) | 18 µg + 103 µg per<br>aerosol actuation |
| Irbesartan | Avapro (Bristol Myers)<br>(also Sanofi) | antihypertensive | tab (75, 150, & 300 mg) |
| Isosorbide mononitrate | Imdur (Key) + generic | coronary vasodilator | extended release tab<br>(30, 60, & 120 mg);<br>tab (30, 60, & 100 mg) |
| Isotretinoin | Accutane (Roche) | prevent and treat acne | tab (10, 20, & 40 mg) |
| Itraconazole | Sporanox (Janssen) | antifungal for oral and<br>esophageal candidiasis | cap (100 mg); oral sol. |
| Lansoprazole | Prevacid (Tap) | proton pump inhibitor (treat<br>duodenal ulcers) | delayed release cap<br>(15 & 30 mg) |
| Latanoprost | Xalatan (Pharmacia) | prostaglandin agonist<br>for glaucoma | opthal. sol. (0.005%) |
| Levofloxacin | Levaquin (McNeil) | fluoroquinolone antibiotic | tab (250 & 500 mg); injection |
| Levothyroxine | Synthroid (Boots)<br>Levoxyl (Daniels)<br>Eltroxin (Roberts)<br>Levothroid (Forest) | management of the thyroid | tablets various strengths<br>(0.025–0.3 mg) |
| Lisinopril | Prinivil (Merck)<br>Zestril (Zeneca) | antihypertensive | tab (2.5, 5, 10, 20, & 40 mg) |
| Lisinopril + HCTZ | Zestoretic (Zeneca) | | 10 + 12.5; 20 + 12.5; 12 + 25 |
| Lithium carbonate | Eskalith (SKB) | treat manic depression | cap (300 mg); controlled<br>release (450 mg) |
| Loratadine | Claritin<br>Claritin-D l2 h | long-acting antihistamine | tab (10 mg)<br>(5 mg + 120 mg PE) + other<br>dosage forms |
| Lorazepam | Ativan (Wyeth) + generic | antianxiety agent | tab (1, 2, & 5 mg); injection |
| Losartan potassium | Cozaar (Merck) | antihypertensive<br>[angiotensin II antagonist] | tab (25, 50, & 100 mg) |
| Losartan potassium + HCTZ | Hyzaar (Merck) | antihypertensive | tab 50 mg + 12.5 mg HCTZ |
| Lovastatin | Mevacor (Merck) | antihyperlipidemic | tab (20 & 40 mg) |
| Medroxyprogesterone | Provera (Upjohn)<br>Cycrin (ESI) + generic | progestin replacement | tab (2.5, 5, & 10 mg) |
| Mesalamine | Asacol (P-G) | anti-inflammatory | tab (400 mg) |
| Metoprolol | Generic<br>Lopressor (Geigy)<br>Toprol XL (Astra) | antihypertensive | tab (50 & 100 mg) & injection<br>extended release tab<br>(50, 100, & 200 mg) |
| Metaproterenol | Alupent (Boehringer) | bronchodilator | tab (10 & 20 mg); inhalation<br>aerosol; syrup |

*(continued)*

## TABLE OF FREQUENTLY DISPENSED DRUGS (cont.)

| Generic Name | Tradename & Company | Category or Use | Dosage Forms & Strengths |
|---|---|---|---|
| Metaxalone | Skelaxin | muscle relaxant | 400 mg tablet |
| Metformin HCl | Glucophage<br>Glucophage XR (BMS) +<br>generic | antidiabetic (a biguanide) | tab (500, 750, 850, & 1000 mg) |
| Metformin + glyburide | Glucovance (BMS) | same | tablets of either 250 or<br>500 mg + 1.25, 2.5 or 5 mg |
| Methylphenidate | Ritalin (Ciba) + generic<br>Concerta (ALZA) | cortical stimulant | tab (5, 10, & 20 mg);<br>SR 20 mg<br>Ext. Rel. (18, 27, 36, & 54 mg) |
| Methylprednisolone | Medrol (Upjohn) | anti-inflammatory | tab (2, 4, 8, 16, 24, & 32 mg)<br>topical; inj. |
| Metoclopramide | Reglan (Robins) | antinauseant; stimulate GI<br>tract motility | 10 mg tab; syrup;<br>inj. (10 mg/2 mL) |
| Metoprolol | Lopressor (Geigy)<br>Toprol XL (Astra) + generic | antihypertensive<br>(adrenergic blocking agent) | tab (50 & 100 mg) |
| Metronidazole | Flagyl (Searle) | trichomonacide | oral tab (250 mg); vaginal tab<br>(500 mg); injection |
| Miconazole | Monistat-7<br>Monistat-3 (*Ortho*) | treatment of vulvovaginal<br>candidiasis | 2% cream; vaginal<br>supp. (100 & 200 mg) |
| Minocycline | Generic<br>Dynacin (Medicis)<br>Minocin (Lederle) | antibiotic | cap (50, 75, & 100 mg) |
| Minoxidil | Rogaine (Upjohn) | stimulate hair growth | solution (20 mg/mL) |
| Mirtazapine | Remeron (Organon) | antidepressant | tab (15, 30, & 45 mg) |
| Mometasone furoate | Elocon (Schering)<br>Nasonex (Schering) | topical corticosteroid | ointment, cream, lotion<br>(all 0.1 %), nasal spray |
| Montelukast | Singulair (Merck) | antiasthmatic | tab (10 mg) &<br>chewable (5 mg) |
| Morphine | MS Contin (Purdue Frederick) | analgesic | tab CR (15, 30, & 100 mg) |
| Mupirocin | Bactroban (SKB) | treat impetigo | 2% ointment |
| Mycophenolate | Cellcept (Roche) | immunosuppressant | cap (250 mg); tab (500 mg);<br>pwd for Inj. |
| Nabumetone | Relafen (SKB) | NSAID | tab (500 & 750 mg) |
| Naproxen | Naprosyn (Syntex) + generic<br>Naprelan (W-A) | antirheumatic | tab (250, 375, & 500 mg);<br>suspension; controlled<br>release (375 & 500 mg) |
| Nedocromil | Tilade (Fisions) | anti-inflammatory | respiratory inhaler |
| Nefazodone HCl | Serzone (Bristol Myers) | antidepressant | tab (100, 150, 200, & 250 mg) |
| Nifedipine | Procardia<br>Procardia XL (Pfizer)<br><br>Adalat (Miles)<br>Adalat CC | antihypertensive<br>(calcium channel blocker) | cap (10 mg)<br>extended release (30, 60, &<br>90 mg)<br>cap (10 & 20 mg)<br>sustained release (30, 60, &<br>90 mg) |
| Nitrofurantoin macrocrystals | Macrodantin (Norwich Eaton)<br>Macrobid (P-G) | urinary tract antibacterial | cap (25, 50, & 100 mg)<br>cap 100 mg |
| Nitroglycerin | Nitroglycerin (Lilly)<br><br>NitroBid (Marion)<br><br>Nitrostat (P-D)<br><br>NitroDur II (Key) | treatment of angina | sublingual tab (0.15, 0.4,<br>& 0.6 mg)<br>cap (2.5 mg); prolonged<br>release 6.5 mg; ointment 2%<br>regular and SR 9 (2.5, 6.5,<br>& 9 mg)<br>ointment 2%; injection, &<br>patches |

*(continued)*

**TABLE OF FREQUENTLY DISPENSED DRUGS (cont.)**

| Generic Name | Tradename & Company | Category or Use | Dosage Forms & Strengths |
|---|---|---|---|
| Nolvadex + generic | Tamoxifen (Zeneca) | treat breast cancer | tab (10 & 20 mg) |
| Norethindrone + ethinyl estradiol | *Ortho*-Novum (*Ortho*) | oral contraceptive | tab (0.5 mg + 35 µg) |
| Norgestimate + ethinyl estradiol | *Ortho*-Cyclen<br>*Ortho*-Tri-Cyclen | same | tab (0.25 mg + 35 µg)<br>3 × 7 tabs |
| Nystatin | Generic<br>Mycostatin (Apothecon)<br>Nilstat (Wyeth) | antifungal | tab (500,000 U);<br>suspension, vaginal<br>supp, cream, ointment |
| Olanzapine | Zyprexa (Lilly) | antipsychotic | tab (2.5, 5, 7.5, & 10 mg) |
| Omeprazole | Prilosec (Merck) | short-term treatment<br>of active duodenal ulcers | sustained-release cap (20 mg) |
| Ondansetron | Zofran (Glaxo) | antiemetic | tab (4 & 8 mg); injection<br>(2 mg/mL) |
| Orlistat | Xenical (Roche) | anti-obesity agent<br>(lipase inhibitor) | cap (120 mg) |
| Oxaprozin | Daypro (Searle) | NSAID for osteoporosis and<br>rheumatoid arthritis | tab (600 mg) |
| Oxybutynin | Ditropan XL (Alza)<br>Oxytrol (Watson) | urinary antispasmodic<br>treat overactive bladder | tab (5, 10, & 15 mg); syrup;<br>transdermal patch (3.9 mg) |
| Oxycodone | Oxycontin (Purdue-Frederick) | narcotic analgesic | tab (10, 20, 40, & 80 mg) |
| Oxycodone HCl + 0.<br>terephthalate + ASA | Percodan (Dupont) | analgesic; antipyretic | tablet |
| Oxycodone HCl + acetaminophen | Percocet-5 (Dupont)<br>Tylox (McNeil)<br>Roxicet (Roxane) | same | tablet |
| Pantoprazole | Protonix (Wyeth) | treatment of GERD | tab (40 mg) |
| Paroxetine | Paxil (SK-B) | antidepressant | tab (10, 20, 30, & 40 mg) |
| Penicillin V potassium<br>(Potassium Phenoxymethyl<br>Penicillin) | Beepen VK (SKB)<br>Betapen VK (Apothecon)<br>Ledercillin VK<br>Pen-Vee K (Wyeth)<br>Veetids (Apothecon) | antibiotic for gram-positive<br>microbes | tablets and suspension<br>of various strengths<br>(usually 125, 250, &<br>500 mg) which are<br>equivalent to 200,000,<br>400,000, & 800,000 units<br>V-Cillin K |
| Phenobarbital | Generic | sedative, hypnotic, antiepileptic | tab (15, 30, 60, & 100 mg) |
| Phenytoin | Dilantin (P-D) | anticonvulsant | cap (30 & 100 mg);<br>infatab (50 mg) |
| Pioglitazone HCl | Actos (Takeda) | antidiabetic | tab (15, 30, & 45 mg) |
| Potassium chloride | K-Tab (Abbott)<br>Klotrix (M-J) + generic<br>Slow-K (Summit)<br>Micro-K (Robins)<br>Klor-Con (Upsher-Smith)<br><br>K-Dur (Key) | potassium supplement | tab (4–10 mEq of K)<br><br>wax matrix tab 8 mEq<br><br>pwd (20 & 25 mEq);<br>tab (8 & 10 mEq)<br>controlled-release tab<br>(10 & 20 mEq) |
| Pravastatin sodium | Pravachol (Squibb) | antihyperlipidemic | tab (10 & 20 mg) |
| Prednisone + generic | Deltasone (P & U) | adrenal corticosteroid | tab (2.5, 5, 10, 20 & 50 mg) |
| Prevacid + Trimox + Biaxin (TAP) | Prevpac | elimination of *H. pylori* | prepack |
| Promethazine HCl | Phenergan + generic | antihistamine; antiemetic | tab (12.5 & 25 mg); supp.<br>(25 & 50 mg) |
| Promethazine + codeine | Generic | antihistamine + antitussive | syrup (6.25 mg + 10 mg<br>per 5 mL) |

*(continued)*

**TABLE OF FREQUENTLY DISPENSED DRUGS (cont.)**

| Generic Name | Tradename & Company | Category or Use | Dosage Forms & Strengths |
|---|---|---|---|
| Propranolol HCl | Inderal (W-A) + generic | treat angina, arrhythmias, etc. | tab (10, 20, 40, 60, & 80 mg); LA cap (80, 120, & 160 mg) |
| Propoxyphene Napsylate + APAP | Darvocet N (Lilly) Propacet (Lemon) + generic | analgesic | tab (50 & 100 mg) + APAP 325 mg |
| Quetiapine Fumarate | Seroquel (AstraZeneca) | antipsychotic | tab (25, 100, & 200 mg) |
| Quinapril | Accupril (P-D) | antihypertensive | tab (5, 10, 20, & 40 mg) |
| Quinapril + HCTZ | Accuretic (P-D) | | tab (10/12.5; 20/12.5; & 20/25 mg) |
| Rabeprazole | Aciphex (Eisai and Janssen) | treatment of GERD, duodenal ulcers, and Zollinger-Ellison Synd. | delayed-release tab (20 mg) |
| Raloxifene HCl | Evista (Lilly) | prevent osteoporosis | tab (60 mg) |
| Ramipril | Altace (Hoechst) | antihypertensive (ACE inhibitor) | cap (1.25, 2.5, 5, & 10 mg) |
| Ranitidine HCl | Zantac (Glaxo) | histamine $H_2$ antagonist | tab (150 & 300 mg); syrup; injection (25 mg/mL); effervescent tab and GELdose cap (150 mg) |
| Risedronate | Actonel (P-G) | prevent osteoporosis treat Paget's disease | tab (5 & 35 mg) |
| Risperidone | Risperdal (Janssen) | antipsychotic | tab (0.25, 0.5, 1, 2, 3, & 4 mg) |
| Rofecoxib | Vioxx (Merck) | NSAID-COX 2 inhibitor | tab (12.5, 25, & 50 mg); suspension (12.5 & 25 mg/5 mL) |
| Rosiglitazone maleate | Avandia (SKB) | antidiabetic | tab (2, 4, & 8 mg) |
| Salmeterol xinafoate | Serevent (GlaxoSK) | bronchodilator | aerosol; diskus (powder) |
| Salmeterol + fluticasone | Advair Diskus (GlaxoSK) | respiratory inhalant | 50 μg salmeterol + fluticasone (100, 250, or 500 μg) |
| Sertraline | Zoloft (Roerig) | antidepressant | tab (50 & 100 mg) |
| Sildenafil | Viagra (Pfizer) | treat erectile dysfunction | tab (25, 50, & 100 mg) |
| Simvastatin | Zocor (Merck) | antihyperlipidemic | tab (5, 10, 20, & 40 mg) |
| Somatropin (Serono Labs) | Serostim | growth hormone | pwd for injection (15 & 18 Int units) |
| Spironolactone | Aldactone (Searle) | potassium-sparing diuretic | tab (25, 50, & 100 mg) |
| Sumatriptan | Imitrex (Cerenex) | treatment of migraine | S.Q. injection (12 mg); tab (25 & 50 mg); nasal spray |
| Tamoxifen | Nolvadex (ICI) + generic | antiestrogen, reduce incidence of breast CA | tab (10 mg) |
| Tamsulosin HCl | Flomax (Boehringer) | benign prostatic hyperplasia (BPH) | cap (0.4 mg) |
| Temazepam | Restoril (Sandoz) + generic | sedative/hypnotic | caps (15 & 30 mg) |
| Terazosin | Hytrin (Abbott) | antihypertensive; treat BPH | tab (1, 2, 5, & 10 mg) |
| Tetracycline HCl | Achromycin V (Lederle) Robitet (Robins) + generic | broad spectrum antibiotic | cap (250 & 500 mg); suspension |
| Tetracycline phosphate | Sumycin (Apothecon) | broad spectrum antibiotic | cap (250 & 500 mg); suspension |
| Timolol maleate | Timoptic (MSD) Betimol (Ciba) | treat glaucoma | ophthalmic solution (0.25 & 0.5%) |
| | Blocadren (MSD) | antihypertensive | tab (5, 10, & 20 mg) |

*(continued)*

## TABLE OF FREQUENTLY DISPENSED DRUGS (cont.)

| Generic Name | Tradename & Company | Category or Use | Dosage Forms & Strengths |
|---|---|---|---|
| Tolterodine tartrate | Detrol<br>Detrol (P&U) | improve urinary tract continence | tab (1 & 2 mg)<br>cap (2 mg); LA capsules (4 mg) |
| Topiramate | Topamax (Ortho-McNeil) | anticonvulsant | 25, 100, & 200 mg tablets |
| Tramadol | Ultram (Ortho-McNeil) | central analgesic | tab (50 mg) |
| Tramadol + APAP | Ultracet (Ortho-McNeil) | analgesic | tab (50 mg) |
| Trazodone | Generic | antidepressant | tab (50 & 100 mg) |
| Triamcinolone acetonide | Kenalog (Squibb) | anti-inflammatory | cream, ointment, and topical aerosol |
| | Azmacort (R-PR)<br>Nasacort (R-PR) | treatment of asthma<br>same | inhalation aerosol<br>intranasal |
| Triamterene + HCTZ | Dyazide (SKF) + generic<br>Maxzide (Lederle)<br>Maxzide-25 | antihypertensive; diuretic | cap (50 + 24 mg)<br>tab (75 + 50 mg);<br>(37.5 + 25 mg) |
| Trimethobenzamide | Tigan (Beecham) | antiemetic | cap (100 & 200 mg);<br>supp. & injection |
| Trimethoprim + sulfamethoxazole | Septra (B-W)<br>Bactrim (Roche) + generic | antibacterial for urinary tract infections | tab (80 + 400 mg);<br>DS = double strength;<br>infusion solution |
| Troglitazone | Rezulin (P-D) | antihyperglycemic | tab (200 & 400 mg) |
| Valacyclovir | Valtrex (G-W) | antiviral | 500 mg, 1 g tablets |
| Valdecoxib | Bextra (P&U) | NSAID (selective COX-2 inhibitor) | tab (10 & 20 mg) |
| Valproic acid | Depakote<br>Depakene (Abbott) | anticonvulsant | tab (125, 250, & 500 mg);<br>liquid |
| Valsartan | Diovan (Novartis) | antihypertensive | cap (80 & 160 mg) |
| Valsartan + HCTZ | Diovan HCT | antihypertensive | tab (80 or 160 mg + 12.5 mg HCTZ) |
| Venlafaxine | Effexor (Wyeth)<br>Effexor XR | antidepressant | tab (25, 37.5, 50, 75, & 100 mg)<br>extended release cap (37.5, 75, & l00 mg) |
| Verapamil | Calan (Searle)<br>Isoptin (Knoll)<br>Verelan (Lederle)<br>Covera HS (Searle) | antihypertensive (calcium channel blocker) | tab (40, 80, & 120 mg)<br>SR = 240 mg; injection<br><br>tab (180 & 240 mg) |
| Warfarin | Coumadin (DuPont)<br>Panwarfin (Abbott)<br>Sofarin (Lemmon) + generic | anticoagulant | tab (2, 2.5, 5, 7.5, & 10 mg) |
| Zafirlukast | Accolate (Zeneca) | treat asthma (lukotriene receptor antagonist) | tab (20 mg) |
| Zolpidem | Ambien (Searle) | non-benzodiazepine hypnotic, sedative, tranquilizer | tab (5 & 10 mg) |

# Top Drugs by Sale Volume in Hospitals

(**Note:** Contains drugs not listed in Appendix A—Frequently Dispensed Drugs)

| Generic Name | Trade Name | Category or Use | Dosage Forms & Strengths |
|---|---|---|---|
| Abciximab | ReoPro | blood former, antithrombotic | Injection (2 mg/mL) |
| Amiodarone HCl | Cordarone IV | treat ventricular arrhythmias | 200 mg tab; injection (50 mg/mL) |
| Amphotericin B lipid-based | AmBisome Abelcet Amphotec | antifungal | injection (50 mg) |
| Ampicillin + sulbactam | Unasyn | antibiotic | injection (1.5 & 3 g) |
| Aprotinin | Trasylol | prophylactic to reduce blood loss during operations | 10,000 units/mL |
| Carboplatin | Paraplatin | antineoplastic (alkylating agent) | injection (50, 150, 450 mg vials) |
| Ceftriaxone | Rocephin | antibiotic | injection (250, 500 mg, & 1 g) |
| Diprivan | Propofol | sedative/hypnotic for anesthesia | injection (10 mg/mL) |
| Docetaxel | Taxotere | metastatic breast cancer | injection (20 & 80 mg) |
| Dolasetron mesylate | Anzemet | antiemetic | tab (50 & 100 mg) injection (20 mg/mL) |
| Drotrecogin alfa | Xigris | antisepsis-activated protein C | injection (5 & 20 mg vials) |
| Enoxaparin | Levonox | anticoagulant | injection (s.c. NOT IM or IV) |
| Epoetin alpha (Human recombinant erythropoietin) | Epogen, Eprex, Procrit | stimulate red blood cell production | injection (several strengths including 2,000–20,000 units/mL) |
| Eptifibatide | Integrilin | inhibit platelet aggregation | injection (0.75 & 2 mg/mL) |
| Filgrastim | Neupogen | increase neutrophil proliferation | injection (300 µg/mL) |
| Gemcitabine | Gemzar | antineoplastic, antimetabolite, immunosuppresent | injection (20 mg/mL) |
| Goserelin Acetate | Zoladex | treat prostate and breast cancer | 3.6 &10.8 mg implant |
| Imipenem + cilastatin | Primaxin | antibiotic | injection (250, 500, & 750 mg vials) |
| Infliximab | Remicade | immunomodulator (Crohn's disease and rheumatoid arthritis) | pwd for injection (300 µg/mL) |
| Irinotecan HCl | Camptosar | antineoplastic | injection (20 mg/mL) |

(continued)

(cont.)

| Generic Name | Trade Name | Category or Use | Dosage Form & Strengths |
|---|---|---|---|
| Leuprolide acetate | Lupron depot | prostatic cancer endometriosis | injection and microspheres for injection |
| Paclitaxel | Taxol | cancer of ovary or breast, Kaposi's sarcoma | injection (6 mg/mL) |
| Palivizumab | Synagis | passive immunity against respiratory syncytial virus | injection (100 mg) |
| Piperacillin + tazobactam | Zosyn | antibiotic | injection (2, 3, & 4 g) |
| Quetiapine fumarate | Seroquel | antipsychotic | tab (25, 100, & 200 mg) |
| Reteplase | Retavase | thrombolytic | injection (10.8 unit vial) |
| Rituximab | Rituxan | immunomodulator, antineoplastic (non-Hodgkin's lymphoma) | injection (10 mg/mL) |
| Zoledronic acid | Zometa | treat hypercalcemia of malignancy, multiple myeloma | injection (4 mg vial) |

# APPENDIX C

# Brand Names (Trade Names) Versus Generic Names

| Trade Name | Generic Name |
|---|---|
| Abelcet | amphotericin B lipid-based |
| Accolate | zafirlukast |
| Accupril | quinapril |
| Accutane | isotretinoin |
| Achromycin V | tetracycline |
| Aciphex | rabeprazole |
| Actonel | risedronate |
| Actos | pioglitazone |
| Adalat CC | nifedipine |
| Adapin | doxepin |
| Adderall | amphetamine salts |
| Advair | salmeterol + fluticasone |
| Aldactone | spironolactone |
| Aldomet | methyldopa |
| Aldoril | methyldopa + HCTZ |
| Alesse | levonorgestrel |
| Allegra | fexofenadine |
| Alphagan | brimonidine |
| Altace | ramipril |
| Alupent | metaproterenol |
| Amaryl | glimepiride |
| Ambien | zolpidem |
| Amcil | ampicillin |
| AmBisone | amphotericin B lipid-based |
| Amoxil | amoxicillin |
| Amphotec | amphotericin lipid-based |
| Ansaid | flurbiprofen |
| Antivert | meclizine |
| Anusol HC | bismuth subgallate, resorcin & hydrocortisone |
| Anzemet | dolasetron |
| Apri | desogestrel + ethinyl estradiol |
| Arava | leflunomide |
| Aricept | donepezil |
| Asacol | mesalamine |

| Trade Name | Generic Name |
|---|---|
| Atarax | hydroxyzine |
| Atenolol | tenormin |
| Ativan | lorazepam |
| Atrovent | ipratropium |
| Augmentin | amoxicillin + clavulanate K |
| Avandia | rosiglitazone |
| Avapro | irbesartan |
| Avonex | interferon Beta-1a |
| Axid | nizatidine |
| Azmacort | triamcinolone acetonide |
| Bactroban | mupirocin |
| Bactrim | trimethoprim + sulfamethoxazole |
| Beconase | beclomethasone dipropionate |
| Beepen VK | potassium phenoxymethyl penicillin |
| Benzamycin | erythromycin + benzyl peroxide |
| Betapen VK | penicillin V potassium |
| Betapace | sotalol |
| Betaserone | interferon beta Ib |
| Betimol | timolol |
| Bextra | valdecoxib |
| Biaxin | clarithromycin |
| Blocadren | timolol |
| Brethine | terbutaline |
| Bricanyl | terbutaline |
| Bumex | bumetanide |
| Buspar | buspirone |
| Calan | verapamil |
| Camptosar | irinotecan |
| Capoten | captopril |
| Carafate | sucralfate |

| Trade Name | Generic Name | Trade Name | Generic Name |
|---|---|---|---|
| Cardizem | diltiazem | Diabeta | glyburide |
| Cardura | doxazosin | Diabinese | chlorpropamide |
| Cartia XT | diltiazem | Diflucan | fluconazole |
| Casodex | bicalutamide | Dilacor XR | diltiazem |
| Catapres | clonidine | Dilantin | phenytoin |
| Ceclor | cefaclor | Dimetapp | brompheniramine maleate |
| Ceftin | cefuroxime | Diovan | valsartan |
| Cefzil | cefprozil | Diprivan | propofol |
| Celebrex | celecoxib | Ditropan XL | oxybutynin |
| Celexa | citalopram | Dopastat | dopamine |
| Cellcept | mycophenolate | Dovonex | calcipotriol |
| Centrax | prazepam | Duragesic | fentanyl |
| Cipro | ciprofloxacin | Duricef | cefadroxil |
| Clarinex | desloratadine | Dyazide | triamterene + HCTZ |
| Claritin | loratadine | Dynacin | minocycline |
| Cleocin | clindamycin | DynaCirc | isradipine |
| Climara | estradiol | | |
| Clinoril | sulindac | Effexor XR | venlafaxine |
| Clozaril | clozapine | Elavil | amitriptyline |
| Combivent | ipratropium + albuterol | Eldepryl | selegiline |
| Combivir | lamivudine + zidovudine | Elixophyllin | theophylline |
| Compazine | prochlorperazine | Elocon | mometasone |
| Coreg | carvedilol | Eltroxin | levothyroxine |
| Cogentin | benztropine | E-Mycin | erythromycin |
| Copaxone | glatiramer | Enbrel | etanercept |
| Corgard | nadolol | Epivir | lamivudine |
| Cordarone IV | amiodarone | Epogen | epoetin alpha |
| Cortisporin | polymyxin B; neomycin; gramicidin; & hydrocortisone | Eprex | epoetin alpha |
| | | ERY-TAB, ERYC | erythromycin |
| | | Erythrocin EES | erythromycin ethyl succinate |
| Cosopt | dorzolamide | | |
| Coumadin | warfarin | Esgic | butalbital + APAP |
| Covera HS | verapamil | Esidrex | hydrochlorothiazide |
| Cozaar | losartan | Eskalith | lithium carbonate |
| Crixivan | indinavir | Estrace or Estraderm | estradiol |
| Cycrin | medroxyprogesterone | Estratest Tab | esterified estrogens + methyltestosterone |
| Cytotec | misoprostol | | |
| | | Evista | raloxifene |
| Dalmane | flurazepam | | |
| Darvocet N | propoxyphene + acetaminophen | Famvir | famciclovir |
| | | Feldene | piroxicam |
| Daypro | oxaprozin | Flagyl | metronidazole |
| DDAVP | desmopressin | Flexeril | cyclobenzaprine |
| Deltasone | prednisone | Flomax | tamsulosin |
| Demulen | estrogens | Flonase | fluticasone |
| Depakene or Depakote | valproic acid | Floxin | ofloxacin |
| | | Flovent | fluticasone |
| Desogen | ethinyl estradiol | Fosamax | alendronate |
| Detrol | tolterodine | | |

| Trade Name | Generic Name | Trade Name | Generic Name |
|---|---|---|---|
| Garamycin | gentamicin | Lasix | furosemide |
| Gemco | gemfibrozil | Lescol | fluvastatin |
| Gemzar | gemcitabine | Levaquin | levofloxacin |
| Glucotrol | glipizide | Levonox | enoxaparin |
| Glucophage | metformin | Levoxyl | levothyroxine |
| Glucovance | metfomin + glyburide | Lidex | fluocinonide |
| Glynase | glyburide | Lipitor | atorvastatin |
| Gyne-Lotrimin | clotrimazole | Lodine | etodolac |
| | | Loestrin-Fe | ethinyl estradiol |
| Halcion | triazolam | Lomotil | diphenoxylate + atropine |
| Haldol | haloperidol | Lo-Ovral 28 | ethinyl estradiol + |
| Hismanal | astemizole | | norgestrel |
| Humulin N & 70/30 | isophane insulin | Lopid | gemfibrozil |
| Humalog | insulin lispro | Lopressor | metoprolol |
| Hydergine | ergoloid mesylates | Lorabid | lorcarbef |
| HydroDIURIL | hydrochlorothiazide | Lorcet Plus | hydrocodone |
| Hygroton | chlorthalidone | Lotensin | benazepril |
| Hytrin | terazosin | Lotrel | amlodipine + benazepril |
| Hyzaar | losartan | Lotrimin | clotrimazole |
| | | Lotrisone | clotrimazole + |
| Ilosone | erythromycin estolate | | betamethasone |
| Imdur | isosorbide | Lorelco | probucol |
| Imitrex | sumatriptan | Lozol | indapamide |
| Imodium | loperamide | Lortab | hydrocodone + APAP |
| Inderal | propanolol | Lupron depot | leuprolide |
| Indocin | indomethacin | Luvox | fluvoxamine |
| Intal | cromolyn | | |
| Integrilin | eptifibatide | Macrobid | nitrofurantoin |
| Intropin | dopamine | Macrodantin | nitrofurantoin |
| Isoptin | verapamil | Maxzide | triamterene |
| Isordil | isosorbide dinitrate | Medrol | methylprednisolone |
| | | Mellaril | thioridazine |
| K-Dur | potassium chloride | Meridia | sibutramine |
| K Lyte | potassium bicarbonate & | Mevacor | lovastatin |
| | citrate | Miacalcin nasal | calcitonin-salmon |
| K-Tab | potassium chloride | Micro-K | potassium chloride |
| Keflex | cephalexin | Micronase | glyburide |
| Keftab | cephalexin | Minipress | prazosin |
| Kenalog | triamcinolone acetonide | Minocin | minocycline |
| Klonopin | clonazepam | Mircette | desogestrel + ethinyl |
| Klor-Con | potassium chloride | | estradiol |
| Kwell | gamma benzene | Monistat | miconazole |
| | hexachloride | Monopril | fosinopril |
| Kytril | granisetron | Monurol | fosfomycin |
| | | Motrin | ibuprofen |
| Lamictal | lamotrigine | MS Contin | morphine sulfate |
| Lamisil oral | terbinafine | Mycelex G | clotrimazole |
| Lanoxin | digoxin | Mycostatin | nystatin |
| Larotid | amoxicillin | | |

| Trade Name | Generic Name | Trade Name | Generic Name |
|---|---|---|---|
| Nalfon | fenoprofen | Percocet-5 | oxycodone HCl + APAP |
| Naprelan | naproxen | Percodan | oxycodone + *O*-terephthalate |
| Naprosyn | naproxen | | + ASA |
| Nasacort | triamcinolone | Peridex | chlorhexidine gluconate |
| Nasalcrom | cromolyn | Persantine | dipyridamole |
| Nasonex | mometasone | Pen-Vee K | potassium phenoxymethyl |
| Neoral | cyclosporine | | penicillin |
| Neosporin | neomycin, polymyxin B, & | Phenergan | promethazine |
| | bacitracin | Plavix | clopidogrel |
| Neupogen | filgrastim | Plendil | felodipine |
| Neurontin | gabapentin | Polycillin | ampicillin |
| Nexium | esomeprazole | Polymox | amoxicillin |
| Nicorette | nicotine polacrilex | Pravachol | pravastatin |
| Nitrobid | nitroglycerin | Premarin | conjugated estrogens |
| Nitrodur II | nitroglycerin | Prempro | conjuated estrogens |
| Nitrostat | nitroglycerin | Prevacid | lansoprazole |
| Nizoral | ketoconazole | Prevpac | Prevacid + Trimox + Biaxin |
| Nolvadex | tamoxifen | Prilosec | omeprazole |
| Normodyne | labetalol | Primaxin | imipenem + cilastatin |
| Norinyl | norethindrone + mestranol | Principen | ampicillin |
| Norlestrin | norethindrone acetate | Prinivil | lisinopril |
| Noroxin | norfloxacin | Polycillin | ampicillin |
| Norvasc | amlodipine | Polymox | amoxicillin |
| Novolin | insulin | Procan SR | procainamide |
| | | Procardia | nifedipine |
| Ogen | estropipate | Procrit | epoetin alfa |
| Omnipen | ampicillin | Prograf | tacrolimus |
| *Ortho*-Cyclen | norgestimate + ethinyl | Pronestyl | procainamide |
| | estradiol | Propacet | propoxyphene + APAP |
| *Ortho*-Novum 7/7/7 | norethindrone + ethinyl | Propine | dipivefrin |
| | estradiol | Proscar | finasteride |
| *Ortho*-Cept | ethinyl estradiol | Protonix | pantoprazole |
| *Ortho*-Tri-Cyclen | estrogens | Proventil | albuterol |
| Orudis | ketoprofen | Provera | medroxy progesterone |
| Oruvail | ketoprofen | Prozac | fluoxetine |
| Ovcon | ethinyl estradiol + | Pulmicort Turbuhaler | budesonide |
| | norethindrone | | |
| Ovral | norgestrel + ethinyl estradiol | Questran | cholestyramine |
| Oxytrol | oxybutynin | | |
| Oxycontin | oxycodone | Rebetron | interferon alfa 2b |
| | | Reglan | metoclopramide |
| Pamelor | nortriptyline | Relafen | nabumetone |
| Panwarfin | warfarin | Remeron | mirtazapine |
| Paraplatin | carboplatin | Remicade | infliximab |
| Patanol | olopatadine | Reopro | abciximab |
| Paxil | paroxetine | Restoril | temazepam |
| PCE | erythromycin | Retavase | reteplase |
| Pepcid | famotidine | Retin A | tretinoin |

| Trade Name | Generic Name | Trade Name | Generic Name |
|---|---|---|---|
| Rezulin | troglitazone | Theo-Dur | theophylline |
| Rhinocort | budesonide | Tigan | trimethobenzamide |
| Risperdal | risperidone | Tilade | nedocromil |
| Ritalin | methylphenidate | Timoptic | timolol |
| Rituxam | rituximab | Topamax | topiramate |
| Rocephin | ceftriaxone | TobraDex | dexamethasone + tobramycin |
| Rogaine | minoxidil | | |
| Robitet | tetracycline | Topex | benzyl peroxide |
| Roxicet | oxycodone | Toprol | metoprolol |
| Rufen | ibuprofen | Toradol | ketorolac |
| | | Totacillin | ampicillin |
| Septra | trimethoprim + sulfamethoxazole | Transderm nitro | nitroglycerin |
| | | Trasylol | aprotinin |
| Serax | oxazepam | Tranxene | chlorazepate |
| Serevent | salmeterol | Trental | pentoxifylline |
| Seroquel | quetiapine | Triavil | perphenazine + amitryptyline |
| Serostim | somatropin | | |
| Serzone | nefazodone | Tricor | fenofibrate |
| Sinemet | carbidopa + levodopa | Tri-Levlen | ethinyl estradiol + levonorestrel |
| Sinequan | doxepin | | |
| Singulair | montelukast sodium | Trimox | amoxicillin |
| Skelaxin | metaxalone | Tri-Norinyl | norethindrone + mestranol |
| Slo-BID | theophylline, anhydrous | Triphasil | ethinyl estradiol + levonorestrel |
| Slow-K | potassium chloride | | |
| Slo-Phyllin | theophylline | Trivora | ethinyl estradiol + levonorgestrel |
| Sofarin | warfarin | | |
| Soma | carisoprodol | Trocal | dextromethorphan + guaifensin |
| Sorbitrate | isosorbide dinitrate | | |
| Sporanox | itraconazole | Tussionex | hydrocodone + phenyltoxamine |
| Stadol NS | butorphanol | | |
| Sublimaze | fentanyl | Tylenol | APAP |
| Sulamyd | sulfonamide | Tylox | oxycodone HCl + APAP |
| Sumycin | tetracycline | | |
| Suprax | cefixime | Ultracet | tramadol + APAP |
| Sustiva | efavirenz | Ultram | tramadol |
| Synagis | palivizumab | Unasyn | ampicillin + sulbactam |
| Synthroid | levothyroxin | | |
| | | Valium | diazepam |
| Tagamet | cimetidine | Valrelease | diazepam |
| Tamoxifen | nolvadex | Valtrex | valacyclovir |
| Tavist | clemastine | Vanceril | beclomethasone dipropionate |
| Taxotere | docetaxel | | |
| Taxol | paclitaxel | Vancenase | beclomethasone dipropionate |
| Tegretol | carbamazepine | | |
| Tenormin | atenolol | Vasotec | enalapril |
| Tequin | gatifloxacin | Vaseretic | enalapril + HCTZ |
| Terazole | terconazole | V-Cillin | potassium phenoxymethyl penicillin |
| Tessalon | benzonatate | | |

| Trade Name | Generic Name | Trade Name | Generic Name |
|---|---|---|---|
| Veetids | potassium phenoxymethyl penicillin | Zantac | ranitidine |
| | | Zerit | stavudine |
| Ventolin | albuterol | Zestoretic | lisinopril + HCTZ |
| Verelan | verapamil | Zestril | lisinopril |
| Viagra | sildenafil | Ziac | bisoprolol |
| Vibramycin | doxycycline | Ziagen | abacavir |
| Vicodin | hydrocodone + APAP | Zinacef | cefuroxime |
| Vicoprofen | hydrocodone + ibuprofen | Zithromax | azithromycin |
| Viracept | nelfinavir | Zocor | simvastatin |
| Viramune | nevirapine | Zofran | ondansetron |
| Vistaril | hydroxyzine pamoate | Zoladex | goserelin |
| Vioxx | rofecoxib | Zoloft | sertraline |
| Vivelle | estradiol patches | Zometa | zoledronic |
| Voltaren | diclofenac | Zomig | zolmitriptan |
| Volmax | albuterol | Zosyn | piperacillin + tazobactam |
| | | Zovirax | acyclovir |
| Wellbutrin SR | bupropion | Zyban | bupropion |
| Wymox | amoxicillin | Zyloprim | allopurinol |
| | | Zyprexa | olanzapine |
| Xalatan | latanoprost | Zyrtec | cetirizine |
| Xanax | alprazolam | | |
| Xenical | orlistat | | |
| Xigris | drotrecogin Alfa | | |

http://secure.rxschool.com/courses/